Trauma, Memory, and Dissociation

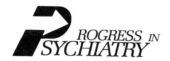

Number 54
David Spiegel, M.D.
Series Editor

Trauma, Memory, and Dissociation

Edited by
J. Douglas Bremner, M.D., and
Charles R. Marmar, M.D.

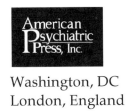

American Psychiatric Press, Inc.

Washington, DC
London, England

Note: The authors have worked to ensure that all information in this book concerning drug dosages, schedules, and routes of administration is accurate as of the time of publication and consistent with standards set by the U.S. Food and Drug Administration and the general medical community. As medical research and practice advance, however, therapeutic standards may change. For this reason and because human and mechanical errors sometimes occur, we recommend that readers follow the advice of a physician who is directly involved in their care or in the care of a member of their family.

Copyright © 1998 American Psychiatric Press, Inc.
ALL RIGHTS RESERVED
Manufactured in the United States of America on acid-free paper
First Edition
01 00 99 98   4 3 2 1

American Psychiatric Press, Inc.
1400 K Street, N.W., Washington, DC   20005
www.appi.org

Library of Congress Cataloging-in-Publication Data
Trauma, memory, and dissociation / edited by J. Douglas Bremner and
    Charles R. Marmar. — 1st ed.
        p.   cm. — (Progress in psychiatry)
    Includes bibliographical references and index.
    ISBN 0-88048-753-4 (alk. paper)
    1. Dissociative disorders.   2. Psychic trauma.
3. Autobiographical memory. 4. Dissociation (Psychology). 5. Post-
traumatic stress disorder.   6. Recovered memory.   I. Bremner, J.
Douglas, 1961–   .   II. Marmar, Charles R., 1945–   .   III. Series.
    [DNLM: 1. Stress Disorders, Post-Traumatic.   2. Dissociative
Disorders.   3. Memory.   4. Unconscious (Psychology)   WM 170
    T77743   1997]
R553.D5T73   1997
616.85′2—dc21
DNLM/DLC
for Library of Congress   97-3211
                                                                                    CIP

British Library Cataloguing in Publication Data
A CIP record is available from the British Library.

Contents

Contributors

Judith Armstrong, Ph.D.
Sheppard Pratt Health System, Baltimore, Maryland

Suzette Boon, Ph.D.
Amsterdam Mental Health Clinic, Amsterdam, The Netherlands

J. Douglas Bremner, M.D.
Assistant Professor, Department of Psychiatry, Yale University School of Medicine, New Haven; Research Psychiatrist, National Center for Posttraumatic Stress Disorder, West Haven Veterans Affairs Medical Center, West Haven, Connecticut

Eve B. Carlson, Ph.D.
Clinical Psychology Associates, Delavan, Wisconsin

Dennis S. Charney, M.D.
Professor and Associate Chair for Research, Department of Psychiatry, Yale University School of Medicine, New Haven; Chief, Psychiatry Service, West Haven Veterans Affairs Medical Center, West Haven, Connecticut

James A. Chu, M.D .
Director, Trauma and Dissociative Disorders Program, McLean Hospital, Belmont; Assistant Professor, Department of Psychiatry, Harvard University School of Medicine, Cambridge, Massachusetts

Janet de Groot, M.D.
Assistant Professor, Department of Psychiatry, University of Toronto; Coordinator, Postgraduate Education, Department of Psychiatry, The Toronto Hospital, Toronto, Ontario, Canada

John H. Krystal, M.D.
Associate Professor, Department of Psychiatry, Yale University School of Medicine, New Haven; Director of Clinical Research, Psychiatry Service, West Haven Veterans Affairs Medical Center, West Haven, Connecticut

Richard Loewenstein, M.D.
Director, Dissociative Disorders Unit, Sheppard Pratt Health System, Baltimore, Maryland

Jose R. Maldonado, M.D.
Assistant Professor and Chief, Medical Psychiatry Section, Department of Psychiatry and Behavioral Sciences, Stanford University; Medical Director, Consultation/Liaison Psychiatry Service, Stanford University Hospital; Director, Medical Psychotherapy Clinic, Stanford University School of Medicine, Stanford, California

Charles R. Marmar, M.D.
Professor and Vice-Chair, Department of Psychiatry, University of California, San Francisco; Chief, Mental Health Service, Department of Veterans Affairs Medical Center, San Francisco, California

Thomas Metzler, M.A.
Department of Psychiatry, University of California, San Francisco; Posttraumatic Stress Disorder Program, San Francisco Veterans Affairs Medical Center, San Francisco, California

John C. Nemiah, M.D.
Professor, Department of Psychiatry, Dartmouth University School of Medicine, Hanover, New Hampshire; Editor Emeritus, *American Journal of Psychiatry*, Washington, D.C.

Frank W. Putnam, M.D.
Director, Laboratory of Developmental Psychology, National Institute of Mental Health, Bethesda, Maryland

Gary Rodin, M.D.
Professor and Head of Psychosomatic Medicine Program,
Department of Psychiatry, University of Toronto;
Psychiatrist-in-Chief, The Toronto Hospital, Toronto, Ontario,
Canada

David Roth, Ph.D.
Clinical Psychologist, Sheppard Pratt Health System,
Baltimore, Maryland

Philip A. Saigh, Ph.D.
Chairman and Professor, School of Psychology, City University
of New York Graduate School; Adjunct Professor of
Psychiatry, Division of Child and Adolescent Psychiatry, New
York University Medical Center, New York, New York

Steven M. Southwick, M.D.
Associate Professor, Department of Psychiatry, Yale University
School of Medicine, New Haven; Director, Posttraumatic Stress
Disorder Program, West Haven Veterans Affairs Medical
Center, West Haven, Connecticut

David Spiegel, M.D.
Professor, Department of Psychiatry and Behavioral Sciences;
Director, Psychosocial Treatment Laboratory, Stanford
University School of Medicine, Stanford, California

Harold Spivak, M.D.
Assistant Professor, Department of Psychiatry, University of
Toronto; Associate Staff, Department of Psychiatry, The
Toronto Hospital, Toronto, Ontario, Canada

Onno van der Hart, Ph.D.
Professor, Department of Psychology, University of Utrecht,
Utrecht, The Netherlands

Bessel A. van der Kolk, M.D.
Professor, Department of Psychiatry; and Chief, Trauma
Clinic, Harvard University School of Medicine, Cambridge,
Massachusetts

Eric Vermetten, M.D.
  Department of Psychiatry, Academic Psychiatric Center,
  Maastricht, The Netherlands

Daniel S. Weiss, Ph.D.
  Professor of Psychiatry, University of California, San Francisco;
  Posttraumatic Stress Disorder Program, San Francisco Veterans
  Affairs Medical Center, San Francisco, California

Introduction to the Progress in Psychiatry Series

The Progress in Psychiatry Series is designed to capture in print the excitement that comes from assembling a diverse group of experts from various locations to examine in detail the newest information about a developing aspect of psychiatry. This series emerged as a collaboration between the American Psychiatric Association's (APA) Scientific Program Committee and the American Psychiatric Press, Inc. Great interest is generated by a number of the symposia presented each year at the APA annual meeting, and we realized that much of the information presented there, carefully assembled by people who are deeply immersed in a given area, would unfortunately not appear together in print. The symposia sessions at the annual meetings provide an unusual opportunity for experts who otherwise might not meet on the same platform to share their diverse viewpoints for a period of 3 hours. Some new themes are repeatedly reinforced and gain credence, whereas in other instances disagreements emerge, enabling the audience and now the reader to reach informed decisions about new directions in the field. The Progress in Psychiatry Series allows us to publish and capture some of the best of the symposia and thus provide an in-depth treatment of specific areas that might not otherwise be presented in broader review formats.

Psychiatry is, by nature, an interface discipline, combining the study of mind and brain, of individual and social environments, of the humane and the scientific. Therefore, progress in the field is rarely linear—it often comes from unexpected sources. Furthermore, new developments emerge from an array of viewpoints that do not necessarily provide immediate agreement but rather expert examination of the issues. We intend to present innovative ideas and data that will enable you, the reader, to participate in this process.

We believe the Progress in Psychiatry Series will provide you with an opportunity to review timely, new information in specific fields of interest as they are developing. We hope you find that the excitement of the presentations is captured in the written word and that this book proves to be informative and enjoyable reading.

David Spiegel, M.D.
Series Editor
Progress in Psychiatry Series

Preface

J. Douglas Bremner, M.D.

In 1993, Frank Putnam and I organized a symposium entitled "Trauma and Dissociation" for the American Psychiatric Association's annual meeting. The symposium was designed to draw together empirical research that had been conducted since the publication of several theoretical papers in 1989 on Pierre Janet's (1889) conceptions of trauma and dissociation (Nemiah 1989; Putnam 1989; van der Kolk and van der Hart 1989). These papers, in addition to David Spiegel's (1984) conceptualization of dissociative disorders as part of the spectrum of psychopathology related to traumatic stress, provided a theoretical framework that galvanized rigorous empirical research in the area. The 1993 symposium had an electric atmosphere that we had not anticipated. There seemed to be a feeling that a reshaping of thinking about a particular area of psychiatry was in progress. Eighty years had passed after Janet's formulations of trauma and dissociation, during which there had been relatively little empirical research on these topics. Freud's theories had a strong influence on the field of psychiatry during that time, which resulted in a relative neglect of other theories, such as those of Janet, as well as topics such as trauma and dissociation, which were more the focus of Janet's writings than of Freud's.

The studies presented during the symposium demonstrated that trauma and dissociation were topics amenable to empirical research. Traumatic stress and dissociative disorders resulted in considerable dysfunction in a large number of patients and therefore represented an important area of clinical psychiatry. Dissociative symptoms were strongly associated with exposure to psychological trauma, whether it was combat exposure, childhood abuse, or other traumas. In addition, there were important relationships with other psychiatric disorders associated with extreme stress, including posttraumatic stress disorder (PTSD). Much of that empirical data is presented in this book.

Many questions that were not answered by the findings in the symposium are considered by several of the authors in this book. There was a traditional assumption that dissociative responses to trauma have a protective effect on the individual, in terms of the development of trauma-related psychopathology. Currently, there is not a clear consensus in the field on this issue, and many questions are left unanswered. Do dissociative responses at the time of trauma protect the individual, or are they an early marker of psychopathology? Or, alternatively, are they a defense mechanism that is only partially effective in preventing psychopathology? Put another way, is dissociation a normal personality trait that varies in the general population and is related to other normal personality traits, such as hypnotizability (as is posited in the dissociative spectrum hypothesis), or is it something only seen in pathological individuals? If dissociation does not represent psychopathology, then why are patients with high levels of dissociative symptomatology made so dysfunctional by their symptoms? On the other hand, if dissociation is not a normal personality variable, then why are episodes of amnesia such an important part of hypnotic induction? Several of the chapters in this book deal with these questions in depth.

Research in psychiatry never remains stationary, and since the time of the original symposium, several important new topics of interest have received attention in the field of psychological trauma. Heightened media attention devoted to delayed recall of memories of childhood abuse (and the so-called false memory syndrome) has focused on the effects of traumatic stress on memory. Dissociation plays an important role in this area because traumatic memories are often encoded, and later recalled, in a dissociated state. Dissociative amnesia is also an important variable in delayed recall of childhood abuse. Other aspects of alterations in memory, including deficits in short-term memory and the overrepresentation of specific traumatic memories, also play an important role in the pathology of trauma victims. The controversy surrounding delayed recall of abuse has threatened the integrity of treatments provided for abuse victims. For these reasons, it makes sense for investigators in the field of trauma and dissociation to study delayed recall, which they have done. As with the field of trauma and dissociation, investigations are needed to replace public fictions with empirically derived data. Finally, because we have learned something about the relationship among trauma, memory, and dissociation, it is time to formulate approaches to treatment for these patients and to understand the pathophysiology of these disorders from a neurobiological perspective. These issues are discussed in several chapters of this book.

The contributions to this book were designed to represent a consolidation of the work of some of the major investigators in the fields of trauma, memory, and dissociation. It is hoped that this book will be a stimulus for future investigations in this important and interesting field.

References

Janet P: l'Automatisme Psychologique. Paris, Balliere, 1889

Nemiah JC: Janet redivivus: the centenary of l'Automatisme Psychologique. Am J Psychiatry 146:1527–1529, 1989

Putnam FW: Pierre Janet and modern views of dissociation. J Trauma Stress 2:413–429, 1989

Spiegel D: Multiple personality as a posttraumatic stress disorder. Psychiatr Clin North Am 7:101–110, 1984

van der Kolk BA, van der Hart O: Pierre Janet and the breakdown of adaptation in psychological trauma. Am J Psychiatry 146:1530–1540, 1989

Chapter 1

Early Concepts of Trauma, Dissociation, and the Unconscious: Their History and Current Implications

John C. Nemiah, M.D.

Historical Considerations

Early Clinical Observations

A Curious Footnote

In one of the earliest psychoanalytic publications there is an apparent misreading that has gone unnoticed since its appearance a hundred years ago. Breuer and Freud's "On the Psychical Mechanism of Hysterical Phenomena: Preliminary Communication," initially printed as a separate paper in 1893, was subsequently incorporated in 1895 as the first chapter in their monograph, "Studies on Hysteria" (Breuer and Freud 1893–1895/1955). It was there that they announced their discovery of the curative effect of cathartic "abreaction" in the treatment of the symptoms of what they termed *traumatic hysteria*.

They wrote:

> We found, to our great surprise at first, that *each individual symptom immediately and permanently disappeared when we had succeeded in bringing clearly to light the memory of the event by which it was provoked and in arousing its accompanying affects, and when the patient had described that event in the greatest possible detail and had put the affect into words.* Recollection without affect almost invariably produces no re-

1

sult. The psychical process which originally took place must be repeated as vividly as possible; it must be brought back to its *status
nascendi* and then given verbal utterance. (Breuer and Freud
1893–1895/1955, p. 6)

After a further brief comment on their procedure, the authors
casually, and as if it were merely an afterthought, refer the reader
to Janet's *l'Automatisme Psychologique* (1889/1989) in a footnote in
which they comment, "In Janet's interesting study on mental
automatism (1889), there is the account of the cure of a hysterical
girl *by a method analogous to ours*" (Breuer and Freud
1893–1895/1955, p. 7, italics added).

A Footnote to a Footnote

Readers who are not familiar with Janet's epoch-making treatise on
psychological automatism will miss the curious fact that in this
short, offhand statement Breuer and Freud seem to attribute to
Janet a discovery that he never made. Not only was that discovery
original with Breuer and Freud themselves, but, in Freud's hands,
it became the kernel of the entire subsequent development of psychoanalytic theory and method. The comparison that follows of the
observations that led Breuer and Freud to their formulation of abreaction with the clinical findings in Janet's "cure of a hysterical girl "
clearly demonstrates the paradoxical nature of that attribution.

The case of Anna O. (Breuer).   At the beginning of the second
section of "Studies on Hysteria," which is devoted to extensive case
presentations, Breuer describes his famous patient, Anna O., and
what came to be called her "talking cure." Breuer had first seen and
treated his patient more than a decade before his collaboration with
Freud. In the course of Breuer's exploration of her multiplicity of
somatic hysterical symptoms, the patient began spontaneously
during therapeutic hypnosis to relive and describe the circumstances of the onset of individual symptoms. To his surprise, Breuer
noted that when the patient recounted in detail the traumatic
events surrounding their development, the symptoms disappeared. Breuer describes his serendipitous discovery as follows:

When this happened for the first time—when, as the result of an accidental and spontaneous utterance of this kind during the evening hypnosis, a disturbance which had persisted for a considerable time vanished—I was greatly surprised. It was in the summer during a period of extreme heat, and the patient was suffering very badly from thirst; for, without being able to account for it in any way, she suddenly found it impossible to drink. She would take up the glass of water she longed for, but as soon as it touched her lips she would push it away like someone suffering from hydrophobia. As she did this, she was obviously in an *absence* for a couple of seconds. She lived only on fruit, such as melons, etc., so as to lessen her tormenting thirst. This had lasted for some six weeks, when one day during hypnosis she grumbled about her English lady companion whom she did not care for, and went on to describe, with every sign of disgust, how she had gone into that lady's room and how her little dog—horrid creature!—had drunk out of a glass there. The patient had said nothing, as she had wanted to be polite. After giving further energetic expression to the anger she had held back, she asked for something to drink, drank a large quantity of water without any difficulty and woke from her hypnosis with the glass at her lips; and thereupon the disturbance vanished, never to return. A number of extremely obstinate whims were similarly removed after she had described the experiences that had given rise to them. (Breuer and Freud 1893–1895/1955, p. 34)

The case of Marie (Janet).   It was shortly after Breuer's clinical experience with Anna 0. in Vienna that Pierre Janet, then an unknown doctoral student in Le Havre, encountered Marie, a young woman, who, as he wrote in his subsequent detailed case report in *l'Automatisme Psychologique* (Janet 1889/1989),

... presented an illness and its cure that were equally curious. . . . The illness consisted of recurrent symptoms regularly accompanying her menses. . . . As her menses approached, Marie's character would change. She would become somber and passionate, which was unusual for her, and would suffer from pains and nervous twitchings in all her limbs. Despite this, everything would go fairly smoothly during the first day, but scarcely twenty hours after its appearance her menstrual flow would suddenly cease, and her whole body would be seized by a shaking chill followed by an acute pain starting in her stomach and rising to her throat, after which she would begin to have major hysterical crises. The convulsions, although very violent, did not last long and never manifested characteristic epileptiform movements, and were followed by an exceedingly long and intense delirium [which] alternated with the convulsions for 48 hours. The episode would end with copious vomiting of blood, following which everything returned pretty much to normal. During the periods between the occurrence of the major symptoms associated with her menses, she maintained . . . a variety of highly changeable anesthesias, and in particular a total and continuous blindness in her left eye.

I wished to have precise information concerning the manner in which her periods began and how they had been interrupted. She did not reply with any clarity since she appeared to have forgotten a large part of the details about which she was questioned. I thought then of putting her into a deep somnambulistic state, capable, as has been seen, of recovering apparently forgotten memories, and I was thus able to recall the exact memory of a scene that she had never been aware of before except in the most incomplete fashion. At the age of 13 she had had her first period, but, either as the result of some childish idea or of a conversation she had overheard, she got into her head that there was something shameful about the process and tried to find a way of stopping her menstrual flow as quickly as possible. Approximately 20 hours after her period had started, she went out secretly and plunged herself into a large tub of cold water. Her action was completely successful, her period was suddenly arrested, and despite a severe shaking chill that followed, she was able to return home. She was ill for some time thereafter and for several days was delirious. Everything quieted down, however, and her periods did not recur for five years. When they did reappear, they were accompanied by the difficulties I have described. Thus, if one compares the sudden arrest of the menses, the shivering, and the pains she now recounts in her waking state, with the account she gave in somnambulism (which, moreover, was indirectly confirmed), one arrives at the following conclusion. Each month the scene of the cold bath is repeated, leading to the same arrest of menses and delirium. . . . In her normal state of consciousness, however, she knows nothing about that and is quite unaware that her shivering is brought on by a hallucination of cold. It is possible, therefore, that the scene occurs below consciousness and brings on all the rest of her difficulty in its train.

Finally, I wished to explore the blindness in her left eye, but Marie objected to it when she was awake, stating that she had always been that way since birth. It was easy to demonstrate by hypnotic somnambulism that she was mistaken. If one changed her into a little girl of five by the usual procedure [i.e., hypnotic age-regression], she recovered the sensation she had had at that age, and one could observe that she saw very well with both eyes. It was when she was six that the blindness had begun. What were the circumstances? Marie persisted in saying when she was awake that she had absolutely no idea. During hypnotic somnambulism, and by means of the successive transformations in which I had her relive the principal scenes of her life at that age, I determined that the blindness had begun at a specific moment in connection with a trifling incident. She had been forced, despite her outcries, to sleep with a child of her own age *the left side of whose face was covered with scabs.* Marie herself sometime afterward developed similar scabs, which appeared almost identical and had exactly the same distribution. These scabs reappeared for several years and then were completely cured, but it was noted from that point on that *the left side of her face was anesthetic and she was blind in her left eye.* She has since always maintained that anesthesia. (Janet 1889/1989, pp. 410–413)

Having thus determined the origins of the patient's symptoms, Janet proceeded to treat them. He wrote:

I tried to remove from her somnambulistic consciousness the absurd fixed idea that her menses had been arrested by the cold bath. . . . I was able to get rid of the idea by a singular procedure. It was necessary to regress the patient by suggestion back to the age of 13 and to place her in the original circumstances of the initial delirium, and then to convince her that her period had lasted three full days and had not been interrupted by any untoward incident. Once that was done, her next menses arrived right on schedule, lasted three full days without being accompanied by any discomfort, convulsions, or delirium. . . . [In the case of her facial symptoms] I used the same therapeutic maneuver. I brought her back [under hypnosis] to the period of contact with the little girl of whom she had such horror. I caused her to believe that the child was very attractive and had no scabs, but she was only half convinced. After making her repeat the same scene a second time, I was successful, and she fearlessly caressed the imaginary child. The sensation in the left side of her face returned without difficulty, and when I woke her up, Marie saw clearly with her left eye.

It is now five months since those experiments were made. Marie no longer manifests the slightest signs of hysteria, she feels well and grows increasingly stronger. Her physical appearance has radically changed. I do not attach any greater importance to this cure than it merits, and I have no idea how long it will last, but I find this history interesting as demonstrating the importance of fixed unconscious ideas and the role they play in certain physical illnesses as well as in emotional disorders. (Janet 1889/1989, pp. 412–413)

Initial Conceptual Formulations

A Comparison of Anna O. and Marie: Abreaction

A critical inspection of these two case vignettes reveals a major similarity and a significant difference. In both instances, the authors agree in attributing the cause and form of their patients' clinical symptoms to pathogenic dissociated memories. "The scene [of Marie's menarche]," says Janet, "occurs below consciousness and brings on all the rest of her difficulty in its train." "Hysterics," comment Breuer and Freud, "suffer mainly from reminiscences." When it comes to treatment, however, Janet and Breuer employed distinctly different therapeutic maneuvers. Janet focused on Marie's cognitive traumatic memories of her little companion's disfigured face and, using hypnotic suggestion, replaced the pathogenic memory images of the actual traumatic event with blandly pleasant, innocuous pseudomemories of the episode. Breuer, however, took a different tack in his treatment of Anna O.; using hypnosis, he focused on bringing into the patient's conscious awareness not only the pathogenic traumatic memories, but also the distressing emotions associated with them and then facilitated the expression of those emotions in a lively cathartic discharge that Breuer and Freud termed *abreaction.* The striking dissimilarity evident in those two different therapeutic approaches rested on a fundamental difference in the theoretical explanations that were advanced independently by Janet in *l'Automatisme Psychologique* and by Freud in "Studies on Hysteria." The more detailed delineation that follows of their respective conceptions of the nature of psychological dissociation and their divergent explanations of its pathogenesis will help us to understand their significance for modern clinical theory and practice.

The Nature of Dissociation

In *l'Automatisme Psychologique,* based on his observations of Marie and a number of other patients with hysterical symptoms, Janet made an original and far-reaching contribution to the understanding of dissociative phenomena. Contrary to the traditional view that human consciousness is a single, unbroken, and unitary continuity, Janet's clinical observations provided convincing evidence that there may coexist within one and the same individual two or more separate, dissociated streams of consciousness, each existing in isolation from the others and each with a wide spectrum of mental contents such as memories, sensations, volitions, and affects. The magnitude and intricacy of those dissociated complexes vary greatly. They may range, for example, from a restricted and limited set of memories of a single past event to a rich and complicated cluster of mental phenomena endowed with a personal identity quite separate and distinct from the primary personality of the individual in whom the dissociation occurs.

Moreover, although the primary consciousness is entirely unaware of the dissociated, unconscious complexes, the latter often engage autonomously in a wide range of mental functions characteristic of ordinary consciousness. They remember; they experience sensations, affects, and desires; they keep track of time, plan ahead, think logically, and solve mental problems; and, when they are endowed with a personal identity, they constitute an independent, self-aware co-conscious personality existing and functioning contemporaneously with, but outside the sphere of awareness of, the primary personality.

Co-consciousness. Related to Hilgard's (1977) conceptualization of the "hidden observer," co-consciousness is better demonstrated than described. It was clearly manifest in BCA, a woman,
age 30 years, with multiple personality disorder observed by
Morton Prince in the early part of this century("B.C.A..,"
1908–1909). The patient's primary personality, C, was a chronic
invalid suffering from a multiplicity of disabling neurasthenic
somatic symptoms. C was totally unaware of the existence of a
secondary personality, B. B, who was fully cognizant of C, was,
on the other hand, quite free of symptoms, cheerful, hale and
hearty, and, when she was in control, an enthusiastic participant
in a variety of lively activities.

In an autobiographical account, B (1908–1909) described the following state of co-consciousness during those times when C, the
primary personality, was in control of the patient's awareness and
external behavior.

> When I am not here as an alternating personality [i.e., dominating
> consciousness], my thoughts still continue . . . although [C is] not
> aware of them. . . . My mental life continues independently. . . .
> When C's mind is concentrated on any one thing, like reading or
> studying, it is closed to every other perception. She does not notice
> the sounds in the house or out of doors, but . . . I do. I hear the
> blinds rattle. I hear the maid moving about the house, I hear the
> telephone ring, etc. She hears none of these things. . . . I know all
> C's thoughts, and think my own besides. When she is talking with
> any one I often disagree with what she says. I think of replies I
> would make quite different from the ones she makes. . . . My train
> of thought may be, and usually is, quite different from C's. When C
> is ill, for instance, she is thinking about her headache and how hard
> life seems and how glad she will be when it is over, and I am think-
> ing how tiresome it is to lie in bed when I am just aching to go for a
> long tramp or do something gay. We rarely have the same opinions
> about any book we are reading, though we may both like it. C, how-
> ever, enjoys some writers whom I find very tiresome, Maeterlinck,
> for instance. She considers him very inspiring and uplifting, but I
> think he writes a lot of nonsense and is extremely depressing. (pp.
> 322–326)

The unconscious and pathogenesis. Although, as B's account graphically demonstrates, the dissociated mental elements may often engage in highly complex autonomous mental activities beneath the surface of the individual's consciousness, they are not entirely encapsulated or barred from having an effect on the individual's primary conscious stream of thought and behavior. On the contrary, their influence is frequently evident in a wide variety of somatic and mental symptoms whose origin is a mystery to the primary consciousness—that is, they are ego-alien. When, for example, the repression of memories of specific events creates a discontinuity in the stream of consciousness, the individual experiences, as the symptom of amnesia, the inability to recall the memories. If, on the other hand, the process of dissociation removes specific sensorimotor functions from conscious awareness and control, the individual will develop a wide variety of localized somatic conversion symptoms, such as the anesthesia, blindness, and shaking chills observable in Marie or the inability to drink in Anna O.—symptoms that represented the somatic expression of the dissociated memory images beneath the consciousness of each patient. And finally the clinical condition of multiple personality disorder ensues when a complex dissociated secondary personality emerges from below to overwhelm and displace the patient's normal personality structure. As William James (1902) commented nearly a hundred years ago,

> In the wonderful explorations by Binet, Janet, Breuer, Freud, Mason, Prince and others of the subliminal consciousness of patients with hysteria, we have revealed to us whole systems of underground life, in the shape of memories of a painful sort which lead a parasitic existence, buried outside the primary fields of consciousness, and making irruptions thereunto with hallucinations, pains, convulsions, paralyses of feeling and of motion, and the whole procession of symptoms of hysteric disease of body and of mind. (pp. 234–235)

It was a striking demonstration of Janet's creative genius to have thus fashioned a psychological model of hysterical symptom formation that incorporated his definition of the nature of dissociation, his description of the mechanisms by which dissociated ideas produced clinical symptoms, and his recognition of the fact that the pathogenic dissociated ideas were often memories of earlier traumatic events.

Similarly, in his initial approach to explaining the origin of hysterical phenomena, Freud agreed with Janet that dissociation was the key element in the pathogenic process. As he and Breuer commented in the introductory chapter of "Studies on Hysteria," "The splitting of consciousness which is so striking in the well-known classical cases of 'double consciousness' is present to a rudimentary degree in every hysteria, and a tendency to such a dissociation . . . is the basic phenomenon of this neurosis" (Breuer and Freud 1893–1895/1955, p. 12). However, when Janet and Freud turned their attention to an explanation of the cause of dissociation itself, they parted company.

Janet's Explanation of Dissociation: La Misère Psychologique

Janet viewed dissociation as the result of a fundamental constitutional flaw in psychological functioning, which he termed *la misère psychologique* (psychological insufficiency). In healthy individuals, Janet proposed, there is a basic quantum of psychological, or mental, energy that enables them to bind together all their mental operations (sensation, memory, cognition, affect, volition) into a unified and firmly integrated synthesis under the domination and control of a personal self with its distinct and persisting identity. In certain individuals, however, as a result of a genetically determined deficiency in the quantity of such binding energy, the personal self is compromised in its capacity to bind together the various mental components in an integrated whole under its control. As a consequence, in the wake of an emotionally draining traumatic experience, the personal self lacks sufficient strength to incorporate into its structure the resulting intense emotions and the memories associated with them, and they become dissociated from the sphere of the primary consciousness.

Freud's Explanation of Dissociation: Psychological Conflict

In "Studies on Hysteria," however, Freud (with Breuer's concurrence) advanced a radically different explanation of the etiology of dissociation with his introduction of the concept of *defense hysteria*. Dissociation occurs, he proposed, when the ego (as he called the personal consciousness) actively *represses* memories of the traumatic event to protect itself from experiencing the painful affects associated with them. "The basis for repression itself," he wrote, "can only be a feeling of unpleasure, the incompatibility between the single idea and the dominant mass of ideas constituting the ego. The repressed idea takes its revenge, however, by becoming pathogenic" (Breuer and Freud 1893–1895/1955, p 116). With this formulation of defense hysteria, Freud introduced the vital concept of psychological conflict that marked the point of his divergence from Janet's views and became the central guiding principle of psychoanalysis and its derivative, psychodynamic psychiatry, in the century ahead. To appreciate the full significance of this most important difference in their respective concepts, we must examine them in somewhat greater detail.

Janet Versus Freud

In Janet's theoretical conception, as I have noted, the personal self, weakened by its genetically determined insufficiency of psychological energy *(la misère psychologique)* is compromised in its ability to bind together its constituent mental functions into the normally integrated synthesis of a healthy personal identity. When a person thus compromised experiences a traumatic life event, the psychological energy expended by the painful emotional reaction to trauma further depletes the quantum of energy available to the personal self, which, thus further weakened, is unable to incorporate the memories of the events and associated feelings into its structure. As a consequence, the memories and associated feelings passively fall away from the conscious awareness and control of the self—that is, they are dissociated.

In Freud's formulation, on the contrary, the personal self, or ego, is viewed as possessing sufficient strength actively to repress the traumatic memories and affects in order to protect itself from experiencing the psychic pain associated with them. A psychological structure is thus created that arises from the ego's defensive repression countering the psychological energy of the unconscious, dissociated traumatic memories and affects striving to return to conscious awareness and expression—the two opposing forces now persisting in a relatively stable psychodynamic equilibrium that sustains the psychological structure.

Psychogenesis.   Given this difference in their conceptions of mental functioning, it is not surprising that Janet and Freud advanced different explanations of symptom formation. In Janet's view, the dissociated mental elements, disengaged from the synthesis of the personal self, now function independently and autonomously outside the sphere of that self, where they indirectly affect the personal self with symptomatic disturbances in its sensorimotor functions. In Marie, for example, the memories and affects of her traumatic encounter with her disfigured little companion, having dropped away from conscious control of her personal self, persist as an unconscious complex of "fixed ideas" that are reflected in her consciousness as a loss of the functions of vision and sensation.

Freud, on the other hand, views the psychogenesis of clinical symptoms as resulting from a compromise between the conflicting forces of the repressed mental elements and the ego's countering defensive repression that results in an indirect, disguised representation of the dissociated complex in the form of consciously experienced, ego-alien symptomatic dysfunction. Thus, in Anna O., the repressed disgust and anger aroused by the behavior of the lady companion's dog achieve a partial but disguised conscious representation in her symptomatic inability to drink. Janet "adhered to an *ego-deficit* model of psychopathology, while Freud's formulation was based on a psychodynamic *conflict* model of symptom-formation" (Nemiah 1989, p.1528).

Therapeutic implications. Against the background of this basic difference in their theoretical conceptions of the origin of dissociation and the psychogenesis of symptoms, we can now understand the rationale for the divergence in the therapeutic maneuvers that Janet and Freud employed—a distinction that Freud apparently failed to detect, as can be seen by examining his footnote in the "Preliminary Communication" in "Studies in Hysteria." Janet, aiming to neutralize the disintegrative effect of the painful emotions attached to the memories of a traumatic event, used hypnotic suggestion to change the content and character of the unconscious memories from unpleasant to innocuous. Thus altered, the memories were deprived of their pathogenic capacity to produce dissociative symptoms. Freud, on the other hand, employing the therapeutic procedure of abreaction (whose effectiveness Breuer had serendipitously discovered in treating Anna O.), aimed at altering the psychodynamic conflict underlying its surface symptomatic manifestations. While the patient was under hypnosis, both the repressed memories and the painful affects associated with them were raised into consciousness, and the patient was thus enabled actively to abreact the affects whose overt discharge over normal pathways of expression had until then been blocked by the ego's defensive repression. The unconscious pathogenic force was thereby dissipated, the conflict between ego defenses and painful affects was resolved, and the symptoms disappeared.

Later Development of Freud's Theoretical Formulations

Although, as I have noted, Freud's innovative concept of psychological conflict was the kernel of subsequent psychoanalytic theory, it should be recognized that its formulation in terms of abreaction was only a first step in the ultimate development of a more comprehensive and sophisticated structure of both theory and practice. In this chapter, I touch only briefly on two of the most significant conceptual changes that occurred in the course of that development. (A more detailed exposition of some of the major stages in that development may be found elsewhere [Nemiah 1984, 1987]).

From External Trauma to Internal Drives

In the early phases of his clinical investigations, Freud, following the lead of Janet, adhered to the idea that traumatic experiences, especially when they occurred early in life, were the source of the pathogenic mental elements leading to psychological conflict and symptom formation. Indeed, in two papers (Freud 1896a/1962, 1896b/1962) published a year after "Studies on Hysteria," he reported the histories of 13 consecutive hysterical patients, in every one of whom their symptoms could be traced back to a childhood sexual trauma. However, Freud's further clinical investigations (1905/1953) led him to the discovery of childhood sexuality as a significant feature of early human psychological development. Libidinal impulses, and the feelings and cognitive fantasies associated with them, far from first appearing at puberty as was then thought, were biologically determined inborn phenomena arising during the early years of the child's development *pari passu* with the development of ego defenses designed to control and modulate them. The sexual conflicts observed in adult patients, it became apparent, rather than reflecting actual childhood sexual traumas, were derived from internal childhood conflicts resulting from distortions in libidinal growth and development. What appeared in adult patients to be memories of early traumatic events were in fact the recurrence of fantasies and feelings directly associated with those early pathogenic developmental distortions. Adult psychogenic conflicts were, in other words, the legacy of disturbances in *internal* psychological processes during early development, not of fortuitous external traumatic experiences. This was a radical shift in the conceptualization of psychological conflict, whose origins were now viewed as being the product of internal, biologically determined factors rather than of accidental environmental causes.

Ego Psychology and the Structural Model

Psychological conflict, as we have seen, involves a clash between two opposing sets of forces: emotions and drives, on the one hand, pushing for overt expression and gratification, and the defensive controlling forces of the ego, on the other, striving to modulate and direct their discharge. Attention thus far has been focused mainly on the emotional and impulsive aspects of the conflict. That, too, was Freud's primary emphasis in the early phase of his work, but it is important to note that right from the start he also was concerned with the nature of the ego as evidenced by his delineation of the ego defense of repression and subsequently of other ego mechanisms of defense as well (Freud 1894/1962, 1896b/1962). Ego psychology, as it came to be called, later became a major focus of Freud's investigations, particularly in his exploration of grief as well as the related phenomena of aggression and narcissistic self-evaluation (Freud 1914/1957, 1917[1915]/1957, 1923/1961)—explorations that led to his formulation of the "structural model" (Freud 1926/1959) of the human psyche that is the basis of modern psychodynamic theory and practice.

In that structural model, the psyche is conceived of as being divided into three major functional components. The *id* is the site of origin of the libidinal and aggressive drives, which motivate much of human behavior. The *ego,* which is the seat of conscious awareness, comprises cognitive, sensory, and volitional functions that control external behavior and the defenses that control and modulate the drives. The *superego,* a special functional component of the ego, consists of a set of internalized values (the ego ideals) and sanctions (the conscience) that guide the ego's self-reflective evaluation of the appropriateness of its actions and determine the nature and degree of the individual's self-esteem. It should be noted, as well, that whereas in the topographic model the term *unconscious* is used to designate a specific component of the psychic structure, in the structural model it merely defines the quality of one aspect of the functioning of all the components of the mental apparatus.

Anxiety: an ego-affect. It is particularly important to recognize that, in the framework of the structural model, anxiety is conceived of as an "ego-affect." It is the ego's response to the threatened escape of unconscious sexual and aggressive drives from its defensive control, it is a signal to the ego of the potentially painful reprisal of guilt arising internally in the superego and of externally derived social disapproval if the drives are not adequately bridled, and it motivates the ego to strengthen its defenses against the emerging forbidden drives. Furthermore, anxiety serves as a marker to outside observers of areas of psychological conflict and, as such, is an important guide to clinicians in their evaluation and treatment of psychiatric patients. I return to that important aspect of anxiety as I review the implications of these historical observations for current psychiatric theory and practice.

Current Implications

Modern Phenomenological Psychiatry

It hardly needs to be said that there has been a major revolution in psychiatric thinking in recent years. To comprehend its magnitude, we need not look back beyond the movement toward a phenomenological view of psychiatric diagnosis that emerged during the formulation in the 1970s of the third edition of the American Psychiatric Association's DSM-III (American Psychiatric Association 1980). In an attempt to be atheoretical, the framers of that document have almost entirely abandoned the psychodynamic understanding of psychiatric phenomena that had dominated psychiatric thought for several decades. In the process, they have generally discarded the empirical psychodynamic observations that had been accumulated over the course of a hundred years in favor of a purely descriptive, phenomenological sorting and classification of the symptoms of psychiatric illness. The term *unconscious* has completely disappeared from their vocabulary, and the traditional concept of hysteria as a disorder with both sensorimotor and mental manifestations has been split apart by assigning the mental symptoms of hysteria, including amnesia, fugue states, and multiple personality disorder (renamed dissociative identity disorder in DSM-IV [American Psychiatric Association 1994]), to the major diagnostic category of dissociative disorders and by allocating the sensorimotor symptoms (designated as conversion disorder) to the entirely different major category of somatoform disorders.

Consequences of Phenomenology

Such a reclassification based purely on surface, descriptive characteristics implies that conversion disorder and the dissociative disorders are totally distinct, unrelated clinical conditions, despite the fact that symptoms referable to both diagnoses frequently appear together and are found to be the result of the underlying process of dissociation. As a consequence, modern clinicians, following the dictates of DSM-III and its sequels, DSM-III-R (American Psychiatric Association 1987) and DSM-IV, are placed in the paradoxical position of having to affirm that individuals manifesting both types of symptoms have two separate illnesses, conversion disorder and (in most instances) multiple personality disorder (now called dissociative identity disorder)—a diagnostic dissociation that the observations of our clinical predecessors demonstrate to be unwarranted. Indeed, what we have now put asunder perhaps Mother Nature meant to be together.

Return of a Dynamic Psychology

A Rent in the Curtain of Phenomenology

Despite contemporary psychiatry's amnesia for its past experiences, there is a beginning rent in the curtain of its phenomenalism. In fashioning its diagnostic categories, the sculptors of DSM-IV have, as is commented on elsewhere (Spiegel et al. 1995, p. 1418), generally followed the lead of their predecessors in DSM-III and DSM-III-R, who adhered to a "descriptive approach that attempted to be neutral with respect to theories of etiology" (American Psychiatric Association 1994, p. xviii). They have defined the major mental disorders in terms of empirically observed symptoms and signs that cluster in apparently naturally occurring categorical syndromes—until, that is, they come to a definition of the dissociative disorders. There, in what would appear to be a shift from their more usual approach, they state, "The essential feature of the Dissociative Disorders is a disruption in the usually integrated functions of consciousness, memory, identity, or perception of the environment" (American Psychiatric Association 1994, p. 477).

In using the word *functions,* the authors intuitively, if perhaps unwittingly, pass from a world of merely empirically observed symptoms and signs to the more dynamic dimension of the psychological *processes* that underlie them. Furthermore, by retaining the word *dissociative* in the diagnostic term *dissociative disorders,* they invoke the nuances of the rich body of psychological fact and theory well-known to clinicians a century ago that I have briefly outlined previously.

Revival of a Traumatic Model

Even more striking in this regard is the fact that modern clinicians investigating both the psychological reactions to traumatic experiences and the dissociative disorders (especially multiple personality disorder) have openly recalled and revived earlier psychological observations and concepts. In particular, they have restored to our awareness Janet's observations concerning psychological trauma and the integration and dissociation of personality (van der Hart and Friedman 1989; van der Kolk and van der Hart 1989), as well as Freud's formulations of psychological conflict and therapeutic abreaction. It is indeed a noteworthy and encouraging feature of the current widespread interest in multiple personality disorder and other dissociative phenomena that it is reviving an appreciation for the importance of unconscious mental processes and their role in the pathogenesis of psychiatric disorders at a time when such psychodynamic concepts have all but disappeared from psychiatric awareness. At the same time, it must be emphasized that the recall is only partial because it focuses attention only on the traumatic model of symptom formation that was a central feature of both Janet's conception and Freud's early formulation of pathogenesis, but quite overlooks the more comprehensive structural model of psychological functioning that Freud developed subsequently.

Implications of a traumatic model.   According to the traumatic model, the production of symptoms is attributed to the underlying effect of undischarged affects of repressed memories of traumatic external events. In his formulation of the psychological processes

involved, Freud initially proposed that the complex of unconscious, dissociated memories and affects persisted as a "foreign
body" until the memories could be recalled to consciousness and
the associated pathogenic affects dissipated through their discharge in overt conscious expression. From that conceptual formulation it followed that therapeutically induced abreaction of the
repressed affects was the treatment of choice. It is not surprising,
therefore, that modern clinicians, in adhering to the traumatic
model, utilize abreaction as an essential therapeutic technique in
the treatment of patients with multiple personality disorder. Indeed, as currently recommended by its proponents (Braun 1986;
Kluft 1991; Putnam 1989), a major phase of treatment, extending
over many months to several years, is devoted to searching out the
many alternating personalities that constitute the dissociated fragments of the patient's personal identity, raising them into consciousness by hypnotic and related measures and facilitating the
emotional abreaction of the pathogenic memories of child abuse associated with them.

As modern investigators have discovered, however, abreaction
alone often does not undo the fractionation of the personality into
isolated alters. Accordingly, once the alters have been recalled to
consciousness and abreacted, their fusion and ultimate integration
into a unified and stable personal identity can be accomplished
only by breaking down the amnestic barriers between the individual alters using active therapeutic maneuvers that appear to rely
heavily on hypnotic suggestion and the systematic desensitization
of anxiety.

Reenter Psychodynamic Psychotherapy

Fusion, moreover, is itself only a stage in the therapeutic process
and must be followed by a final phase of therapy in which the
now-integrated patient is enabled to work through the long-
standing conflicts underlying the patient's characterological distortions and disturbed personal relationships. Thus, as Kluft (1991)
comments, once integration has been accomplished, the patient
must learn *"new coping skills . . .* and be helped to negotiate the cir-

cumstances that once were handled in a dissociative manner in more constructive ways. . . . *Solidification of gains and working through* may require as much therapy as reaching integration or resolution" (p. 179).

It is evident from the treatment recommendations offered by Kluft and others that the final phase of solidification of gains is an essential and often lengthy component of the therapeutic process. It is interesting to note, however, that in their current, extensive writings most modern investigators of multiple personality disorder have very little to say about that vital aspect of clinical management. Although recognizing the importance of the working through of psychological conflicts and of developing new coping skills, they do so in principle only and fail to elaborate on the details of the concepts and specific procedures required to reach those ultimate therapeutic goals. The major focus of their attention has been directed toward the traumatic and dissociative aspects of psychopathology and psychological treatment. That focus provides a useful basis for the integrative phase of the overall treatment program of patients with multiple personality disorder, but achieving the final stage of consolidation requires a thorough understanding of the structural model and the therapeutic techniques of psychodynamic psychotherapy derived from it—an approach whose importance Marmer (1991) has underscored and that Gabbard (1994) has recently made explicit. "Following integration," Gabbard writes, "traditional psychodynamic psychotherapy is possible in which gains can be solidified, losses can be mourned, and interpretive resolution of conflict is addressed" (p. 305). Therefore, I conclude with a brief consideration of the psychodynamic understanding and treatment of multiple personality disorder.

Trauma and the Structural Model

The proper and effective application of psychodynamic psychotherapy, as I have suggested in this chapter, requires of the therapist a conceptual understanding that goes beyond the traumatic model to include the structural model of psychological functioning on which such therapy is based. A central feature of the structural model, as noted earlier, is the presence of psychological conflicts between biologically derived libidinal and aggressive drives and their affects arising in the id, and ego defenses countering their emergence into conscious awareness.

Furthermore, the anxiety experienced by the ego when pressured by the underlying drives represents its reaction to the threatened reprisals of superego guilt and external social condemnation that determine the ego's degree of awareness and behavioral expression of those drives. Based on this conceptual model, treatment is aimed at modifying the internal psychological structure through psychotherapeutic procedures designed to moderate the pathogenic conflict between the drives and defenses. When that occurs, the ego becomes better able to permit the drives to emerge into conscious awareness without experiencing anxiety and to facilitate their discharge in behavior that is both gratifying and personally and socially acceptable.

It must be emphasized that although the focus of attention of the structural model is on *internal* psychodynamic processes, these are not viewed as occurring in a vacuum. On the contrary, the internal conflicts are sensitive to external stressful events that often increase their intensity and set in motion pathogenic psychological processes leading to the appearance of clinical symptoms. Childhood abuse constitutes an especially important case of such an interaction between environmental stresses and internal psychological processes. The abusive act is particularly traumatic in its own right because of its inherently overpowering, terrifying, often violent aggressiveness. Its pathogenic potential is further intensified by the fact that the child experiences the abusive assault when his or her internal psychological structure is in the early phases of its development. The first glimmerings of inborn sexual and aggressive drives are prematurely aroused to overwhelming intensity, guilt and self-criticism are pathologically magnified, and primitive ego defenses, including the proclivity for dissociation, are fixated. As a consequence of that combination of extreme trauma impinging on its developing, still immature psychological organization, the individual carries into adulthood especially severe distortions of psychic structure and psychological conflicts that need to be taken into account in understanding and treating the psychiatric disorders that may result.

Complementarity of the Traumatic and Structural Models

When viewed in the light of this larger conceptual framework, it is evident that the traumatic model and the structural model are not mutually exclusive. Indeed, the traumatic model is specifically applicable to the phenomena associated with the trauma of child abuse. It allows us to understand how the child, when confronted with the terrifying experience of physical or sexual violence, defends himself or herself with the special psychological defense of repression, which is particularly designed to spare the child from experiencing psychological distress by removing from consciousness the cognitive memory images of the external events that produce that distress. It also allows us to see how the defensive repression produces a pathological fractionation of the ego into multiple dissociated fragments that, along with the pathological defense of dissociation itself, is carried into adulthood in the form of a dissociative disorder. Furthermore, the traumatic model provides a rational basis for the abreactive phase of treatment of adult patients with multiple personality disorder designed to achieve a unification and permanent integration of the dissociated ego as a prelude to engaging the patient in traditional psychodynamic psychotherapy.

However, the pathogenic effect of child abuse extends beyond its role in producing the dissociative fragmentation of ego functions and results in severe developmental distortions of the entire psychological structure that persist into adulthood as pathogenic psychological conflicts leading to psychiatric disorders and pathological disturbances in behavior and personal relationships. These broader psychopathological ramifications of the earlier effect of child abuse on internal psychological structure can be understood only in terms of the structural model. The structural model, as I have suggested, is not in conflict with the traumatic model but complements and amplifies it. Taken together, the two models constitute a more encompassing conceptual basis than either one alone for understanding and treating not only the dissociative disorders but also other common psychiatric disorders.

Conclusion

Much more, of course, remains to be learned about the psychodynamic factors underlying clinical dissociation and the therapeutic procedures based upon them. When viewed in the light of the structural model, many questions concerning the nature and treatment of the dissociative disorders are immediately apparent. What is the relation of ego-anxiety to the fear aroused by external trauma? In what ways do fear and anxiety differ from sexual and aggressive feelings with regard to their place in the psychodynamic structure, and what are the implications of such differences for the application of therapeutic procedures? What, for example, are the comparative effects of the abreaction of anxiety and fear, on the one hand, and of anxiety-producing aggressive and libidinal impulses on the other? What are the respective roles of childhood traumatic experiences and the concurrent, biologically determined, developmental sexual and aggressive fantasies in determining the content of adult memories of early life? Is the tendency of adult individuals to dissociate the result of genetic predisposition or of early trauma? Is psychodynamic psychotherapy indicated in all patients with multiple personality disorder after the integration of the ego has been achieved, or is it precluded in some by remaining deficits in ego function? And how does one determine whether the individual thus integrated is capable of engaging in such dynamic psychotherapy?

Those and the many other unanswered questions can be elucidated only by a more detailed investigation of the psychological structure and conflicts of patients with dissociative disorders than has as yet been accomplished. The recent recall of the traumatic model of psychogenesis from psychiatry's current amnesia for psychodynamic fact and theory is a first step in that direction, and one may hope that the recollection of the still dissociated structural model, with its more sophisticated concepts and methods of exploration of human psychology, will follow suit.

References

American Psychiatric Association: Diagnostic and Statistical Manual of Mental Disorders, 3rd Edition. Washington, DC, American Psychiatric Association, 1980

American Psychiatric Association: Diagnostic and Statistical Manual of Mental Disorders, 3rd Edition, Revised. Washington, DC, American Psychiatric Association, 1987

American Psychiatric Association: Diagnostic and Statistical Manual of Mental Disorders, 4th Edition. Washington, DC, American Psychiatric Association, 1994

"B": An introspective analysis of co-conscious life. J Abnorm Psychol 3:311–334, 1908–1909

"B.C.A.": My life as a dissociated personality. J Abnorm Psychol 3: 240–260, 1908–1909

Braun B: Issues in the psychotherapy of multiple personality disorder, in Treatment of Multiple Personality Disorder. Edited by Braun B. Washington, DC, American Psychiatric Press, 1986, pp 3–28

Breuer J, Freud S: Studies on hysteria (1893–1895), in The Standard Edition of the Complete Psychological Works of Sigmund Freud, Vol 2. Translated and edited by Strachey J. London, Hogarth Press, 1955, pp 1–319

Freud S: The neuro-psychoses of defence (1894), in The Standard Edition of the Complete Psychological Works of Sigmund Freud, Vol 3. Translated and edited by Strachey J. London, Hogarth Press, 1962, pp 41–68

Freud S: The etiology of hysteria (1896a), in The Standard Edition of the Complete Psychological Works of Sigmund Freud, Vol 3. Translated and edited by Strachey J. London, Hogarth Press, 1962, pp 189–221

Freud S: Further remarks on the neuro-psychoses of defence (1896b), in The Standard Edition of the Complete Psychological Works of Sigmund Freud, Vol 3. Translated and edited by Strachey J. London, Hogarth Press, 1962, pp 157–185

Freud S: Three essays on the theory of sexuality (1905), in The Standard Edition of the Complete Psychological Works of Sigmund Freud, Vol 7. Translated and edited by Strachey J. London, Hogarth Press, 1953, pp 125–243

Freud S: On narcissism: an introduction (1914), in The Standard Edition of the Complete Psychological Works of Sigmund Freud, Vol 14. Translated and edited by Strachey J. London, Hogarth Press, 1957, pp 67–102

Freud S: Mourning and melancholia (1917 [1915]), in The Standard Edition of the Complete Psychological Works of Sigmund Freud, Vol 14. Translated and edited by Strachey J. London, Hogarth Press, 1957, pp 237–260

Freud S: The ego and the id (1923), in The Standard Edition of the Complete Psychological Works of Sigmund Freud, Vol 19. Translated and edited by Strachey J. London, Hogarth Press, 1961, pp 8–66

Freud S: Inhibitions, symptoms and anxiety (1926), in The Standard Edition of the Complete Psychological Works of Sigmund Freud, Vol 20. Translated and edited by Strachey J. London, Hogarth Press, 1959, pp 75–175

Gabbard G: Psychodynamic Psychiatry in Clinical Practice. Washington, DC, American Psychiatric Press, 1994

Hilgard E: Divided Consciousness: Multiple Controls in Human Thought and Action. New York, Wiley-Interscience, 1977

James W: The Varieties of Religious Experience. New York, Longmans, Green, & Co., 1902

Janet P: l'Automatisme Psychologique (1889), Nouvelle Édition. Paris, la Société Pierre Janet, 1989

Kluft R: Multiple personality disorder, in American Psychiatric Press Review of Psychiatry, Vol 10. Edited by Tasman A, Goldfinger SM. Washington, DC, American Psychiatric Press, 1991, pp 161—188

Marmer S: Multiple personality disorder: a psychoanalytic perspective. Psychiatr Clin North Am 14:677–693, 1991

Nemiah J: The unconscious and psychopathology, in The Unconscious Revisited. Edited by Bowers K. New York, Wiley-Interscience, 1984, pp 49–87

Nemiah J: The psychoanalytic view of anxiety, in Diagnosis and Classification in Psychiatry. Edited by Tischler G. Cambridge, England, Cambridge University Press, 1987, pp 209–222

Nemiah J: Janet redivivus: the centenary of l'Automatisme Psychologique. Am J Psychiatry 146:1527–1529, 1989

Putnam F: Diagnosis and Treatment of Multiple Personality Disorder. New York, Guilford, 1889

Spiegel D, Liebowitz M, Nemiah J: Introduction to anxiety disorders, dissociative disorders, and adjustment disorders, in Treatments of Psychiatric Disorders, 2nd Edition, Vol 2. Edited by Gabbard GO. Washington, DC, American Psychiatric Press, 1995, pp 1416–1420

van der Hart O, Friedman B: A reader's guide to Pierre Janet on dissociation: a neglected intellectual heritage. Dissociation 2:8–16, 1989

van der Kolk B, van der Hart O: Pierre Janet and the breakdown of adaptation in psychological trauma. Am J Psychiatry 146:1530–1540, 1989

Chapter 2

Hypnosis, Dissociation, and Trauma: Myths, Metaphors, and Mechanisms

Frank W. Putnam, M.D., and Eve B. Carlson, Ph.D.

The renewal of interest in dissociation and the dissociative disorders has once again raised the fundamental question of the relationship between hypnosis and dissociation. This question persists across two centuries of clinical interest in these unusual disorders. Definitions and phenomenological descriptions of hypnosis and clinical dissociation suggest that both processes involve a lack of integration of thoughts, feelings, and experiences into the normal stream of consciousness. However, the two terms are often used to refer to different phenomena. Hypnosis generally occurs in a controlled context and involves the intentional evocation of a special state characterized by focused attention, distortions in perception, and the subjective experience of involuntariness. Clinical or pathological dissociation, on the other hand, is typically used to describe behaviors and experiences that spontaneously appear in uncontrolled contexts. Clinical dissociation involves experiences of loss of memory (amnesia) and disturbances in the sense of self (e.g., depersonalization, alter personality states).

Although many clinicians and theoreticians regard hypnosis and clinical dissociation as essentially synonymous processes, recent research suggests that their relationship is more complex and may be very narrowly confined to specific groups of subjects. In this chapter, we seek to sort out the myths, metaphors, and mechanisms regarding the hypnotic basis of pathological dissociation.

Brief History of the Association Between Hypnosis and the Dissociative Disorders

Dissociative disorders, especially multiple personality disorder (MPD), have been conceptually associated with hypnosis since the early clinical formulations of Eberhard Gmelin in 1789 (Bliss 1986). Subsequent reports of the use of mesmerism/hypnosis with dissociative patients appeared throughout the 1800s (E. T. Carlson 1989). At the end of the nineteenth century, the seminal work of Pierre Janet brought a new perspective on dissociation (Putnam 1989b). Janet regarded clinical dissociation as a form of hypnosis, remarking that "Hypnosis may be defined as the momentary transformation of the mental state of an individual, artificially induced by a second person, and sufficing to bring about dissociations of personal memory" (as quoted in Haule 1986, p. 86). Janet recognized the association of pathological dissociation with trauma and viewed dissociation as adaptive in the context of an overwhelming traumatic experience (Putnam 1989b). Morton Prince (1890), a contemporary of Janet and well-known for his pioneering work with MPD patients, was among the first to speculate on the possible creation of alter personalities by hypnosis, suggesting that if a patient were " . . . hypnotized sufficiently often and under sufficiently varied circumstances, the conscious experiences of her second self . . . would become extensive" (p. 51).

Modern interest in the relationship between dissociation and hypnosis has received impetus from two major areas of investigation. The first is the neodissociation theory of E. R. Hilgard (1986), who generated a series of studies on the effects of hypnosis on cognitive control functions. The neodissociative model of hypnosis postulates that there is a hierarchical system of cognitive controls for behavior and that hypnosis alters the relationship of these levels of control so that higher levels of cognitive control have less influence on the initiation and monitoring of behavior. As a result, a hypnotized individual experiences his or her own behavior as involuntary. Alternative formulations of the nature of hypnosis include the social psychological models of Sarbin and Coe (1972) and Spanos (1986). However, social psychological models do not account for much experimental data and, as yet, have had little impact on clinical formulations of the dissociative disorders (Bowers 1990; Kihlstrom and Hoyt 1990).

The second major catalyst for the increase of interest in dissociation and hypnosis has been the rise over the last decade in the numbers of reported cases of MPD and other dissociative disorders. Reports of an MPD "epidemic" are exaggerated, although the concerns underlying this hyperbole are sometimes justified by overdiagnosis and by serious deficiencies in DSM criteria. Nevertheless, the increased attention to MPD has stimulated theories and therapeutic interventions that directly or indirectly involve hypnosis. In particular, the "autohypnotic" model is frequently offered in training workshops as the explanatory mechanism for the development of MPD and as a justification for the use of hypnosis in treatment.

The autohypnotic model of MPD postulates that a traumatized individual (usually thought to be a child) uses his or her innate hypnotic capacities to induce "self-hypnosis" as a defensive response to overwhelming traumatic events (Bliss 1984; Frischholz 1985; Kluft 1984; Putnam 1986; Spiegel 1986). The traumatized individual is said to enter into an autohypnotic or self-induced hypnotic state that produces amnesia for the painful experience. With repetitive trauma, the autohypnotic state is somehow transformed over time into an alter personality, giving rise to MPD. The details of the process of transformation from an autohypnotic state to an alter personality state have not been specified.

Because most proponents of the autohypnotic model only address the creation of MPD, it is not clear how this theory applies to the other dissociative disorders, which are also linked to traumatic antecedents (Putnam 1985). Dissociative amnesia and dissociative fugue frequently occur in the immediate context of the traumatic experience and are time limited, whereas MPD, a chronic condition, appears to emerge over time and with development in the context of early childhood trauma (Putnam 1989a). Although one often hears workshop leaders lump all dissociative disorders together under the mechanistic umbrella of the autohypnotic model, the application of the autohypnotic model to the other dissociative disorders is not well worked out.

Five lines of argument are usually made in support of the auto-hypnotic theory of MPD. The first is the often-made statement that patients with dissociative disorders have increased levels of hypnotizability compared with psychiatric patients and other comparison groups. This statement is based on only two studies using standard scales of hypnotizability (Bliss 1984; Frischholz et al. 1992). Bliss (1984) reported on a sample of 28 MPD subjects who averaged 10.1 on the Stanford Hypnotic Susceptibility Scale Form C (SHSS-C; Weitzenhoffer and Hilgard 1962), compared with a control group of 49 cigarette smokers who averaged 6.0. Frischholz et al. (1992) reported on a study of the hypnotizability of 12 MPD patients and 5 patients with dissociative disorder not otherwise specified (DDNOS) compared with schizophrenic, mood disorder, and anxiety disorder patients and college students. The mean hypnotizability score of the DDNOS patients on the SHSS–C was 8.94 (Frischholz et al. 1992). Although this score was significantly elevated compared with the scores for the other groups, it is slightly below the cutoff score of 9 often used to designate the lower boundary of high hypnotizability in laboratory studies. Thus, two small sample studies indicate that the hypnotizability scores of dissociative disorder patients are in the upper range of the SHSS–C, but these mean scores are not "off the scale" as they are sometimes portrayed in explications of the autohypnotic model of MPD.

The second line of argument used to support the autohypnotic model is the observation that analogues of some of the symptoms common to MPD patients can be produced under hypnosis in highly hypnotizable healthy subjects (Putnam 1986). Auditory hallucinations, motor paralyses, automatic writing, age regression, and posthypnotic amnesias can be induced by hypnotic suggestion in some susceptible subjects (E. R. Hilgard 1986). Analogies have been made between these experimental phenomena, respectively, and auditory hallucinations, conversion symptoms, passive influence experiences, child alter personality states, and the array of amnesias and other memory disturbances that are common clinical features of MPD. However, apparent similarities in behavioral phenomena do not constitute proof that the underlying mechanism is the same.

A third argument is that hypnosis is therapeutic for MPD; therefore, it must be acting upon the basic pathological mechanism. There is no question that the judicious use of therapeutic hypnosis is an efficacious intervention that can ameliorate distress and transiently contain some of the troublesome symptoms and behaviors in MPD patients (Bliss 1986; Kluft 1982; Putnam 1989a). But it is worth noting that two studies have found that the therapeutic use of hypnosis did not change the basic clinical features of MPD patients (Putnam et al. 1986; Ross and Norton 1989). If autohypnosis were the fundamental mechanism underlying the dissociative symptoms of MPD, one might expect therapeutic hypnosis to influence strongly the clinical features of the condition by eliminating or significantly transforming dissociative symptoms—but this is *not* the case.

The fourth line of argument that MPD is based on an autohypnotic mechanism cites initial reports of increased hypnotizability following childhood trauma (Nash and Lynn 1985–1986; Nash et al. 1984). These preliminary findings were seized upon by MPD theorists (including the aforementioned authors) as support for the autohypnotic model. In subsequent studies, Nash and his colleagues were not able to replicate their initial findings and now believe that the apparent differences in hypnotizability between abused and nonabused subjects were spurious and resulted from a "context" effect produced by the paired administration of the measures (M. R. Nash, personal communication, November 1993). We will examine this issue in more detail later in the chapter.

The last line of argument is based on reports of creating, under hypnosis, alter personality–like phenomena in highly hypnotizable healthy subjects. Several old reports claimed that alter personality–like entities could be created under hypnosis (Harriman 1943; Kampman 1976; Levitt 1947). Reanalysis of these reports by Braun (1984) suggests that these hypnotically created entities are transient "ego-state" phenomena that do not clinically resemble MPD. The term *ego-states* refers to "a body of behaviors and experiences which are bound together by some common principle and separated from other such states by a boundary which is more or less permeable" (Watkins and Watkins 1979–1980, p. 5).

E. R. Hilgard (1984) likewise cautions against equating the time-limited phenomenon of the hypnotically created hidden-observer function in highly hypnotizable healthy subjects with the alter personality states of MPD patients. He notes that the dissociative aspects of the hidden observer " . . . bear some resemblance to those of multiple personality, but it is a mistake to extrapolate too quickly to the more profound and enduring changes found in clinical cases of multiple personality" (E. R. Hilgard 1984, p. 252). Thus, authorities on both MPD and hypnosis reject the analogy between hypnotically created transient "ego-state" or "hidden-observer" phenomena and the persistent alter personality states of MPD patients.

The autohypnotic theory of MPD (and by extension here to the other dissociative disorders) is largely based on argument by analogy rather than on empirical data. Moreover, several of the lines of argument are at least partially contradicted by recent research. Nonetheless, the autohypnotic theory of MPD has given rise to highly elaborated hypnotic treatment protocols currently circulating in continuing education workshops and other training forums. The explicit or implicit assertion that hypnosis and clinical dissociation are synonymous processes is frequently given as the justification for using hypnotic treatment in dissociative disorders. This assertion demands that we critically reexamine the theoretical assumptions about the "hypnotic" nature of clinical dissociation in the light of recent research findings.

Issues in the Conceptualization of Hypnosis and Dissociation

Nature of the Measures and Research Samples

We have pointed out elsewhere (E. B. Carlson and Putnam 1989) that hypnosis scales and dissociation measures tap very different experiential and response domains. Standard hypnosis scales— such as the Stanford Hypnotic Susceptibility Scale (SHSS-A, B,

Weitzenhoffer and Hilgard 1959; SHSS-C, Shor and Orne 1962) and the Harvard Group Scale of Hypnotic Susceptibility (HGSHS; Shor and Orne 1962)—feature items sampling motor and cognitive alterations induced by hypnosis in a clinical or laboratory setting. Typical hypnosis scale items include suggestions of hand lowering; inability to separate clasped hands; hallucination of a mosquito; hallucination of sweet and sour taste; age regression; eye catalepsy; and posthypnotic amnesia (E. R. Hilgard 1986). Motor items are heavily represented on most hypnotizability scales and are objectively scored by observing the subject's responses.

In contrast, measures of clinical dissociation, such as the Dissociative Experiences Scale (DES; Bernstein and Putnam 1986), Bliss Dissociation Scale (M. Wogan, "The Bliss Scale: Development, Reliability, and Validity," unpublished document, 1992), Perceptual Alteration Scale (PAS; S. Sanders 1986), and the Questionnaire of Experiences of Dissociation (QED; Riley 1988), inquire about spontaneous experiences of alterations in memory, identity, and awareness and subjective experiences, such as depersonalization and derealization, occurring in the context of daily activities. Examples include the experience of finding oneself in a place and having no idea of how one got there; having no memory for important life events, such as one's wedding or graduation; and feeling as if one is standing outside of one's body and watching oneself as if watching another person. Dissociation scale items tap subjective experiences and ask the individual to estimate the frequency or extent of these experiences in daily life.

A second area of difference lies in the subject samples typically used in hypnosis and dissociation research. Much hypnosis research is based on samples of healthy undergraduate and graduate students, who generally score in the low range on dissociation scales. In contrast, research on clinical dissociation is generally conducted with clinical samples and with traumatized subjects. These differences can produce confounding effects. First, the relatively restricted range of dissociation scores in healthy population samples constrains the magnitude of correlation coefficients between hypnosis and dissociation measures. Second, it is possible that traumatized persons with posttraumatic symptoms, such as hypervigilance and hyperarousal, and with emotional reasons for being distrustful of authorities and wishing to remain in control may have more difficulty establishing rapport in experimental hypnosis studies. Difficulty with rapport and trust could produce lower scores on hypnosis measures. However, our own experience in repeated assessment of hypnotizability at yearly intervals with sexually abused girls and the hypnotizability studies of combat veterans suggest that rapport problems are probably not a major confound in research with traumatized subjects (Putnam et al. 1995; Spiegel et al. 1988; Stutman and Bliss 1985).

Different Types and Dimensions of Hypnosis?

Within the field of hypnosis research there is a long-standing question about the possibility that there are two or more types of hypnosis. A related hypothesis is that hypnosis is a multidimensional process and individuals may excel along certain dimensions but not others, giving rise to different hypnotic capacities and experiences. A full discussion of this subject is beyond the scope of this chapter; however, the hypothesis that there may be more than one type and dimension of hypnosis emerges from two lines of evidence. The first is that in clinical settings, individuals who score in the low to moderate range on standard hypnotic measures may nonetheless demonstrate surprisingly powerful clinical responses to hypnotic interventions for pain and anxiety (Barber 1980; Frankel 1978, 1990). Some authorities have interpreted this finding as indicating that there may be *laboratory* and *clinical* contextual forms of hypnosis. This observation is relevant clinically in that hypnotizability scale scores do not necessarily predict therapeutic response to hypnotic interventions.

The second line of evidence emerges from laboratory studies of highly hypnotizable subjects. A number of hypnotic tasks can be used to divide highly hypnotizable subjects (as measured by standard scales) into two groups. Hypnotic tasks believed to yield dichotomous cleavages include creating a hidden observer, displaying duality of experience during age regression, and generating imagery during hypnotic analgesia. Based on the small sample studies conducted to date, duality of experience during age regression (i.e., the subject's sense of the simultaneous copresence of a child and adult self) is related to the subject's ability to create a hidden observer, a hypnotic capacity restricted to approximately half of all highly hypnotizable subjects (E. R. Hilgard 1984). Pekala (1991) found evidence that highly hypnotizable subjects differ in their use of imagery during the administration of the HGSHS. A series of research studies under the direction of Kenneth Bowers (1991) strongly supports a multidimensional conceptualization of hypnosis. Barrett (1992) has identified dichotomous differences among highly hypnotizable subjects in time to enter deep trance, amnesia for trance experiences, and similarity/dissimilarity between trance experiences and nontrance fantasy states. Thus, bimodality of highly hypnotizable subjects has been found for a number of different hypnotic tasks.

These two lines of evidence suggest that either two or more types of hypnosis exist or that hypnotizability is a multidimensional capacity and scores on standard scales only measure part of the clinical and experimental variance. The dichotomous responses of highly hypnotizable subjects to the same task (e.g., age regression or image generation) are a particularly important observation supporting the position that hypnosis is at the very least a multidimensional construct (Bowers 1991). Concerns about the persistent bimodality of hypnosis score distributions across many scales and tasks have troubled researchers for decades and remain to be satisfactorily explained (Balthazard and Woody 1989; E. R. Hilgard 1965). Frankel (1990) has cautioned that despite current dimensional conceptualizations, qualitative differences in hypnotizability and dissociation at some point on their respective continuums remain a distinct possibility.

Relationship Between Hypnosis and Dissociation

Correlations Between Measures of Hypnotizability and Dissociation

Following the publication of valid and reliable dissociation measures such as the DES (Bernstein and Putnam 1986), researchers began to explore the relationships between dissociation and hypnotizability. The first test of the autohypnotic model of disso-ciative disorders is to determine the statistical relationship between measures of hypnotizability and clinical dissociation. Table 2–1 summarizes the results of studies to date. Inspection of Table 2–1 reveals that, in most studies, scores on standard hypnosis scales are not significantly correlated with scores on a variety of dissociation scales. Even when the correlations reach statistical significance as a result of a large sample size, their magnitude is low and only ex-plains a very small percentage of the variance. Several studies (de-noted by the [a] in Table 2–1) compared the relationship between dissociation score and hypnotizability when the two measures were administered together (" in context") and separately (" out of context"). When the dissociation measure was administered to-gether with the hypnosis measure, there was usually a small in-crease in the correlation coefficient, sometimes achieving statistical significance. This context effect has been studied for a number of attributes thought to be relevant to hypnotizability (Spanos et al. 1993).

The data in Table 2–1 demonstrate that standard measures of hypnotizability and dissociation are only weakly related, even in samples that include identified victims of trauma. Hypnotizability and dissociativity, as measured by current instruments, are clearly not synonymous processes. In fact, they are largely independent, and changes in one account for little of the variance in the other.

Although it seems clear that hypnotizability and dissociativity, as measured by current instruments, are not the same phenome-non, there are methodological aspects of these studies that may be acting to minimize their relationship. In many of these studies, un-dergraduate students are used as subjects. Although a convenient sample, undergraduates are not typical of the larger population and represent levels of psychological health necessary to remain in college and therefore may not be representative of the range of dissociation and/or hypnotizability found in the population as a whole. Restriction in the range of scores for either hypnosis or dis-sociation will reduce the size of correlations between the two measures.

Table 2–1. Correlations between measures of hypnotizability and dissociation

Author/date	N	Hypnosis measure	Dissociation measure	Pearson r, P value
Segal and Lynn 1992–1993	85	HGSHS	DES	.17, P = NS
J. P. Green and S. J. Lynn, "Dissociative Experiences in a Sample of Male and Female College Students," unpublished manuscript, Ohio University, Athens, OH, 1990	218	HGSHS	DES	.09, P = NS[a]
Nadon et al. 1991	475	HGSHS	DES	.08, P = NS[a]
Frischholz et al. 1992	309	HGSHS	DES	.12, P < .05
Putnam et al. 1995	105	SHCS Child	CDC	11, P = NS[a]
M. Nash, personal communication, December 1992	98	SHSS-A	IDS	.16, P = NS
M. Nash, personal communication, December 1992	47	SHSS-A	DES	.27, P = NS
M. Nash, personal communication, December 1992	98	SHSS-A	PAS	.12, P = NS
Spanos et al. 1993	75	CURSS-O	DES	.11, P = NS[a]
DiTomasso and Routh 1993	312	HGSHS	DES	.16, P < .01
Silva and Kirsch 1992	190	CURSS-O	DES	.15, P = NS[a]

(continued)

Table 2–1. Correlations between measures of hypnotizability and dissociation (*continued*)

Author/date	N	Hypnosis measure	Dissociation measure	Pearson r, P value
G. Johnson, I Kirsch, and H. Wasch, "Dissociation, hypnotizability and fantasy proneness in survivors of abuse," unpublished manuscript, University of Connecticut, Storrs, CT, 1992	148	SHSS-A	DES	.20, P < .05[a]
Tanabe and Kasai 1993	107	HGSHS[b]	DES[b]	.15, P = NS
Faith and Ray 1994	886	HGSHS	DES	.09, P = NS
Covino et al. 1994	37	SHSS-C	DES	.41, P < .02

Note. HGSHS = Harvard Group Scale of Hypnotic Susceptibility; DES = Dissociative Experiences Scale; SHCS Child = Stanford Hypnotic Clinical Scale for Children; CDC = Child Dissociative Checklist (Putnam et al. 1993); SHSS-A = Stanford Hypnotic Susceptibility Scale—Form A; PAS = Perceptual Alteration Scale; CURSS-O = Carleton University Responsiveness to Suggestion Scale—Objective Dimension; IDS = Indiana Dissociation Scale.
[a]Hypnosis and dissociation measures administered in different contexts.
[b]Japanese translation.

Interrelationships of Hypnotizability, Dissociativity, Fantasy Proneness, and Absorption

Research suggests that the constructs of absorption (Roche and McConkey 1990; Tellegen and Atkinson 1974) and fantasy proneness (Lynn and Rhue 1986; Wilson and Barber 1983) are interrelated with those of hypnotizability and dissociativity. Absorption, defined as an individual's openness to absorbing and self-altering experiences, is conceptualized as a trait, present to a greater or lessor degree in all individuals. Fantasy-prone persons were originally described by Wilson and Barber (1981) as individuals who " . . . live much of the time in a world of their own making—in a world of imagery, imagination and fantasy" (p. 133). Fantasy proneness, although usually measured with dimensional instruments, is often viewed as a personality type variable apportioned at low, moderate, and high levels (Lynn et al. 1988; Silva and Kirsch 1992).

A number of studies link absorption and fantasy proneness with each other and with dissociativity and hypnotizability (e.g., see Barrett 1992; Glisky et al. 1991; LeBaron et al. 1988; Lynn and Rhue 1986; Lynn et al. 1988; Plotnick et al. 1991; Roche and McConkey 1990; Segal and Lynn 1992–1993; Silva and Kirsch 1992; Wilson and Barber 1981, 1983). A less than exhaustive review of studies correlating two or more of these four constructs suggests the following trends: Absorption is moderately to strongly correlated with measures of fantasy proneness ($r = .40–.74$). Absorption is moderately correlated with dissociation ($r = .35–.45$). Absorption is moderately correlated with hypnotizability ($r = .22–.44$). Fantasy proneness is moderately to strongly correlated with dissociation ($r = .42–.63$). Fantasy proneness is moderately correlated with hypnotizability ($r = .29–.53$). Thus, absorption and fantasy proneness are most strongly correlated with each other. Hypnotizability and dissociativity tend to have stronger correlations with absorption and fantasy proneness than they do with each other. Preliminary data suggest that fantasy proneness and absorption are also elevated in traumatized individuals compared with nontraumatized individuals (Johnson and Kirsch 1990; Lynn et al. 1988), a

feature also found for dissociativity but not necessarily hypnotizability (see below).

Hypnosis, Dissociation, and Trauma

Hypnosis and Trauma

A second test of the autohypnotic model of MPD and the dissociative disorders involves the postulated increase in hypnotizability
following traumatic experiences. Early work by J. R. Hilgard (1979)
suggested that the severity of childhood experiences of punishment and discipline was correlated (r (185) = .30, $P <$ .001) with
SHSS–C (Weitzenhoffer and Hilgard 1962) scores. Studies by
Nowlis (1969) and London (1962) appeared to lend further support
to the hypothesis that childhood stress and punishment are associated with increased hypnotizability scores. As mentioned previously, preliminary reports of increased hypnotizability in abuse
victims were also cited in support of the thesis that stress and
trauma increase hypnotizability.

   However, results from subsequent carefully controlled studies
do not support this hypothesis. Studies by DiTomasso and Routh
(1993), Johnson and Kirsch (1990), Nash et al. (1993), Putnam et al.
(1995), and Rhue et al. (1990) compared abused with nonabused
subjects and found no differences in hypnotizability. Table 2–2 details these negative studies. The Putnam et al. (1995) study, which
compared sexually abused girls, ages 6–15 years, with carefully
matched healthy control girls at two points in time found no significant differences on the Stanford Hypnotic Clinical Scale for
Children (SHCS Child; Morgan and Hilgard 1979) scores either
initially or 1 year later. In fact, the Putnam et al. (1995) study actually found significantly more highly hypnotizable subjects in the
age, gender, socioeconomic, race, and family constellation–matched comparison group than in the abused group.
Within the abused sample analyses in all of the Table 2–2 studies,
there were no significant associations between hypnotizability
scores and various abuse variables (e.g., frequency of abuse, duration of abuse, type of abuse, relationship with perpetrator).

However, two studies have linked elevated levels of hypnotizability with posttraumatic stress disorder (PTSD) in Vietnam combat veterans. In a small sample study, Stutman and Bliss (1985) found that veterans with high PTSD ratings scored significantly higher on the SHSS–C than did veterans with low PTSD ratings. This finding was replicated using the Hypnotic Induction Profile (HIP; Spiegel et al. 1988) with a larger sample of veterans with PTSD compared with clinical and nonclinical subjects. Given the negative results summarized in Table 2–2, the findings with combat veterans require replication before they are accepted. There may be several factors confounding these two studies of combat veterans, including sample sizes and choice of the comparison groups.

Traumatized subjects who fulfill diagnostic criteria for PTSD or MPD also may be qualitatively different from the more heterogeneous pool of trauma subjects included in the Table 2–2 studies. Johnson and Kirsch (1990) observed that the original data from Nash et al. (1984) and Nash and Lynn (1985–1986) on child abuse and hypnotizability, as well as their own data, suggest the possibility of a bimodal distribution of hypnotizability scores in the traumatized sample. Putnam et al. (1995) identified the existence of a small subgroup of subjects who were both highly dissociative and highly hypnotizable, 90% of whom were in the abuse group. In this study, the concurrence of high hypnotizability and high dissociativity was associated with significantly earlier onset of abuse and greater abuse severity on several trauma indexes. These observations suggest the possibility of a latent-type variable, perhaps related to specific features of trauma, which is obscured by current dimensional analyses.

Dissociation and Trauma

The relationship between antecedent trauma and clinical dissociation is better established. To date, every study that has investigated this relationship has found significant associations between measures of trauma and clinical dissociation. Research studies of the association between dissociativity and trauma fall into four broad

Table 2–2.　Hypnotizability and trauma: studies comparing hypnotizability between trauma and nontrauma groups

Author/date	N	Hypnosis measure	Trauma group	Comparison group	Increased hypnotizability
DiTomasso and Routh 1993	312	HGSHS	Abused undergraduates	Nonabused undergraduates	No
Putnam et al. 1995	105	SHCS Child	Sexually abused girls ages 5–15 yrs	Matched, nonabused girls	No
Johnson et al. 1992	148	SHSS-A	Abused undergraduates	Nonabused undergraduates	No
Nash et al. 1993	105	SHSS-A	Abused adults	Nonabused adults	No
Johnson and Kirsch 1990	40	SHSS-A	Abused outpatients	Nonabused outpatients	No
Rhue et al. 1990	99	HGSHS	Abused undergraduates	Nonabused undergraduates	No
Spiegel et al. 1988	245	HIP	Combat veterans with PTSD	Patients with other psychiatric disorders and healthy subjects	Yes
Stutman and Bliss 1985	26	SHSS-C	Combat veterans with PTSD	Combat veterans without PTSD	Yes

Note.　HGSHS = Harvard Group Scale of Hypnotic Susceptibility; SHCS Child = Stanford Hypnotic Clinical Scale for Children; SHSS-A = Stanford Hypnotic Susceptibility Scale—Form A; SHSS-C = Stanford Hypnotic Susceptibility Scale—Form C; HIP = Hypnotic Induction Profile; PTSD = Posttraumatic Stress Disorder.

methodological categories: 1) studies reporting rates of trauma in patients meeting DSM-III-R (American Psychiatric Association 1987) diagnostic criteria for dissociative disorders (e.g., see Coons et al. 1988; Loewenstein and Putnam 1990; Putnam et al. 1986; Ross et al. 1991), 2) studies comparing levels of dissociation between traumatized and nontraumatized samples (see Table 2–3), 3) within-trauma-sample studies correlating the severity of trauma indexes with dissociation scores (e.g., see Branscomb 1991; Cardena and Spiegel 1993; E. B. Carlson and Rosser-Hogan 1991; Kirby et al. 1992), and 4) studies of the relationship of peritraumatic dissociation to the development of PTSD (e.g., see Koopman et al. 1994; Marmar et al. 1994). Within-trauma-group analyses of trauma indexes and dissociation scores are also often included in the comparison group studies.

Table 2–3 summarizes research studies that report significantly higher levels of dissociation in traumatized individuals compared with nontraumatized comparison samples. In aggregate, these studies, which include different sources of trauma and use different measures of dissociation and comparison groups, demonstrate that antecedent traumatic experiences are associated with significantly higher levels of dissociation compared with nontraumatized samples.

The within-trauma-group analyses give us some idea of the degree of this association, generally reported in the form of correlations between various indexes of trauma severity and dissociation. Although most studies report significant correlations between dissociation and trauma measures, the magnitude of these correlations is generally only in the moderate range (i.e., $r = .20–.45$). In part, this may reflect the methodological complexities of the quantification of the many dimensions of trauma. Our own experience with the quantification of maltreatment in sexual abuse victims suggests that many of the dimensions of trauma are confounded. For example, incest involving force and coercion is typically disclosed sooner than incest not involving force. Stepfather-stepdaughter incest is more likely to include penetration abuses and coercion than is father-daughter incest. Thus, duration may be confounded with type of abuse, relationship to perpetrator,

Table 2–3. Dissociation and trauma: studies reporting significantly higher levels of dissociation in the trauma group versus comparison group

Author/date	N	Dissociation measure	Trauma group	Comparison group
DiTomasso and Routh 1993	312	DES	Abused undergraduates	Nonabused undergraduates
Putnam et al. 1995	105	CDC	Sexually abused girls	Matched nonabused girls
Nash et al. 1993	105	IDS, DCS	Abused women	Nonabused women
Sandberg and Lynn 1992	66	DES	Abused undergraduates	Nonabused undergraduates
Bremner et al. 1992	85	DES	Veterans with PTSD	Veterans without PTSD
Briere and Runtz 1989	195	TSC-33	Patients with CSA	Patients without CSA
Briere and Runtz 1988	251	HSCL	Women with CSA	Women without CSA
Chu and Dill 1990	98	DES	Psychiatric inpatients with CSA	Psychiatric inpatients without CSA
Goff et al. 1991	61	DES	Psychotic patients with CSA	Psychotic patients without CSA
Sanders and Giolas 1991	47	DES	Adolescent inpatients with CSA	Adolescent inpatients without CSA
Strick and Wilcoxon 1991	84	DES	Female outpatients with CSA	Female outpatients without CSA

Warshaw et al. 1993	711	DES	Patients with PTSD	Patients without PTSD
Pribor et al. 1993	99	DES	Patients with abuse histories	Patients without abuse histories
Johnson et al. 1992	148	DES	Abused undergraduates	Nonabused undergraduates

Note. DES = Dissociative Experiences Scale; CDC = Child Dissociative Checklist (Putnam et al. 1993); IDS = Indiana Dissociation Scale; DCS = Dissociation Content Scale; PTSD = Posttraumatic Stress Disorder; TSC-33 = Trauma Symptom Checklist—33; CSA = Childhood Sexual Abuse; HSCL = augmented version of the Hopkins Symptom Checklist.

and use of force or coercion. However, it is likely that there are other relevant factors (e.g., family environment and nonabusive child-rearing practices) that account for significant amounts of the presently unexplained variance (Nash et al. 1993; Tillman et al., in press).

Discussion

Autohypnosis as the Mechanism Underlying Multiple Personality Disorder and Dissociative Disorders?

In this chapter, we review the current arguments and data linking hypnosis, dissociation, and trauma. An examination of the five lines of conceptual argument commonly offered in continuing education workshops to support the autohypnotic theory of pathological dissociation reveals that they are largely based on argument by analogy and are, in some instances, contradicted by empirical data. In both general population and traumatized samples, hypnotizability and dissociativity, as measured by current scales, are only weakly related constructs and share stronger relationships with absorption and fantasy proneness than they do with each other. The sample size–weighted mean correlation coefficient between standard measures of hypnotizability and dissociativity is only $r = .12$ and explains less than 2% of the variance (see Table 2–1). These data indicate that hypnosis, as operationally defined by current standard measures, is not the mechanism underlying the increased levels of dissociation found in traumatized individuals.

Recent research indicates that in most studies, a history of trauma is not associated with significant increases in hypnotizability. However, two studies do report significant differences in hypnotizability between trauma and nontrauma groups, and a trend toward bimodality of hypnotizability scores in other traumatized samples has been observed (Table 2–2). These discrepancies remain to be accounted for, and the trauma-hypnotizability question should remain open to active investigation. Nonetheless, the weight of the current data indicates that trauma does not alter hypnotizability in most individuals.

However, a history of trauma is significantly associated with increased dissociation in all studies to date. Although dissociation and trauma are significantly associated, the moderate correlations between indexes of trauma severity and dissociativity indicate that a substantial percentage of the variance of this relationship remains to be accounted for.

Hypnosis as a Heuristic Metaphor for the Experience of Pathological Dissociation

In addition to being invoked as the mechanism underlying dissociative disorders, the autohypnotic model also has served as a metaphor for empathically conveying the subjective experience of clinical dissociation. Dissociative individuals are frequently described as entering into and/or existing in "hypnotic" or "trance" states. The metaphoric use of *hypnotic trance* to describe the psychological experience of dissociative states has legitimate but limited heuristic value. It is useful for helping clinicians, who are often personally familiar with hypnosis, develop empathy for the subjective experiences of clinical dissociation. It also builds a sense of therapeutic confidence by redefining an unfamiliar condition, pathological dissociation, in terms of a familiar and more benign process, hypnosis.

However, metaphors have powerful ways of influencing our thinking and often limit our ability to conceptualize processes in new and more meaningful ways. The autohypnotic metaphor has become the standard, and all too often only, way in which the dissociative disorders are conceptualized. A generation of clinicians has seized upon this theoretical model as "the explanation." Given the data reviewed in this chapter, this explanation is, at best, problematic. At this point in our understanding, workshop leaders, supervisors, and other authorities should be careful to draw clear distinctions between the use of hypnosis as a teaching metaphor for clinical dissociation and hypnosis as an explanatory mechanism. It is far better to admit that we are unsure of the underlying mechanism (as is the case with most psychiatric illness) than to promulgate an unsupported model that has powerful implications for clinical formulation and intervention. A related proposition is that expertise in hypnosis does not necessarily translate into expertise with dissociative disorders and vice versa.

Future Directions for Research

It should be apparent from this review that much research is required to better understand the nature of dissociation, hypnosis, absorption, and fantasy proneness and the impact of traumatic antecedents on these four constructs and their interrelationships. We identify four general approaches to these problems. The first approach echoes suggestions initially made by Nash et al. (1993) and Tillman et al. (in press) that the role of nontraumatic factors, such as family process and environmental variables (e.g., child-rearing practices, attachment types, and genetic factors), be explored and controlled for in future studies of dissociation, hypnosis, and trauma. These factors may be much more important than we have appreciated to date.

The second approach is to tackle the persistent problem of bimodality more aggressively. In particular, the possibility of bimodality of hypnosis scores in traumatized samples must be explored further. Gangestad and Snyder (1985) and Strube (1989) have discussed the problems inherent in the presumption of dimensionality and the prejudice against class variables existing in modern analyses of personality factors. Powerful new statistical methods exist for exploring latent class variables that may be obscured by dimensional analyses (Golden 1982). The existence of a dissociative "type," characterized by high hypnotizability with a high vulnerability to traumatically induced pathological dissociation, would provide a parsimonious explanation for much of the data.

A third approach is to utilize the rich array of cognitive, metacognitive, and memory encoding/retrieval paradigms developed by neuropsychologists for the study of memory and cognition (Lister and Weingartner 1991). Comparison of dissociative disorder patients with nondissociative, highly hypnotizable subjects could elucidate similarities and differences in the cognitive mechanisms underlying amnesia, involuntariness, and other "dissociative" features supposedly shared by these two populations.

Finally, prospective, longitudinal, developmentally informed research is necessary to elucidate the developmental pathways and trajectories for normal nonpathological dissociation, pathological dissociation, hypnotizability, absorption, and fantasy proneness. This approach may be especially informative regarding the interrelationships of these constructs and the possibility that environmental events (e.g., trauma) produce significant differences in degree or type of dissociation through developmental mechanisms such as divergent causality (Gangestad and Snyder 1985).

References

American Psychiatric Association: Diagnostic and Statistical Manual of Mental Disorders, 3rd Edition, Revised. Washington, DC, American Psychiatric Association, 1987

Balthazard CG, Woody EZ: Bimodality, dimensionality, and the notion of hypnotic types. Int J Clin Exp Hypn 37:70–89, 1989

Barber J: Hypnosis and the unhypnotizable. Am J Clin Hypn 23:4–9, 1980

Barrett D: Fantasizers and dissociaters: data on two distinct subgroups of deep trance subjects. Psychol Rep 71:1011–1014, 1992

Bernstein E, Putnam FW: Development, reliability and validity of a dissociation scale. J Nerv Ment Dis 174:727–735, 1986

Bliss EL: Spontaneous self-hypnosis in multiple personality disorder. Psychiatr Clin North Am 7:135–148, 1984

Bliss EL: Multiple personality, allied disorders and hypnosis. New York, Oxford University Press, 1986

Bowers K: Dissociated control, imagination, and the phenomenology of dissociation, in Dissociation: Culture, Mind and Body. Edited by Spiegel D. Washington, DC, American Psychiatric Press, 1994, pp 21–38

Branscomb L: Dissociation in combat-related posttraumatic stress disorder. Dissociation 4:13–20, 1991

Braun BG: Hypnosis creates multiple personality: myth or reality? Int J Clin Exp Hypn 32:191–198, 1984

Bremner JD, Southwick S, Brett E, et al: Dissociation and posttraumatic stress disorder in Vietnam combat veterans. Am J Psychiatry 149: 328–332, 1992

Briere J, Runtz M: Symptomatology associated with childhood sexual victimization in a non-clinical sample. Child Abuse Negl 12:51–59, 1988

Briere J, Runtz M: The trauma symptom checklist (TSC-33): early data on a new scale. Journal of Interpersonal Violence 4:151–163, 1989

Cardena E, Spiegel D: Dissociative reactions to the San Francisco Bay area earthquake of 1989. Am J Psychiatry 150:474–478, 1993

Carlson EB, Putnam FW: Integrating research on dissociation and hypnotizability: are there two pathways to hypnotizability? Dissociation 2:32–38, 1989

Carlson EB, Rosser-Hogan R: Trauma experiences, posttraumatic stress, dissociation and depression in Cambodian refugees. Am J Psychiatry 148:1548–1552, 1991

Carlson ET: Multiple personality and hypnosis: the first one hundred years. J Hist Behav Sci 25:315–322, 1989

Chu JA, Dill DL: Dissociative symptoms in relation to childhood physical and sexual abuse. Am J Psychiatry 147:887–892, 1990

Coons PM, Bowman ES, Milstein V: Multiple personality disorder: a clinical investigation of 50 cases. J Nerv Ment Dis 176:519–527, 1988

Covino N, Jimerson D, Wolfe B, et al: Hypnotizability, dissociation and bulimia nervosa. J Abnorm Psychol 103:455–459, 1994

DiTomasso MJ, Routh DK: Recall of abuse in childhood and three measures of dissociation. Child Abuse Negl 17:477–485, 1993

Faith M, Ray W: Hypnotizability and dissociation in a college age population: orthogonal individual differences. Personality and Individual Differences 17:211–216, 1994

Frankel FH: Scales measuring hypnotic responsivity: a clinical perspective. Am J Clin Hypn 21:208–218, 1978

Frankel FH: Hypnotizability and dissociation. Am J Psychiatry 147: 823–829, 1990

Frischholz EJ: The relationship among dissociation, hypnosis, and child abuse in the development of multiple personality, in Childhood Antecedents of Multiple Personality. Edited by Kluft RP. Washington, DC, American Psychiatric Press, 1985, pp 99–126

Frischholz EJ, Lipman LS, Braun BG, et al: Psychopathology, hypnotizability and dissociation. Am J Psychiatry 149:1521–1525, 1992

Gangestad S, Snyder M: "To carve nature at its joints": on the existence of discrete classes in personality. Psychol Rev 92:317–349, 1985

Glisky ML, Tataryn DJ, Tobais BA, et al: Absorption, openness to experience, and hypnotizability. J Pers Soc Psychol 60:263–272, 1991

Goff DC, Brotman AW, Kindlon D, et al: Self-reports of childhood abuse in chronically psychotic patients. Psychiatry Res 37:73–80, 1991

Golden RR: A taxometric model for the detection of a conjectured latent taxon. Multivariate Behavioral Research 17:389–416, 1982

Harriman PL: The experimental induction of a multiple personality. Am J Orthopsychiatry 13:179–186, 1943

Haule JR: Pierre Janet and dissociation: the first transference theory and its origins in hypnosis. Am J Clin Hypn 29:86–94, 1986

Hilgard ER: Hypnotic Susceptibility. New York, Harcourt, Brace & World, 1965

Hilgard ER: The hidden observer and multiple personality. Int J Clin Exp Hypn 32:248–253, 1984

Hilgard ER: Divided Consciousness: Multiple Controls in Human Thought and Action. New York, John Wiley & Sons, 1986

Hilgard JR: Personality and Hypnosis: A Study of Imaginative Involvement, Revised Edition. Chicago, University of Chicago Press, 1979

Johnson G, Kirsch I: Dissociation, hypnotizability, and fantasy proneness in a clinical sample of survivors of abuse. Paper presented at the annual meeting of the American Psychological Association, Washington, DC, 1990

Kampman R: Hypnotically induced multiple personality: an experimental study. Int J Clin Exp Hypn 24:215–227, 1976

Kihlstrom JF, Hoyt IP: Repression, dissociation and hypnosis, in Repression and Dissociation. Edited by Singer JL. Chicago, University of Chicago Press, 1990, pp 181–208

Kirby JS, Chu JA, Dill DL: Correlates of dissociative symptomatology in patients with physical and sexual abuse histories. Compr Psychiatry 34:258–263, 1992

Kluft RP: Varieties of hypnotic interventions in multiple personality. Am J Clin Hypn 24:230–240, 1982

Kluft RP: Multiple personality disorder in childhood. Psychiatr Clin North Am 7:121–134, 1984

Koopman C, Classen C, Spiegel D: Predictors of posttraumatic stress symptoms among survivors of the Oakland/Berkeley, California, firestorm. Am J Psychiatry 151:888–894, 1994

LeBaron S, Zeltzer LK, Fanurik D: Imaginative involvement and hypnotic susceptibility in childhood. Int J Clin Exp Hypn 36:284–295, 1988

Levitt HC: A case of hypnotically produced secondary and tertiary personalities. Psychoanal Rev 34:274–295, 1947

Lister R, Weingartner H: Perspectives on Cognitive Neuroscience. New York, Oxford University Press, 1991

Loewenstein R, Putnam F: The clinical phenomenology of males with multiple personality disorder: a report of 21 cases. Dissociation 3:135–143, 1990

London P: Hypnosis in children: an experimental approach. Int J Clin Exp Hypn 10:79–91, 1962

Lynn SJ, Rhue JW: The fantasy prone person: hypnosis, imagination and creativity. J Pers Soc Psychol 51:404–408, 1986

Lynn SJ, Rhue JW, Green JP: Multiple personality and fantasy proneness: is there an association or dissociation? British Journal of Experimental and Clinical Hypnosis 5:138–142, 1988

Marmar CR, Weiss DS, Schlenger WE, et al: Peritraumatic dissociation and posttraumatic stress in male Vietnam theater veterans. Am J Psychiatry 151:902–907, 1994

Morgan AH, Hilgard JR: The Stanford Hypnotic Clinical Scale for Children. Am J Clin Hypn 21:148–155, 1979

Nadon R, Hoyt IP, Register PA, et al: Absorption and hypnotizability: context effects re-examined. J Pers Soc Psychol 60:144–153, 1991

Nash MR, Lynn SJ: Child abuse and hypnotic ability. Imagination, Cognition and Personality 5:211–218, 1985–1986

Nash MR, Lynn SJ, Givens DL: Adult hypnotic susceptibility, childhood punishment, and child abuse: a brief communication. Int J Clin Exp Hypn 32:6–11, 1984

Nash MR, Hulsey TL, Sexton MC, et al: Long-term sequelae of childhood sexual abuse: perceived family environment, psychopathology, and dissociation. J Consult Clin Psychol 61:276–283, 1993

Nowlis DP: The child-rearing antecedents of hypnotic susceptibility and of naturally occurring hypnotic-like experience. Int J Clin Exp Hypn 17:109–120, 1969

Pekala RJ: Hypnotic types: evidence from a cluster analysis of phenomenal experience. Contemporary Hypnosis 8:95–104, 1991

Plotnick AB, Payne PA, O'Grady DJ: Correlates of hypnotizability in children: absorption, vividness of imagery, fantasy play, and social desirability. Am J Clin Hypn 34:51–58, 1991

Pribor EF, Yutzy SH, Dean JT, et al: Briquet's syndrome, dissociation and abuse. Am J Psychiatry 150:1507–1511, 1993

Prince M: Some of the revelations of hypnotism, in Morton Prince: Psychotherapy and Multiple Personality, Selected Essays. Edited by Hale NG. Cambridge, MA, Harvard University Press, 1890, pp 37–60

Putnam FW: Dissociation as a response to extreme trauma, in Childhood Antecedents of Multiple Personality. Edited by Kluft RP. Washington, DC, American Psychiatric Press, 1985, pp 65–98

Putnam FW: The scientific investigation of multiple personality disorder, in Split Minds, Split Brains: Historical and Current Perspectives. Edited by Quen J. New York, New York University Press, 1986, pp 109–125

Putnam FW: Diagnosis and treatment of multiple personality disorder. New York, Guilford, 1989a

Putnam FW: Pierre Janet and modern views of dissociation. J Trauma Stress 2:413–429, 1989b

Putnam FW, Guroff JJ, Silberman EK, et al: The clinical phenomenology of multiple personality disorder: review of 100 recent cases. J Clin Psychiatry 47:285–293, 1986

Putnam FW, Helmers K, Trickett PK: Development, reliability, and validity of a Child Dissociation Scale. Child Abuse Negl 17:731–741, 1993

Putnam FW, Helmers K, Horowitz LA, et al: Hypnotizability and dissociativity in sexually abused girls. Child Abuse Negl 19:1–11, 1995

Rhue JW, Lynn SJ, Henry S, et al: Child abuse, imagination and hypnotizability. Imagination, Cognition and Personality 10:53–63, 1990

Riley KC: Measurement of dissociation. J Nerv Ment Dis 176:449–450, 1988

Roche SM, McConkey KM: Absorption: nature, assessment and correlates. J Pers Soc Psychol 59:91–101, 1990

Ross CA, Norton GR: Effects of hypnosis on the features of multiple personality disorder. Am J Clin Hypn 32:99–106, 1989

Ross CA, Miller SD, Bjornson L, et al: Abuse histories in 102 cases of multiple personality disorder. Can J Psychiatry 36:97–101, 1991

Sandberg DA, Lynn SJ: Dissociative experiences, psychopathology and adjustment, and child and adolescent maltreatment in female college students. J Abnorm Psychol 101:717–723, 1992

Sanders B, Giolas MH: Dissociation and childhood trauma in psychologically disturbed adolescents. Am J Psychiatry 148:50–54, 1991

Sanders S: The perceptual alteration scale: a scale measuring dissociation. Am J Clin Hypn 29:95–102, 1986

Sarbin TR, Coe WC: Hypnosis: A Social Psychological Analysis of Influence Communication. New York, Holt, Rinehart & Winston, 1972

Segal D, Lynn SJ: Predicting dissociative experiences: imagination, hypnotizability, psychopathology, and alcohol use. Imagination, Cognition and Personality 12:287–300, 1992–1993

Shor RE, Orne EC: Harvard Group Scale of Hypnotic Susceptibility. Palo Alto, CA, Consulting Psychologists Press, 1962

Silva CE, Kirsch I: Interpretative sets, expectancy, fantasy proneness, and dissociation as predictors of hypnotic response. J Pers Soc Psychol 63:847–856, 1992

Spanos NP: Hypnotic behavior: a social-psychological interpretation of amnesia, analgesia and "trance logic". Behavioral and Brain Sciences 9:449–502, 1986

Spanos NP, Arango M, de Groot HP: Context as a moderator in relationships between attribute variables and hypnotizability. Personality and Social Psychology Bulletin 19:71–77, 1993

Spiegel D: Dissociation, double binds, and posttraumatic stress in multiple personality disorder, in Treatment of Multiple Personality Disorder. Edited by Braun BG. Washington, DC, American Psychiatric Press, 1986, pp 61–78

Spiegel D, Hunt T, Dondershine HE: Dissociation and hypnotizability in posttraumatic stress disorder. Am J Psychiatry 145:301–305, 1988

Strick FL, Wilcoxon SA: A comparison of dissociative experiences in adult female outpatients with and without histories of early incestuous abuse. Dissociation 4:193–199, 1991

Strube MJ: Evidence for the "type" in type A behavior: a taxometric analysis. J Pers Soc Psychol 56:972–987, 1989

Stutman RK, Bliss EL: Posttraumatic stress disorder, hypnotizability, and imagery. Am J Psychiatry 142:741–743, 1985

Tanabe H, Kasai H: Hypnotic susceptibility and the dissociative experiences scale. Paper presented at the 57th annual meeting of the Japanese Psychological Association. Tsukuba City, Japan, April 1993

Tellegen A, Atkinson G: Openness to absorbing and self-altering experiences (" absorption"): a trait related to hypnotic susceptibility. J Abnorm Psychol 83:268–277, 1974

Tillman JG, Nash MR, Lerner PM: Does trauma cause dissociative pathology? in Dissociation: Clinical and Theoretical Perspectives. Edited by Lynn SJ, Rhue JW. New York, Guilford, in press, pp 395–414

Warshaw MG, Fierman E, Pratt L, et al: Quality of life and dissociation in anxiety disorder patients with histories of trauma or PTSD. Am J Psychiatry 150:1512–1516, 1993

Watkins JG, Watkins HH: Ego states and hidden observers. Journal of Altered States of Consciousness 5:3–18, 1979–1980

Weitzenhoffer AM, Hilgard ER: Stanford Hypnotic Susceptibility Scale: Forms A & B. Palo Alto, CA, Consulting Psychologists Press, 1959

Weitzenhoffer AM, Hilgard ER: Stanford Hypnotic Susceptibility Scale: Form C. Palo Alto, CA, Consulting Psychologists Press, 1962

Wilson SC, Barber TX: Vivid fantasy and hallucinatory abilities in the life histories of excellent hypnotic subjects (" somnambules"): preliminary report with female subjects, in Imagery, Vol 2: Concepts, Results, and Applications. Edited by Klinger E. New York, Plenum, 1981, pp 133–149

Wilson SC, Barber TX: The fantasy-prone personality: implications for understanding imagery, hypnosis, and parapsychological phenomena, in Imagery: Current Theory, Research, and Application. Edited by Sheikh AA. New York, Wiley, 1983, pp 340–387

Chapter 3

Trauma, Dissociation, and Hypnotizability

Jose R. Maldonado, M.D., and David Spiegel, M.D.

Trauma can be understood as the process of being made into an object, the victim of someone else's rage, of organized aggression, of nature's indifference. The helplessness engendered by such situations creates sudden challenges to normal ways of processing perception, cognition, affect, and relationships. Trauma in the form of both natural disaster and human assault causes disruption to normal cognitive and affective process. The traumatic experience forces the victim to reorganize mental and psychophysiological processes in order to buffer the immediate impact of the trauma (Maldonado and Spiegel 1994). This reorganization may take the form of fostering separation from painful surroundings and realities (derealization) or from the victim's own body (depersonalization). Even though such defenses may initially be adaptive, directed at maintaining control of, at times, overwhelming stress, some trauma victims develop persistent dissociative, amnestic, and anxiety-like symptoms. The ultimate sequelae of trauma for a substantial minority of its victims may be the development of acute stress disorder, posttraumatic stress disorder (PTSD), or a dissociative disorder (American Psychiatric Association 1994).

Components of the hypnotic phenomena are, in many aspects, similar to symptoms presented by patients who have been victims of intense trauma. Traumatic flashbacks resemble the intense experiences elicited during hypnotic absorption. Highly hypnotized individuals may experience a suggested scene as real, with all the sensations (i.e., smells, sounds, and sights) that are appropriate to it. Likewise, victims of trauma can become so absorbed in their traumatic memories that they lose touch with their present surroundings and even forget that these events are in the past, so they respond to them as if they are happening all over again. As such, given a simple environmental cue, memories of a traumatic experience can be triggered.

Dissociative defenses serve to compartmentalize various aspects of consciousness, memory, and identity. Under hypnosis, individuals are capable of dissociating a given part of their body from the rest. Examples are a subject unable to recognize his leg as such and a subject who finds herself unable to walk after the inability to perform this common bodily function is suggested during trance. Likewise, trauma victims are able to dissociate memories and feelings, as well as memories from bodily sensations. When the latter occurs these patients may subsequently present with somatic complaints for which there is no organic explanation.

Even more dramatically, trauma victims may use their dissociative abilities to disconnect affect from their current experiences. By doing this, they can prevent current feelings from triggering past memories. Lastly, hypnotic suggestibility is to some extent similar to the hypersensitivity or responsivity to environmental cues observed in trauma survivors. Highly hypnotizable individuals may experience a number of emotions or somatic sensations (or lack thereof) if suggested. Traumatized victims also may behave as if their traumatic memories were being relived if they misinterpret environmental cues (e.g., flashbacks).

Many victims of traumatic events, especially childhood physical and sexual abuse, will suffer long-standing sequelae. Severe traumatic experiences disrupt every belief system the victim has had an opportunity to develop. It can profoundly disrupt the victim's beliefs about what is safe, secure, and predictable. This is particularly true in cases of physical and sexual abuse in which the perpetrator happens to be a family member. Victims are left with a damaged sense of themselves. Likewise, patients lose their sense of control over their bodies and future. Their memories become distorted, distant, and incomplete. Suddenly, the world is no longer safe, and for many of them it will never be safe again. Finally, many victims see themselves as defective, unwanted, and filthy objects. Their perceptions seem to match the extent of the traumatic experience or the perpetrator's actions.

Dissociation

Dissociation can be understood as the separation of mental contents that would ordinarily be processed together. The process of dissociation can be seen as an attempt to preserve some form of control, safety, and identity in the face of overwhelming stress. Dissociative defenses may give the victim a false sense of control and relief from the experience. That is why some trauma victims act as if the event is not happening and later as if it had never happened. The ultimate goal of dissociation is to separate oneself from the full impact of the trauma.

Hypnosis

Hypnosis is a natural psychophysiological state of aroused, attentive, and receptive focal concentration with a corresponding relative suspension of peripheral awareness (H. Spiegel and Spiegel 1987). Depending on the degree of natural ability to enter a trance state, subjects will require more or less guidance entering such a state; that is, highly hypnotizable individuals enter trance states with ease, on many occasions even without being fully aware of it. Low-hypnotizable individuals require more direction or help from the therapist who facilitates the trance experience. Hypnosis can be conceptualized as having three main components: absorption, dissociation, and suggestibility (H. Spiegel and Spiegel 1987).

Absorption is the tendency to alter our perceptions and surroundings while in a state of highly focused attention with complete immersion in a central experience at the expense of contextual orientation (Hilgard 1970; Tellegen 1981; Tellegen and Atkinson 1974). It is possible for a highly hypnotizable individual to become so deeply involved in a central focus of consciousness (trance experience) that he or she may ignore more peripheral perceptions, thoughts, memories, or motor activities.

This ability of hypnotized individuals to become so intensely absorbed in their trance experience facilitates the phenomenon known as *trance logic*. Trance logic is a way of reasoning that does not follow the rules of "normal" logical processes or tolerance of logical inconsistencies. An example of trance logic is when it is suggested to an individual that he or she will open his or her eyes and observe a tennis game without leaving the therapist's office. A highly hypnotizable subject will hallucinate the experience without thinking about its absurdity. Extreme forms of pathological absorption are seen in cases of traumatic flashbacks. During these episodes, subjects become so absorbed in the experience that has been triggered by an environmental cue that they act as though they are reliving the whole trauma all over again, despite the impossibility of it. Tellegen and Atkinson (1974) have demonstrated a positive correlation between hypnotizability and a spontaneous tendency for people to undergo absorbing or self-altering experiences.

The mechanism of dissociation allows us to carry on more than one complex task or action simultaneously by keeping out of consciousness routine experiences or tasks. This process is mediated by the intense absorption characteristic of hypnotic states. Normally, dissociation is a very useful mechanism, and when working properly it allows us to carry out several complex tasks simultaneously. Not only can hypnotized individuals dissociate motor functions, but they also may be able to separate completely from an emotion or a somatic sensation while under trance. Highly suggestible individuals can achieve a level of dissociation to the extent of not recognizing a body part as belonging to their own body or not remembering a piece of information previously known to them (e.g., forgetting someone's name or the inability to recall their own name).

The intense absorption experienced during trance allows hypnotized individuals to have a heightened responsiveness to ideas (suggestions). These may include social cues as well as verbal suggestions. It is not true that hypnotized individuals are deprived of their will, but it is true that they are less likely to judge instructions critically; therefore, highly hypnotizable individuals may be more likely to act upon suggested ideas. This enhanced suggestibility allows hypnotized subjects to easily accept and follow instructions given. This quality of the hypnotic process allows subjects to suspend the usual conscious curiosity that makes people question the reasons for their actions and allows hypnotized individuals to accept suggestions no matter how irrational they might be (e.g., trance logic).

Likewise, the level of suggestibility may be such that some subjects under hypnosis may have difficulty distinguishing instructions coming from an outside source (i.e., therapist) from those coming from within themselves or they may confuse reality (i.e., past memories) with primary process experiences (i.e., dreams and fantasies). This is known as *hypnotic source amnesia.* This plasticity allows highly suggestible individuals to act on another person's ideas as though they were their own. In good hands, this aspect of hypnosis may be utilized by conscientious therapists to bypass the patients' defenses, uncover buried memories, and mobilize their strengths. Unfortunately, hypnotized patients are less likely to correct therapists' mistakes and could become confused by hypnotic instructions or even confabulate memories suggested by their therapists.

Trauma and Hypnotizability

Many trauma victims describe experiencing a sense of detachment from their surroundings occurring at the time of the trauma. These episodes have a dramatic resemblance to what can better be described as spontaneously induced self-hypnosis. This sense of detachment is particularly true in individuals who have undergone repeated trauma, such as victims of childhood physical and sexual abuse. We believe that some trauma victims may accidentally learn how to use hypnotic-like techniques in order to avoid the full impact of a traumatic experience.

Case Example

A woman was admitted to the hospital because of severe weight loss and medical problems related to starvation. The patient had been in therapy for some time before her admission and was diagnosed as suffering from an eating disorder. After a few months of treatment, it was discovered that she had been the victim of severe childhood sexual abuse. During the course of her hospitalization, it was determined that her inability to eat reflected her inability to have anything in her mouth. Having an object in her mouth triggered somatic flashbacks associated with having been forced to perform oral sex during the course of her sexual abuse. During one psychotherapy session, she seemed to stare off toward the corner of the room as if she were able to look through the examiner. Later, she talked about the incident and casually mentioned the "lace on the window." She also mentioned hearing nursery rhymes being "sung in my head." These are the same rhymes she sings in her head when she mutilates her body at present. Indeed, there was a window in the office, but there was no lace curtain. We believe that as she was discussing an incident related to her previous sexual abuse, she entered a spontaneous self-hypnotic state similar to the one she produced in the past. As a child, she would stare out of the window, through the lace covering it. That would be her "focusing point." Then she would begin singing songs in her head. Next, she knew "everything was over. I would crawl in my corner and cry."

There may be a relationship between stress during childhood trauma and high hypnotizability. Multiple authors have described an extraordinarily high incidence of dissociative-like defenses and pathological symptoms in victims of early childhood abuse (Coons et al. 1989; A. Freud 1946; Kilhstrom 1984, 1990; Kluft 1985, 1990, 1991; Maldonado and Spiegel 1994, 1995; Nash and Lynn 1986; Nash et al. 1984; D. Spiegel 1984, 1988, 1990; D. Spiegel and Cardena 1991; D. Spiegel and Fink 1979; D. Spiegel et al. 1982, 1988). Indeed, exposure to stressful events may be one of the paths that naturally leads toward the development of high hypnotizability. Several authors have reported a positive correlation between severity of punishment undergone during childhood and hypnotizability levels (Chu and Dill 1990; Hilgard 1970, 1984; Nash and Lynn 1986; Nash et al. 1984; Putnam 1993; D. Spiegel 1988, 1990; D. Spiegel and Cardena 1991; D. Spiegel et al. 1988). As the case example above illustrates, it is possible that the impact of the stress suffered by victims of early abuse forces or encourages victims toward a more effective use of their self-hypnotic abilities (Kluft 1984, 1992; D. Spiegel et al. 1982).

The natural history of hypnotic capacity in a given individual varies throughout the life cycle. Individuals are more highly hypnotizable during their late childhood years, with a peak in hypnotic capacity around age 12 years. This peak is followed by a moderate decline with stabilization later in middle age (Morgan and Hilgard 1973; H. Spiegel and Spiegel 1987). Repeated exposure to abuse may prevent the decline or extinction later in life of high hypnotizability and other dissociative defenses seen in adults who were once victims of abuse (Kluft 1984, 1992; Nash et al. 1984; Putnam 1985; D. Spiegel et al. 1982).

Extensive review of clinical cases suggests that victims of intense trauma use their dissociative defenses to guard themselves from the full impact of the traumatic experience (Putnam 1985; D. Spiegel 1984, 1986, 1988, 1990; D. Spiegel et al. 1988; van der Kolk and van der Hart 1989). We also know that, later in life, many of them will again use their already mastered hypnotic-like capacities in the face of further traumatization. The process by which they elicit these defenses can be volitional, but some are completely unconscious.

Case Example

A young woman who was repeatedly sexually abused as a child was an only child of immigrant parents. Both parents needed to work outside of the home, which forced her to be alone at home frequently. She used to go back and forth from school on her own by age 8 years. One day, as she walked up the steps of her home, she found her neighbor waiting for her there. This was not an uncommon occurrence. Unfortunately, this time he forced himself into her life forever. He took her into her parents' house and brutally raped her. She wanted to tell her parents but was afraid. She feared not only their reaction but also her assailant, who had warned her that he would "hurt them too" if she were to tell. Convinced that "it would be best that way," she never spoke a word. Unfortunately, the abuse did not stop there. It continued over a number of years until the family finally moved away. Having no one whom she could safely talk to, she had no other source of help or escape than her own imagination.

As in the previous example, this woman also learned how to enter a self-hypnotic trance and mentally transport herself to a beautiful meadow where she ran after butterflies and picked flowers. Meanwhile, her body was being repeatedly raped in her parents' bedroom. Soon she recognized that to survive she needed to maintain composure. So, when it was safe to return, she would "come back from the dream," run to the bathroom to wash herself, and then continue with her life "as if nothing ever happened." In therapy, she described how she initially "found this place" (hypnotic state) rather accidentally. But later, she learned how to elicit it in a semiunconscious manner.

Years later, as an adult, she continued to utilize this once-useful dissociative defense. Not completely conscious of what she was doing, she would induce a self-hypnotic state whenever an emotionally charged experience elicited feelings that somehow resembled the initial trauma. By the time she began treatment with us, her now pathological defenses had turned against her. She was being repeatedly admitted to the acute inpatient unit. Her psychiatric records revealed that she had received multiple psychiatric diagnoses. In fact, at different times she appeared to have different syndromes, including frank psychosis. She seemed to enter a self-hypnotic state every time she felt overwhelmed. As such, some of her symptoms represented a state of "hysterical psychosis" (Spiegel and Fink 1979). These episodes appeared to be the result of spontaneous dissociative states, not unlike the ones she entered during episodes of early abuse.

Her "psychotic" episodes were characterized by grandiose fantasies. In these fantasies, she had the power to care for people, especially children. At times, she believed that she was God. On other occasions, she was plagued with fear of demonic voices that haunted her for the perversity of her sexual actions. Rather than having discrete "switches" among distinct personalities, she would just transform (dissociate) into a "crazy" person who appeared to make no sense but if listened to carefully was telling the story of the abuse she endured during childhood.

Many victims of abuse continue to utilize hypnotic-like phenomena when faced with the threat of a traumatic experience. Some patients will completely block significant parts of their memories at the expense of losing personal information, as in cases of dissociative amnesia. Others will develop a complicated system in which "somebody else" recalls and suffers the pain of the memories, as in cases of dissociative identity disorder (DID).

Trauma and Dissociation

At the time of trauma, some victims experience radical disintegration of their experience, polarization of their sense of self, and fragmentation of their memory. Later, these victims' mood states alternate between vivid, painful experiences and a sense of detachment. The intense reliving of memories may represent an attempt to process the recollection of the traumatic events. In other cases, the apparent lack of emotions can be conceptualized as a kind of "artificial normality" by which the victims avoid the full impact of the experience. It is likely that patients utilize the process of dissociation to achieve this apparent normality. Years after the initial trauma, these victims maintain memories and images associated with the traumatic event away from awareness by utilizing a similar mechanism to that utilized at the time of initial trauma. These dissociative behaviors exhibited by trauma victims may be linked to heightened hypnotic responsivity. As several authors have reported, combat veterans with PTSD and other victims of severe trauma usually have higher scores on hypnotizability scales (D. Spiegel 1988; D. Spiegel et al. 1988; Stuntman and Bliss 1985) and measures of dissociation (Bremner et al. 1992, 1993; Marmar et al. 1994).

Indeed, many trauma victims may later experience a multitude of dissociative syndromes. For example, dissociated perception of the internal or external world may result in feelings of depersonalization or derealization. Others who may exhibit restricted access to facts and memories may have dissociative amnesia or dissociative fugue. The dissociative episodes may include motor dysfunctions such as those seen in cases of conversion disorder.

Although dissociated memories may be temporarily unavailable to consciousness, they may continue to influence conscious (or unconscious) experiences and behavior (Hilgard 1977; Kilhstrom 1984). Just because trauma victims cannot consciously remember a memory does not mean that it does not affect them. In fact, many of the symptoms experienced by trauma victims can be explained by the influence exerted by dissociated memories (Kilhstrom 1984, 1990).

But not everyone exposed to trauma will develop dissociative symptoms. Keane and Fairbank (1983) reported that slightly less than 25% of soldiers exposed to combat go on to develop severe dissociation or posttraumatic syndrome. Therefore, other factors must be involved in producing dissociative-like symptoms. The developmental stage during which the trauma occurs will markedly influence the intensity and extent of psychological damage produced. As a rule, the earlier in life the trauma occurs, the greater the psychological sequelae. This result is probably due, in part, to the defense mechanisms and coping styles that the individual has had an opportunity to develop before the occurrence of the trauma, which in turn will modulate the way in which he or she perceives the experience (Maldonado and Spiegel 1994).

Childhood trauma will influence the development of distorted cognitive patterns, defective self-images, and erratic self-organization. By nature, children do not fully understand the notion of independent causation; therefore, they are inclined to blame themselves for the insult suffered even when this insult is inflicted upon them. The result is a pervasive sense of unworthiness. This psychological reaction should be labeled "survivor shame" rather than "survivor guilt" because these individuals come to see their abuse as justified rather than unwarranted. This justification makes them direct their anger at themselves rather than toward the perpetrator and results in a variety of syndromes ranging from depression, to generalized feelings of worthlessness, to PTSD, and ultimately, to dissociative disorders (Finkelhor 1984;

Frischholz 1985; Gelinas 1983; Kluft 1985, 1990; Maldonado and Spiegel 1995; D. Spiegel and Cardena 1991; Stein et al. 1989). Indeed, several authors have found that between 74% and 97% of the patients diagnosed with DID have reported histories of sexual abuse during childhood (Coons and Milstein 1986; Kluft 1984, 1993; Putnam et al. 1986; D. Spiegel 1984; D. Spiegel and Cardena 1991). Likewise, many of them also have reported a high incidence of dissociative-like phenomena.

Dissociation as a common response to traumatic events has already been described by numerous researchers (Coons et al. 1989; A. Freud 1946; S. Freud 1914/1958; Kihlstrom 1984, 1990; Kluft 1985, 1990, 1991; Nash and Lynn 1986; Putnam 1985, 1991; D. Spiegel 1984, 1988; D. Spiegel and Cardena 1990, 1991; D. Spiegel and Fink 1979; D. Spiegel et al. 1988; H. Spiegel and Spiegel 1987). They report instances during which individuals undergoing severe stress reported the occurrence of spontaneous dissociative experiences, both at the time of the trauma and later (D. Spiegel 1986, 1988, 1990; D. Spiegel et al. 1988; van der Kolk and van der Hart 1989).

Trauma and Psychiatric Disease

Traumatic events induce a separation of the individual's mind from the surrounding environment in an attempt to separate himself or herself from the full impact of the trauma. Unfortunately, this defense (i.e., dissociation) carries with it devastating consequences. Because the content of these memories is not readily available to the patient, he or she is unable consciously to work through the meaning of the stressful event and put into perspective the facts surrounding the traumatic experience.

Trauma then becomes the common denominator to a number of phenomena listed under dissociative disorders and related syndromes (Cardena and Spiegel 1993; Classen et al. 1993; Coons et al. 1989; Keane and Wolfe 1990; McFarlane 1986, 1988; Solomon et al. 1989; Putnam 1985, 1993b; D. Spiegel 1984, 1986, 1990; van der Kolk and van der Hart 1989; Wilkinson 1983). These include depersonalization disorder, in which patients feel detached from their own mental processes or bodies. Depersonalization disorder has at times been described as robotlike or out-of-body experiences. In dissociative amnesia, patients exhibit an inability to recall important personal information. The memory loss may be for a part (localized) or all (selective) of the traumatic experience and may develop gradually over the days and weeks following the trauma. In extreme cases, the deficits in memory may include personal information regarding their entire life (generalized amnesia). In dissociative fugue, patients suddenly "get away," usually traveling far from home and developing a "new identity" while remaining amnestic to their past personal histories. Patients who have DID usually exhibit two or more identities or personality states accompanied by frequent memory gaps (amnesia) (American Psychiatric Association 1994).

By definition, a traumatic experience is a predecessor in the development of PTSD. PTSD is triggered by exposure to a traumatic event involving actual or threatened injury, intense fear, and helplessness (American Psychiatric Association 1994). A history of intense traumatic experiences (usually childhood physical and sexual abuse) is also commonly found in patients who have borderline personality disorder (BPD) (Brown and Anderson 1991; Brooks 1982; Bryer et al. 1987; Herman 1981; Herman et al. 1989; Nigg et al. 1991; Pribor and Dinwiddie 1992; Salzman et al. 1993; Saunders and Arnold 1993; Stone 1981; van der Kolk et al. 1991; Weaver and Clum 1993; Westen et al. 1990; Zanarini et al. 1989). Likewise, the vast majority of patients who have DID report histories of childhood traumas (Brown and Anderson 1991; Chu and Dill 1990; Kluft 1985, 1993; Pribor and Dinwiddie 1992; Putnam et al. 1991; Rowan et al. 1994; Silberman et al. 1986; Terr 1991).

Indeed, there are striking similarities among all three disorders (i.e., PTSD, BPD, and DID). These disorders are always (in the case of PTSD) or often (BPD and DID) the result of intense trauma, especially childhood abuse. In all three, individuals find themselves powerless and violated. The frequent and sometimes disabling use of dissociative defenses is also a common sequela to all three disorders (Cardena and Spiegel 1993; Chu and Dill 1990; Classen et al.

1993; Coons et al. 1989; Keane and Wolfe 1990; Kluft 1993; Maldonado and Spiegel 1995; McFarlane 1986, 1988; Pribor and Dinwiddie 1992; Ross et al. 1989; Solomon et al. 1989; D. Spiegel 1984, 1986, 1990; van der Kolk and van der Hart 1989; van der Kolk et al. 1991; Wilkinson 1983). Herman et al. (1989) have suggested that some symptoms exhibited by BPD patients reflect a history of trauma severe enough to cause PTSD. Furthermore, many of the dissociative-like symptoms exhibited by borderline patients are similar to those exhibited by DID patients. Self-destructive behavior, frequent suicidal ideation, lability of affect, defective self-images, and interpersonal difficulties also may be present. Conversely, the intense reliving of traumatic experiences witnessed in patients with PTSD is remarkably similar to the intense episodes of dissociation seen in flashbacks and dreams in DID (and BPD) patients.

These three disorders may be seen as a triad in a continuum of psychiatric sequelae to intense trauma. Many patients diagnosed with DID have previously been misdiagnosed as having (and exhibiting many of the characteristics of) BPD. Likewise, most patients diagnosed with BPD have a background history common to (and exhibit many of the symptoms of) PTSD.

Hypnotizability, Dissociation, and Psychopathology

Throughout the years, many researchers have associated hypnotizability with dissociative phenomena, both normal and pathological. Early on, Charcot (1890) described a relationship between dissociated bodily sensations and functions (i.e., conversion disorders) and hypnotizability. He theorized that both phenomena were due to a pathological disorder afflicting the central nervous system. His rationale implied that only sick (hysterical) people could be hypnotized. His contemporaries and followers, including Bernheim (1889/1964), Breuer and Freud (1893–1895/1955), and Janet (1920, 1925), refuted his ideas, attributing the symptoms of conversion to unconscious mechanisms rather than true neurological conditions. They also saw the therapeutic potential of hypnosis.

Although patients "may not be able to remember" dissociated memories, the dissociated information continues to exert its effects on current life events (Kihlstrom 1984, 1990). In fact, dissociated information continues to affect patients' moods, behavior, and cognitive processes. It is common for these patients to realize that something is wrong, but they are unable to identify what. Many patients will experience a sense of discomfort or sometimes even panic when in specific situations.

So, what is the relationship between hypnotizability and dissociative psychopathology? Several studies have demonstrated significantly higher hypnotizability scores among individuals who have various psychiatric disorders. Among them are patients with PTSD (Kluft 1993; Putnam 1992; D. Spiegel 1992; D. Spiegel et al. 1988; Stuntman and Bliss 1985); dissociative disorders (Allen and Smith 1993; Bliss 1986; Braun and Sachs 1985; Carlson and Putnam 1989; Coons and Milstein 1986; Frischholz 1985; Frischholz et al. 1992; Kluft 1985, 1993; D. Spiegel 1984; D. Spiegel et al. 1989); anxiety disorders, particularly phobias (Bodden 1991; Frankel and Orne 1976; Gerschman et al. 1987; Menzies and Clarke 1993; Rodolfa et al. 1990; Smith 1990); and impulse control behaviors characteristic of eating disorders (Evans and Staats 1989; Kranhold et al. 1992) and personality disorders, especially BPD (Baker 1983; D. R. Copeland 1986; Murray-Jobsis 1991; Pettinati et al. 1990).

Most of these disorders have in common an early onset of dissociative defenses triggered by a traumatic event. Therefore, patients have enhanced their natural ability to dissociate in order to separate themselves from the initial painful experience. Later, the dissociative defenses that allowed them to tolerate overwhelming fear and pain earlier in life become an ongoing part of their personality structure. The excessive use of dissociative or self-hypnotic defenses facilitates the compartmentalization of memories and experiences. The end result is the splitting of memory, personality, and consciousness into multiple dissociated selves.

Bulimic patients not only demonstrate higher hypnotizability scores compared with restrictor patients (i.e., anorexia nervosa), but many of them also report being in a trancelike state when they engage in their compulsive bingeing and purging behavior (Petti-nati et al. 1990). Similarly, patients who exhibit self-destructive be-havior (e.g., cutting, burning) describe dissociative or trancelike states surrounding the periods of self-mutilation. All of these be-haviors are associated with the diagnoses of DID and BPD.

Even some psychotic-like phenomena may be the result of self-hypnotic or dissociative events. However, schizophrenic patients, by virtue of their decreased attention and concentration, may prove to have low hypnotizability (Lavoie and Elie 1985; Lavoie and Sabourin 1980; Pettinati 1982; Pettinati et al. 1990; D. Spiegel et al. 1982; Weitzenhoffer and Hilgard 1962). Therefore, a "psy-chotic" patient who proves to be highly hypnotizable may have been misdiagnosed as schizophrenic (M. D. Copeland and Kitch-ing 1937; Kluft 1993; D. Spiegel and Fink 1979; Steingard and Frankel 1985).

Because of their ability to identify highly suggestible subjects and dissociative disorder patients, hypnotizability tests can be used to assist in the differential diagnosis of several psychiatric conditions (Kluft 1993; D. Spiegel and Fink 1979; Steingard and Frankel 1985). As in any other test used in medicine, the presence or absence of hypnotic capacity should be interpreted within the context of a patient's presenting symptoms, past medical and psychiatric histories, and genetic background. In the case of an acute psychosis, where there is no familial background, presenting symptoms occur later in life than normal, a history of physical or sexual abuse exists, and the hypnotizability score is very high, a di-agnosis of hysterical psychosis or a dissociative disorder (in par-ticular DID) should be strongly considered when evaluating the possibility of schizophrenia (Kluft 1993; Maldonado and Spiegel 1995).

Clinical Hypnosis

As described earlier, hypnosis is a natural psychophysiological state of aroused, attentive, and receptive focal concentration. It in-volves relative suspension of peripheral awareness. There are many myths about the usefulness and capabilities of this treatment technique. Hypnosis is neither an infallible technique nor a destructive treatment method. Like all other tools available to therapists, its utility depends upon how it is applied and the context in which it is used.

When considering using hypnosis in clinical practice, therapists can use several guiding principles. Keeping these in mind will help therapists maintain a clear perspective of this treatment technique.

First and foremost, all hypnosis is self-hypnosis; therefore, hypnosis is something that the therapist does *with* a patient, not something done *to* a patient. The function of the therapist is to help the patient use his or her own hypnotic capacity to enter a trance state. Indeed, one of the most important aspects of using hypnosis is helping the patient understand the degree of control he or she has over his or her mental processes. In essence, the therapist is trying to help the patient discover what he or she already knows. This approach is a good way to foster mastery and control of mental processes in patients.

The purpose of using this approach is to allow patients to understand the extent to which the "unconscious" use of their hypnotic abilities may create or contribute to their dissociative psychopathology. This approach is particularly helpful in treating patients who have dissociative disorders and conversion phenomena (Bliss 1980, 1984; D. Spiegel and Fink 1979; H. Spiegel 1974).

Contrary to what many people believe, hypnosis is not sleep. Hypnotized subjects are awake and alert during trance, although they appear to be asleep because of their decreased reactivity to their surroundings. This decreased reactivity, in turn, is due to the subjects' increased absorption to hypnotically elicited material. Thus far, there appear to be no gender differences in hypnotic capacity (Hilgard 1965; Stern et al. 1979).

Hypnotizability is a stable and measurable trait that is not universal. In other words, not everyone is hypnotizable, but those who demonstrate some degree of hypnotic capacity will exhibit stable performance levels over time (Hilgard 1965; H. Spiegel and Spiegel 1987). Indeed, hypnotizability is as consistent over time in adulthood as is intelligence (Piccione et al. 1989). About 75% of the population have some usable hypnotic capacity, with only about 10% exhibiting high hypnotic capacity. Therefore, about 25% of our adult patients have no usable hypnotic capacity (H. Spiegel and Spiegel 1987).

The dangers of hypnosis reside not in the process itself, but in whom applies it and how it is used. In and of itself, hypnosis is not therapy. The entry into a hypnotic state does not have any therapeutic effects, although some may find the experience pleasant and relaxing. The therapeutic value of the process comes not from the state itself, but from what occurs during it. Hypnosis is thereby a facilitator for a variety of treatment strategies, including enhancing control over dissociative states, facilitating the recovery and restructuring of repressed or dissociated memories, and allowing for control of conversion symptoms or fugue states.

There are a number of brief, objective tests that can be used to assess the natural level of hypnotizability. The latest tests, developed specifically for clinical use, such as the Hypnotic Induction Profile (H. Spiegel and Spiegel 1987), can require as little as five minutes. The use of such a measure of hypnotic capacity has several advantages: it objectively assesses patients' natural ability to utilize their own hypnotic capacity, and it provides objective data about patients' ability to respond to treatment employing suggestion. Therefore, it can accurately predict patients' capacity to respond to psychological treatment.

Hypnosis in the Treatment of Traumatic and Dissociative Experiences

Rationale

A traumatic experience may trigger sudden discontinuity of physical and mental contents. This spontaneous dissociation is intended to buffer the immediate impact of the trauma in order to maintain psychological control during a time of enormous physical and emotional stress. Unfortunately, a number of trauma victims go on to suffer acute or chronic symptoms, such as intrusive thoughts, anxiety, hyperarousal states (e.g., posttraumatic phenomena), and dissociation.

It has been theorized that patients suffering from disorders characterized by dissociative phenomena are highly hypnotizable (Kluft 1984; Maldonado and Spiegel 1994, 1995; D. Spiegel 1988, 1989; D. Spiegel et al. 1982, 1988; Stuntman and Bliss 1985). Many trauma victims may unknowingly be using their hypnotic capacities to remain unaware of the content of their traumatic memories while creating different types of psychopathology (Maldonado and Spiegel 1994, 1995; Sanders and Giolas 1991; D. Spiegel 1984, 1986, 1989; Spiegel et al. 1988; Terr 1991).

If patients who have dissociative disorders and other posttraumatic disorders are, years later, unknowingly using their own hypnotic capacities, it makes sense then to teach them how to enter, access, and control their now-pathological trancelike defenses. If an uncontrolled use of their hypnotic capacity is the source of their symptoms (i.e., flashbacks, alter personalities), appropriate use of hypnosis in the present can become a tool to access previously dissociated material during the course of therapy. The ability to achieve a controlled mobilization of their dissociative mechanisms and the resemblance between some of the symptoms found in traumatized patients and individuals in hypnotic-like states make the use of hypnosis especially relevant in the treatment of dissociative disorders.

As we have previously discussed, many patients who have experienced trauma respond to the traumatic event by using dissociative-like defenses during or after the trauma. In instances of repeated trauma, it is likely that patients "learn" how to trigger these dissociative responses (self-hypnosis) to avoid further trauma. If hypnotic-like states are spontaneously elicited during traumatic experiences, it makes sense that the very entry into this same state will lead to the retrieval of memories and affects associated with the original trauma as predicted by the theory of state-dependent memory (Bower 1981). The transition from normal consciousness into a hypnotic trance can facilitate access to memories related to a dissociated state, similar to what might have happened at the time of the original trauma.

Any psychotherapeutic treatment of posttraumatic and dissociative disorders must focus on helping patients acknowledge and bear the extent of the psychic damage caused by the trauma. This acknowledgment is then followed by helping patients develop more mature and adequate coping mechanisms that will assist them in putting their lives into perspective. A comprehensive treatment approach, including cognitive restructuring, will allow patients to adapt to a new life incorporating memories of the traumatic experience, worked through in a manner that interferes as little as possible with their daily living activities.

Trauma patients "choose to forget" memories related to the trauma because reality is too painful to be faced. In many instances, this forgetting is encouraged by the fact that retaining memories may make them liable to cause damage. For example, in the case of the abused child, the abuser warns that "terrible things will happen to your parents if you speak." The options are to risk causing damage or to "forget" that anything happened. But there is no perfect defense. Many memories are stored at a conscious and/or unconscious level. Some patients always remember. Some remember only parts of it. Yet in some cases, many memories are transformed and others interspersed with fantasy (i.e., some cases of ritual abuse or alien abduction).

The feelings of fear and shame associated with the amnestic events slowly leak into the conscious mind. Because many of the memories are not available, it is difficult for patients to make sense of them, thereby creating a state of panic. Many victims experience some of the leaked memories in the form of flashbacks or dreams. Many trauma patients isolate themselves because of the shame they feel in relation to the suspected trauma. Individuals who have experienced traumatic events often see themselves the same way they see the object that the trauma temporarily made them into. For example, they believe they are filthy, just as "what they made me do" or "what they did to me" was filthy.

Many patients fear that if they allow traumatic memories to surface, they will once again lose control. In essence, losing control is what happens every time they experience a flashback. Trauma patients have a difficult time separating themselves and their surroundings from their memories. At the time of a flashback and during episodes of dissociation, many of our patients see themselves as they were at the time of the trauma. They believe they are as defenseless and vulnerable as when the trauma occurred.

On Using Hypnosis

There are a number of clues that may indicate that a patient may benefit from the therapeutic use of hypnotic techniques. First, during the course of working in psychotherapy, memories of a traumatic experience may be elicited, resulting in the reactivation of the formerly repressed memories. Second, patients may experience dreams or nightmares in which traumatic material is implicitly (i.e., disguised in fantasy) or explicitly revealed. Third, patients may re-experience elements of the traumatic event in the form of cognitive or somatic flashbacks. Fourth, patients may overtly develop pathological ways to dissociate the content of the memories while still acting on the newly discovered material. They do this by developing alter personalities and the amnestic episodes associated with them.

The therapists' task is to help patients retrieve the painful memories, express them in ways that do not foster self-destructive behaviors (i.e., self-mutilation, high-risk behaviors), encourage the development of mature defenses, and restructure the ways they think about themselves, while allowing them to develop improved self-esteem and self-image.

Many traumatic memories may be elicited during the course of psychotherapy without requiring methods of memory enhancement. Nevertheless, hypnosis can facilitate access to repressed memories that have not emerged using other techniques. This is true not only of painful, repressed memories, but also is true of situations when both the patient and the therapist have worked on resistance issues and feel that some additional leverage is necessary (Maldonado and Spiegel 1995).

Breuer and Freud (1893-1895/1955) first described the usefulness of hypnosis in the treatment of trauma-related disorders. They described how abreactions were accompanied by the release of psychic tension and, on occasion, relief of physical symptoms. This approach was the precursor of the cathartic method. The belief was that some intense affect associated with the traumatic event needed to be released. Therefore, facilitating recall of the event, along with its associated emotion, during a trance state would result in symptom resolution.

The idea that recollection alone (i.e., catharsis) would cause a cure did not last long. Soon afterward, S. Freud (1914/1958) realized that conscious cognitive work needed to be done on the recovered material for it to be successfully worked through. For psychotherapy to be effective, patients must experience an enhanced sense of control over the memories being abreacted. In fact, every time patients go through a flashback, they experience an uncontrolled abreaction. Therefore, there is a risk of further retraumatization in the continuous reliving of traumatic experience without adequate restructuring before new defenses are in place (Kluft 1992, 1993; Maldonado and Spiegel 1995; D. Spiegel 1981; H. Spiegel and Spiegel 1987).

Properly done, hypnosis effectively facilitates symbolic restructuring of the traumatic experience under hypnosis (Spiegel 1981). As an adaptation of the techniques used for the treatment of PTSD, hypnosis can be used to provide controlled access to the dissociated or repressed memories and then help patients restructure their memories (Maldonado and Spiegel 1995; D. Spiegel 1992).

What makes hypnosis one of the most helpful tools in the treatment of patients who have dissociative disorders is its ability to be used both as a diagnostic tool and a powerful therapeutic technique. Victims of traumatic events experience their symptoms (i.e., fugue states, dissociated identities, amnestic episodes, flashbacks) as occurring unexpectedly and beyond their control. In contrast, the hypnotic state can be seen as a controlled form of dissociation (Nemiah 1985). Hypnosis facilitates the recovery of memories while allowing for some of them to remain dissociated from cognition until the time when the patient is ready to deal with them. Finally, hypnosis also allows for the recovery and reprocessing of recovered memories at a pace the patient can tolerate.

When hypnosis is used correctly, a therapist demonstrates to patients the amount of control they have over these states of mind that they experience as automatic, uncontrollable, and unpredictable. The purpose is to teach patients that they can control their episodes of dissociation and allow the development of improved patterns of communication, which will lead to a reduction in spontaneous dissociative symptoms. The goal is for trauma patients to recognize their dissociative states and learn how to master their capacity to control them.

Hypnosis Applied

Hypnosis during the treatment of patients who have experienced trauma and patients who have dissociative disorders has as its primary objective an assessment of the patients' memories, cognitive restructuring of their self-image, and a working through that may be similar to grief work. As mentioned before, hypnosis is just another tool therapists can use to facilitate trauma work. The art of hypnosis work does not lie in the induction process but rather in what happens after trance is induced. In other words, what really counts is not how to get there but what happens once you are there. Remember that all hypnosis is really self-hypnosis; therefore, therapists are only tapping into their patients' natural ability to enter a trance state. What patients need then is guidance and sometimes "permission" to use it appropriately.

The initial phase involves memory retrieval or recovery. Therapists using hypnosis during this phase need to remember two things: 1) these patients are highly suggestible, and 2) these patients need help achieving a controlled abreaction. The purpose of hypnotic retrieval is not limited to helping patients remember the trauma. Every flashback, every traumatic nightmare, even every unstructured hypnotic retrieval could represent an uncontrolled abreaction. Each of these exposes patients to further retraumatization. Therefore, adequate hypnotic retrieval involves using techniques that promote physical levels of relaxation and a sense of mental and emotional control. Recovery of traumatic memories should proceed at a pace patients can tolerate. Because of the need for patients to regain control over their physical and mental lives, the hypnotic technique should be tailored to patients' particular needs, with a special emphasis on utilizing the occasion to enhance patients' sense of control over their mental state and the working through of traumatic memories.

There are a number of hypnotic techniques that can facilitate the process of recovery of traumatic memories while still allowing patients to feel in control. Many patients fear that if they allow traumatic memories to surface, they will once again lose control, symbolically reenacting the helplessness experienced during the traumatic episode. To some extent, this is not an unreasonable fear. Many patients do indeed have their memories take over their mental life every time they experience a flashback. Therefore, one of the advantages of using hypnosis is that it allows patients to separate themselves from their memories. Part of the therapist's role is to help patients control and structure the retrieval and expression of painful memories and feelings associated with them. Hypnotic techniques that can be used to facilitate this controlled recovery include relaxation, projection, age regression, and the affect bridge.

After inducing a trance state, the therapist may instruct patients to imagine themselves in a place that they associate with feelings of relaxation and calmness to achieve a level of physical relaxation. This could be a place they have been before or a place they construct in their mind. In some patients, a greater level of physical relaxation can be achieved by having them imagine they are floating in a hot tub, a pool, or in space. Once the desired level of relaxation is achieved, patients are instructed to maintain this state while they are asked to confront emotionally charged traumatic memories. The objective is to process, within the context of therapy, traumatic memories at a pace that can be tolerated while maintaining the same level of physical and, if possible, emotional relaxation.

The second method involves projective techniques. It implies that patients will "project" images, sensations, and thoughts away from themselves onto an imaginary screen. Depending on your patients' inclinations, this could be a movie screen, a computer screen, the surface of a calm lake, a mirror, or a blue sky. This technique facilitates the process of separating memories from physically painful sensations in order to minimize traumatic abreaction or retraumatization. The screen allows for the manipulation of the affect that invariably is mobilized during the retrieval of traumatic memories. Patients are taught that they can control the intensity of the content by making the images larger or smaller or by moving the screen closer or farther away from them. Patients can further manipulate the images by changing the color (e.g., making images black and white rather than color), the sounds (e.g., lowering the volume or completely eliminating the sound), and the speed (e.g., slowing or fast-forwarding images), or they can choose to turn off the images if they become uncontrollable at any given time. Patients are reminded that, as in a frightening movie, some scenes are difficult or even repulsive. But they do not have to reexperience the pain associated with the traumatic memories or images. This technique allows patients to have an enhanced sense of control and a feeling of safety.

A variation of this technique calls for patients to divide the screen in half. While doing this, patients are then asked to project on the left (sinister) side of the screen images of what they need to work on (i.e., memories of the trauma). On the right side of the screen, they picture something they did to protect themselves. On occasion, some patients may have difficulty remembering anything good about themselves or what they did. Some may even blame themselves for not having done enough, which translates into "it was my fault." The therapist encourages them to recall anything they might have done to protect themselves and restructure their perception of powerlessness into a useful survival technique. Fighting back, screaming for help, or just "lying still" in order to avoid further abuse are some examples of common defensive acts. The idea at this stage is to facilitate traumatic memories to become more bearable as the patients see that part of themselves that attempted to protect themselves or others and maintain dignity.

At the end, the two images serve to restructure the memory of the trauma. The image on the left side of the screen symbolizes the summary or condensation of the trauma. The images on the right side of the screen help patients to realize that although they were indeed victimized, they were also attempting to master the situation and displayed courage during a time of overwhelming terror and pain. This process also allows them to realize that the humiliation of the trauma is only one aspect of the experience.

A third method involves age regression. Different from projective techniques, age regression may not provide patients with the protective advantage of being able to "project" memories away from themselves. Because of this lack of protective advantage, age regression may prove to be a more intense experience. It is very useful in helping patients understand the origin of long-forgotten bodily symptoms, such as conversion symptoms and somatic flashbacks. Age regression may even help them recall dissociated memories. Highly hypnotizable individuals are able to use this technique as a form of "role-playing" the events, as if they are happening all over again. This role-playing allows for the associated affects to surface, which in turn may facilitate the recovery of yet more repressed memories. Age regression may even help explain some present behaviors, such as patients' disproportionate reactions to seemingly benign stressors.

A fourth technique is the "affect bridge" (Watkins 1987). This technique is particularly useful in cases in which patients have phobiclike symptoms. In using this technique, the therapist produces a hypnotic trance. Then, after achieving a state of physical and emotional relaxation, patients are instructed to "go back to the very first time you felt this way before." Usually, highly hypnotizable individuals respond by recounting a past experience associated (literally or figuratively) with the current fearful feelings. This recounting a past experience then allows the therapist to help patients figure out associations or explanations for current inappropriate responses, such as phobias.

Cognitive Restructuring

Any of the above techniques allow access to repressed or forgotten material and, more importantly, allow insight into many questions these patients ask themselves over and over again, such as why they never told anyone or why the abuse lasted as long as it did. These techniques also help explain to them why they could not stop the abuse, which is usually accomplished by making them relate again to the fear that paralyzed them as children and did not allow them to escape. Patients may remember their fear when they believed that if they did not do as they were told, something horrible would happen to them or their loved ones. They may remember having being convinced by the perpetrator that their parents would never believe them if they told the truth or that their parents would punish them further if they found out.

After the recovery of long-forgotten memories, patients may be able to reassess their situation from a dual perspective: the point of view at the time of trauma and now from their current perspective. Their traumatic perspective was influenced by infantile feelings and fantasies. The current perspective should be more realistic as they find themselves distanced from the threat, with more information and more control. Before knowing the facts, many trauma patients blamed themselves for not having done something differently, for "allowing" the trauma to happen. Some even fantasize about somehow having provoked it. After traumatic memories have been retrieved, aided by hypnosis, and the facts analyzed from a different perspective, patients realize that in most instances they did the best they could under the circumstances. At this point, most patients have a more realistic view of the traumatic experience and themselves.

After the stage of memory retrieval comes the phase of memory restructuring. During this stage, trauma patients can be guided under hypnosis through an exercise in which they can allow themselves to accept the victimized self. They need to acknowledge the events that led to where they are now. Patients learn that the intrusive memories, the flashbacks, the nightmares, and their bodily symptoms are ways in which the unconscious attempts to communicate and express painful and overwhelming memories.

More importantly, they recognize and give themselves credit for what they did, as a child, in order to survive. This way of approaching their traumatic past allows them to change their self-image from that of a victim to that of a survivor. Patients also learn that they are able to use self-hypnosis to access the memories, thus controlling the way past events affect their present.

Several methods can be used to accomplish the cognitive restructuring. An advantage of using hypnosis is that the affect elicited during the trance state can be so powerful that patients do not need to remember every single event of abuse or trauma. In fact, hypnosis may help patients consolidate the memories in a constructive and orderly way, facilitating later reprocessing. The fact that patients will now have a method that allows them to control the access and retrieval of traumatic memories gives them an enhanced sense of control. It also provides them with a new and more appropriate method for managing the traumatic memories and their manifestations.

During hypnotic imagery, therapists can help patients visualize a scene in which they (current image) join the "victimized" memory, similar to the approach used in the fusion of alter states in cases of dissociative disorders. It is the intense state of absorption (concentration) associated with the hypnotic state that serves to reverse the fragmentation of the mind initially elicited by the traumatic experience.

Yet another method involves the use of self-mothering techniques in which patients are able to go beyond the anger toward a parent or perpetrator and provide for themselves the nurturing and protection that they needed but never received. So, during the hypnotic exercise, the patients, usually recounting their experiences as children, are comforted, cared for, and loved by the adult self. This method fosters the process of increased self-acceptance and self-esteem.

These approaches involve helping patients acknowledge the extent of the emotional pain caused by the trauma. Then, through therapy, patients are assisted in developing mature and adequate coping mechanisms that will allow them to put the experience into proper perspective. The final goal is to allow patients to come to terms with the trauma and redefine themselves in view of the past, but with a firm hold on the realities of the present.

The Hypnotic "Condensed Approach"

Psychotherapeutic treatment of PTSD need not necessarily be extensive. Hypnosis can be used as an adjunct to intensify and speed the therapeutic process. When the above principles are sequentially applied in the treatment of trauma patients who have post-traumatic or dissociative symptoms, a condensed method is available to facilitate the treatment process.

This condensed approach using hypnosis as a facilitator has two major treatment goals: 1) to make *conscious* previously repressed traumatic memories and 2) to develop a sense of *congruence* between memories associated to the traumatic experience and patients' current realities and self-images. These goals can be achieved by using six consecutive and interdependent steps or stages, described later in this discussion. Each of them allows patients to work through previously repressed memories, therefore giving them the opportunity to regain control of their mental processes. Regaining control in turn helps them understand the why and how of what happened, accept the past with a better sense of perspective, and restructure their ideas of self and their current existence (Maldonado and Spiegel 1994, 1995; D. Spiegel 1992).

Using this condensed approach, therapists can help their patients recognize and understand factors involved in the development of their symptoms. Hypnosis may help define one or several particularly frightening memories during the review of the patients' history, which summarizes or condenses the main conflicts. The focused concentration characteristic of the hypnotic state can facilitate both the recall of traumatic material and the development of well-defined boundaries around them. Hypnosis can then facilitate the process of restructuring recovered memories and, more importantly, help patients move from the position of victim to that of survivor by helping them remember everything they did in order to survive. Patients benefit from learning how to think about the trauma rather than attempting to negate its existence.

If a sense of congruence is achieved among the content and feelings associated with the traumatic experience and the patients' ongoing feelings and views of self, the need to dissociate memories vanishes. Thereafter, a reduction in dissociative symptoms, such as decreased frequency and intensity of amnestic episodes, acting out by alters, and self-destructive behaviors, usually follows. The adequate recovery and restructuring of memories associated with the trauma are also followed by a diminution in posttraumatic symptoms (i.e., flashbacks, intrusive recollections, nightmares, anxiety) that were initially associated with the threat posed by the presence of repressed traumatic memories.

The six treatment stages used in the condensed approach are confrontation, condensation, confession, consolation, concentration, and control. The first stage is *confrontation* of the trauma. Patients must recognize that there were important factors and events in their lives that resulted in the development of their symptoms. It helps to keep in mind that most patients have been told "forget it . . . it is all in the past . . . there is nothing you can do about it . . . just let go of it . . . why can't you just snap out of it?" Comments like these only add to patients' guilt and their sense that there must be something wrong with themselves. It also makes them believe that those memories should be eliminated, further promoting repression and dissociation. Therefore, the therapist's role should be one of a supportive, nonjudgmental listener, who avoids suggesting or implanting facts.

Hypnosis then is used in the process of *condensation* of the traumatic memories. There may be little need to force patients to purge or recount every episode or traumatic detail. Many patients will have the compulsion to retell and sometimes abreact traumatic experiences over and over again. Therapists can use hypnosis to define particularly frightening segments or episodes during the review of traumatic memories and help patients summarize or condense them. Later, hypnosis can be used to help restructure these condensed memories. Usually, trauma patients feel as if they can never do anything right. The restructuring of these memories may help patients realize what they did at the moment of trauma in order to survive.

After condensing the traumatic material, many patients feel the need for *confession* of the feelings and experiences that they are profoundly ashamed of and may have never told anyone before. During this stage, it is imperative that the therapist convey a sense of "being present" for the patient while remaining neutral. Judgments that patients attribute to the actions they are able to recall must be dispelled. These self-judgments (e.g., "I am filthy") are usually ego-dystonic cognitions that have been integrated from external sources (e.g., parents, church).

Once patients have "purged" or confessed the content of the traumatic, and in many cases secret, memories, they feel an immense sense of shame and sorrow. These feelings of shame and sorrow require the therapist to be more active during the next stage, *consolation*. During this phase, the therapist must be emotionally available to patients. It is appropriate, and even recommended, that the therapist make empathic comments about the impact the experience must have had on the patient. This consolation must be done in a respectful and professional manner. The therapist should keep in mind, at all times, that past traumatic experiences in patients have caused tremendous violations of physical and emotional boundaries. Because of these violations, caution is recommended regarding the method used to display empathy.

Hypnosis is a state of intense *concentration*. It is this focused level of attention that facilitates selective therapeutic work on traumatic memories. The hypnotic trance allows patients to "turn on" memories in the secure environment created by the safety of the therapy session. It will also allow patients to "shut them off" once the intended work has been completed at the end of the session. Likewise, it provides flexibility to work on one aspect of the memory without requiring patients to recall the entire trauma. In other words, under the guidance of the therapist, the hypnotic process promotes concentration on the desired goal while helping patients remain in control. This is a refreshing change for patients who are fearful of remembering because in the past these attempts resulted in emotions such as terror and pain. Many patients fear that memories will take over and they will be defenseless once again. Using the structured experience of the hypnotic trance, patients learn that rather than not thinking about the trauma, they can learn how to think about it constructively.

At the end of hypnotic treatment, patients must feel an enhanced sense of *control*. The sense of mastery and order must be restored. The traumatic experiences have rendered patients defenseless, impotent, and shattered. Most experiences involving extreme trauma are accompanied by a sense of helplessness and loss of physical and emotional control. It was this lack of control that initially triggered the need for dissociative defenses as an attempt to master the traumatic experience. Therefore, it is critical that therapists guide the therapeutic interaction in such a way that patients' sense of control over their memories is enhanced. This sense of self-control can be enhanced by instructing patients to "remember as much as can safely be remembered now" rather than pushing them to remember the entire event. Used adequately, self-hypnosis can teach patients that they are in charge of their experiences and therefore their memories. By modeling this sense of trust, therapists teach their patients to believe in themselves. It allows patients to learn, once again, to trust their own feelings, perceptions, and intuitions. An important aspect of enhancing patients' sense of mastery is for them to learn not only how to control memories and symptoms, but also when to ask for help.

Limitations and Therapeutic Precautions

The intense emotions characteristic of hypnotic retrieval of traumatic memories may facilitate the expression of inner fantasies and deep personal experiences. In some patients, the hypnotic state will facilitate a sense of *infantile dependency* in which the transference expectations are intensified. As in any other therapeutic relationship, the quality and affective content of this transference reaction will be based on the patients' early object relations. A difference may be the intensity of the feelings developed due to the strong emotions that arise during trance. Therapists may erroneously foster these infantile dependency feelings, or they may use the transference to foster patients' ability to help themselves and create an environment of control and self-mastery.

The hypnotic trance may allow for such an intense experience during the recovery process that some patients may have a sensation or feeling that the therapist had "been there" with them at the moment of trauma. The presence and intensity of transference reactions during the psychotherapy of trauma patients are enormous. Hypnosis does not prevent development of these reactions.

On the contrary, hypnosis may facilitate their emergence. In many instances, the development of transference reactions may occur earlier than in conventional therapy because of the intensity in which the material is expressed and the speed at which memories are recovered.

From a therapeutic point of view, the intense perception some patients experience of having the therapist there with them at the moment of trauma allows the therapist to provide guidance, support, protection, and comfort as patients go through the difficult task of reprocessing and restructuring traumatic memories. But the same intense experience may turn against the therapist in the form of *traumatic transference* (Maldonado and Spiegel 1995; D. Spiegel 1989). This special kind of transferential reaction involves the transference of feelings not related to early object relations, but feelings related to the abuser or the circumstances associated with the traumatic experience (D. Spiegel 1992).

Therapists can be more helpful if they interpret this anger (and other feelings) as an attempt to experience anger toward the perpetrator rather than assuming it represents primitive feelings about parents or other early figures in their patients' lives. These feelings should not be minimized or shut off. Doing so would only confirm the patients' beliefs that there was something wrong with them for having them. These beliefs would then further activate the use of primitive defenses, including dissociation and acting out.

An even more detrimental complication of using hypnosis in the treatment of trauma patients is the possible creation of what has been termed *false memories*. Hypnosis can enhance memory recall because of the heightened concentration that allows patients to focus intensely on a given time or place. The principle of state-dependent memory may explain why merely entering into a trance state can facilitate retrieval of memories associated with a similar state of mind as may have occurred at the time of trauma (Bower 1981). To the extent that trauma patients were in a dissociated state at the time of the trauma, entering the structured dissociation of hypnosis may well facilitate access to trauma-related memories. But not all recovered memories are true. Hypnosis will facilitate improved recall of both true and confabulated material

(Dywan and Bowers 1983). High suggestibility is inherent to the hypnotic process, and this high suggestibility facilitates the possibility that information may be implanted or imagined. Furthermore, patients may have such an intense experience that they may enhance their conviction that their memories are veridical regardless of their accuracy—the problem of "confident errors" (Laurence and Perry 1983; McConkey 1992; Orne 1979).

Because of the possibility of confabulation and contamination, therapists are warned about believing everything a patient recalls. Therapeutic judgment should be used when analyzing and interpreting patients' hypnotically recovered material. This approach is similar to the way with which (nontraumatic) childhood memories, fantasies, and dreams are dealt. Some of them are accurate representations of reality, whereas others are created fantasies that need to be interpreted before an accurate picture can be obtained.

Hypnosis and the Law

Hypnosis is a useful tool for the recovery of repressed and dissociated material. Patients do dissociate at the time of trauma. Because of this dissociation, many years later, they are incapable of remembering events of the trauma, even if they were "fully conscious" as it happened (Cardena and Spiegel 1993; Koopman et al. 1994; D. Spiegel and Cardena 1991). This failure to remember may persist years after the traumatic event takes place (Williams 1994). Because of the ability of hypnosis to promote age regression and other states of mind that enhance remembering, one of the most common applications of hypnosis in the court and other legal settings has been to refresh the recollection of witnesses and victims of crimes. A widely publicized case was the Chowchilla school bus hijacking (*People v. Schoenfeld* 1980). In this case, the driver of the bus was hypnotized to help recover details associated with the incident. Under hypnosis, the bus driver was able to recall the license plate number of the car driven by the kidnappers. The accurate recovery of this information led to the arrest and conviction of the criminals.

In this case, the information recovered by using hypnosis had not been consciously available to the driver before the hypnotic intervention.

On the other hand, anyone treating patients in whom prior trauma may be an issue must keep in mind recent developments in the legal system. Because of so many discrepancies among experts and difficulties, if not impossibilities, proving most or any of the allegations brought forth by victims, courts and society in general look upon this matter with considerable suspicion. Therefore, when therapists use hypnosis to treat their patients, the level of suspicion increases and in many instances the credibility of the victim decreases. Used improperly, hypnosis may render a witness incapable of testifying in court (*People v. Guerra* 1984; *People v. Shirley* 1982).

When using hypnosis in the treatment of trauma patients or patients with dissociative disorders, the following factors must be considered: the patients' ability to testify in court, the possibility of contamination, the phenomena of concreting and confabulation, and the way the mind stores and processes memory. An instruction to a patient that "the mind is like a video recorder" amounts to a suggestion to create information that is not remembered. Information that patients provide, whether the patients are lying on the couch, sitting on the chair, or deep in a hypnotic trance, may simply be the product of further retrieval efforts, may be influenced by the hypnotic context, and may not necessarily be true. What patients remember in the context of therapy may seem true to the patient; however, that does not mean that the information is true. On the other hand, the mere fact that hypnosis was used does not mean that the results are the product of suggestion or confabulation. The process of memory retrieval is affected by multiple factors, such as early object relations, comorbid psychiatric illnesses, current psychosocial stressors, patients' primary and secondary goals, and nature of the therapeutic relationship.

Therapists must be aware that using hypnosis may compromise patients' ability to testify in court. Many states, such as Arizona (*State ex rel Collins v. Superior Court* 1982), California (*People v. Guerra* 1984; *People v. Shirley* 1982), New Jersey (*People v. Hurd*

1980), and New York (*People v. Hughes* 1983), limit the testimony of victims or witnesses who have undergone hypnosis as a method of memory enhancement. Their rationale is a combination of the real and exaggerated dangers and limitations of using hypnosis (D. Spiegel 1987). Revisions to this question and several legal battles have made it possible for some courts (California Legislature 1985) to allow witnesses to testify after hypnosis has been employed, provided that certain guidelines have been followed. The restrictions primarily relate to the credentials and independence and training of the therapist (or other professional) conducting the hypnotic interrogation, as well as having the entire process electronically documented (D. Spiegel and Spiegel 1986).

In 1985, the Council on Scientific Affairs of the American Medical Association convened a panel of experts to examine the research evidence relevant to addressing the controversy surrounding hypnotic retrieval of memories. The report concluded that existing evidence confirms that the use of hypnosis increases the productivity of witnesses, resulting in new memories, some of which are true and some of which are incorrect. Some of the studies reviewed showed an increased level of confidence expressed by hypnotized subjects for the memories retrieved, despite the fact that their percentage of correct responses had not improved. The panel pointed out the differences inherent to the experimental situations in which tests are conducted, in a laboratory setting, and the real life situation existing in courtroom cases. Because of the differences in "reality" in these two scenarios, great caution should be used when drawing any conclusions. Those situations where extreme emotional and physical trauma have occurred differ markedly from the simulated experimental cases. The panel's final recommendations call for the use of careful guidelines similar to those adopted by the state of California to be followed when hypnosis is used in the forensic setting (California Legislature 1985).

Because of possible limitations involved in the application of hypnosis in legal cases, patients and attorneys must be cautioned that its use might result in a challenge of the victims' credibility as witnesses or even the admissibility of their testimony in a court of law (Scheflin and Shapiro 1989; D. Spiegel and Scheflin 1994).

Hypnosis is not a truth serum. Because of its fallibility, courts must weigh the effects of any hypnotic procedure on a witness versus the risks of contamination and credibility. Situations in which potential benefits of the use of hypnosis outweigh the risks include cases of traumatic amnesia from events of a crime or those instances in which all other avenues of exploration have been exhausted.

It is difficult to avoid potential contamination using any memory enhancement procedure (Loftus 1975, 1993; Loftus and Burns 1982). Therefore, three simple steps should be followed to decrease the amount of contamination while increasing the chances of admissibility in a court of law. First, obtain the patients' permission to consult with their attorney. If an investigation is in progress or court proceedings are likely, it may be desirable to contact the district attorney's office or the police. Second, make video recordings of all contact with the patients so the court can examine them for possible suggestive influences. These recordings should include the initial interview, hypnotic and nonhypnotic treatment interventions, and any other interaction with patients. If it is not possible to make a videotape of the sessions, obtain an audiotape recording of all contacts. Voices of the patients, therapist, and anyone else participating in the process should be clearly heard. Third, use a neutral attitude throughout the entire procedure. Guide patients through the experience but at all times avoid using leading or suggestive questions. The goal is to avoid contamination by introducing or suggesting information during the interrogation. Ask open-ended questions based on information already known and provided by the patients, for example, "Who else was there?" rather than "Was he there?" or "What is happening now?" rather than "Did he rape you?"

The hypnotic phenomenon involves a suspension of critical judgment, and therefore a state of heightened suggestibility or responsivity to social cues can be created. This heightened state of suggestibility is the main concern of the courts. Indeed, hypnosis can distort memory by any of three ways: 1) through confabulation, which involves creating pseudomemories that are then reported as real (Laurence and Perry 1983); 2) through concreting, an unwarranted increased sense of confidence with which hypnotized individuals report their memories, whether these are true or false (Diamond 1980; McConkey 1992; Orne 1979; D. Spiegel and Scheflin 1994; D. Spiegel and Spiegel 1986); or 3) as the result of an additional recall trial (Erdelyi and Kleinbard 1978).

In 1980, H. Spiegel described the so-called "honest liar." This is a hypnotized witness who, wanting to please the hypnotist or simply as a result of being in the suggestible state of hypnosis, will make up material and later believe the newly created story as real. Witnesses can then mislead a jury by producing confident errors (McConkey 1992) because they usually do not exhibit obvious signs of discomfort or insecurity when presenting their stories.

Finally, some authors have suggested that the hypnotic process yields new and true information along with facts that may have been distorted by any of the above mentioned methods (American Medical Association 1985; Orne 1979). Recent controversies surrounding so-called false memory syndrome have intensified questions regarding the accuracy and veracity of hypnotically recovered material.

Because of all these limitations, courts have restricted the admissibility of the testimony of hypnotized witnesses. Not only have they banned patients from being hypnotized in court, but they also have ruled that the testimony of witnesses who have been previously hypnotized may also be excluded. Even subjects acting in good faith can produce nontruthful material. Indeed, hypnosis can amplify both truth and falsehood. When used as a method of memory enhancement, hypnosis increases the recovery of memories, both true and confabulated.

There is no doubt that hypnosis can facilitate the recall of repressed or dissociated memories (Dywan and Bowers 1983). This is especially true when recall is inhibited by the strong affect associated with the traumatic nature of its content (D. Spiegel et al. 1982; Kardiner and Spiegel 1947). Nevertheless, research indicates that the most clearly reproducible problem is the production of confident errors, that is, exaggerating the truth value of memories recovered by hypnosis. Confident errors are not a problem limited to the hypnotic process. Victims and witnesses repeatedly interrogated by police and other investigators are subject to the same degree of suggestibility and concreting as hypnotized individuals. This is especially true when the person being interrogated happens to be a highly hypnotizable subject.Recommended guidelines for using hypnosis in the forensic setting include adequate coordination with the patients' counsel before any procedures take place, careful documentation of the subjects' knowledge of possible traumatic events before hypnosis is employed, the use of nonleading questions during hypnotic interrogation, complete electronic recording of all contacts with the patients, and careful debriefing after completion of the process (Maldonado and Spiegel 1995; D. Spiegel and Spiegel 1986).

A point of further debate is how to proceed when memories of possible abuse are recovered. First of all, we begin by warning our patients of the facts surrounding hypnotically recovered memories, including the possibilities of confabulation and concreting, as well as the difficulties in differentiating between fantasized or remembered memories. If memories of abuse are recovered, we do not encourage our patients to take legal action. There is no scientific evidence indicating that confrontation with alleged perpetrators of childhood abuse provides any therapeutic benefit to patients. The same is true for the pursuit of legal action or retribution toward perpetrators. It is impossible for therapists or the courts to be certain of the veracity of the memories recovered by either conventional therapy or hypnosis. Without objective external confirmation, therapists cannot distinguish memories that are real, those that result from confabulation, and those that result from a combination of both.

Furthermore, our experience in legal cases is that not only would it be difficult to substantiate many of our patients' allegations, but also little can be done to protect patients from the embarrassment, humiliation, and further abuse that would be imposed on them by virtue of the legal proceedings. It has been emphasized throughout this chapter that one of the primary goals of therapists is to help patients achieve control. Therefore, despite warning their patients of the potential repercussions of the decision to pursue legal action, it is the duty of therapists to be supportive of their patients' final decision.

Conclusion

The challenge in treating patients who have a dissociative disorder or who have experienced overwhelming trauma is to help them achieve a new sense of integration or unity and heal the fragmentation caused by the traumatic experience. Traumatic experiences cause sudden and radical discontinuities in consciousness that leave patients with a polarized sense of themselves. On the one hand, they visualize the old self (i.e., before the trauma), and, on the other, they see themselves as soiled, defenseless, and helpless victims incapable of doing much to alter their present or future. This aspect of treatment is a form of grief work.

Patients are encouraged to acknowledge the content of the traumatic memories rather than avoid (dissociate) or repress them. Acknowledgment is followed by therapy work that allows them to put into proper perspective these painful life events. Successful completion of these two tasks will allow for the conscious awareness of painful realities. The same shift in concentration elicited at the time of trauma can now be controlled with the help of hypnosis. Hypnosis can be helpful in mobilizing affect and defenses and putting traumatic memories into perspective, with the subsequent reduction of symptoms.

Because hypnosis is a controlled form of dissociation, its use provides boundaries for the psychotherapeutic mourning process. Rather than telling patients not to ruminate over the details of a traumatic experience, therapists should instruct patients on how to think and deal with the traumatic experience. In time, patients slowly separate themselves from the victim's role and step into the role of survivor. Different from the powerless role of the victim, being a survivor involves mastering rather than being mastered by their memories and the dissociative defenses associated with the aftermath of trauma.

To achieve this new sense of unity, the condensed hypnotic approach can be used. First, patients must confront the trauma. Hypnosis is then used to help patients condense the traumatic memories. Once memories are recovered, patients usually need to confess feelings and experiences of which they are profoundly ashamed. Confession is followed by consolation, during which the therapist needs to be emotionally available to patients. Next is concentration, which allows patients to access or turn on the traumatic memories during the psychotherapeutic session and eventually obtain an image symbolic of the entire traumatic experience, thereby preventing the need to dwell on every detail associated with the trauma. The final stage assumes patients will be able to define themselves as being in control once again.

During this treatment process, the patients' task is to acknowledge and place into perspective painful life events, thereby making them acceptable to conscious awareness. The therapist's task is to help patients retrieve these painful memories, express them in ways that prevent self-destructive feelings and acts, and restructure the ways they think about themselves by reframing their memories and their self-perception. Hypnosis may allow patients to take an objective look at the facts surrounding the trauma. Then, the therapeutic process should help them restructure their memories and realize that they actually did the best they could under the circumstances.

Finally, therapists must be aware of the legal ramifications of trauma work, whether hypnosis is used or not, and must remember the limitations inherent in the use of hypnotic enhancement of memories. To protect therapists and patients, the following guidelines are recommended: 1) inform the patients' counsel of your plans before any procedures take place, 2) carefully document the subjects' knowledge of possible traumatic events before hypnosis is employed, 3) use nonleading questions during hypnotic interrogation, 4) obtain electronic recordings of all contacts with patients, and 5) carefully debrief both counsel and patients after completion of the process.

Definitions

The following definitions are adapted from *Webster's Tenth New Collegiate Dictionary*:

Absorption (*ab*-**sawrp**-*shen*), noun: the process of absorbing or being absorbed; great interest; entire occupation of the mind. From the Latin *absorbere* (*ab*, meaning away + *sorbere*, meaning drink in, to suck), to suck up, to assimilate, to interest greatly, to take in and not reflect, to engage one's whole attention.

Dissociation (*di-so-***se-a-***shen*), noun: the act of dissociating or state of being dissociated; separation. In psychology, the term used to describe the separation of whole segments of the personality (as in multiple personality) or of discrete mental processes (as in the schizophrenias) from the mainstream of consciousness or of behavior. From the Latin *dissociare* (*dis*, meaning asunder + *sociare*, meaning to unite), to separate, to disunite.

Hypnosis (*hyp-***no-***sas*), noun: the state of being hypnotized; abnormal sleep. From the Greek *hypnos* (meaning sleep). There is no formal definition in the dictionary for *hypnotizability* or *hypnotic capacity*. These could properly be defined as a subject's ability to use a natural state of mind known as hypnosis.

Suggestibility (*seg-***jes-***te-***bil-***et-e*), noun: the ability to influence by suggestion. From the Latin *suggest* (*sub*, meaning under + *gerere*, meaning to carry), to seek to influence, to bring to the mind for consideration, to call to mind by thought or association of ideas, to mention or imply as a possibility, to propose as desirable or fitting, to offer for consideration or as a hypothesis.

Trauma (**traw-***ma*), noun: bodily injury caused by violence; emotional shock (psychic trauma) with a lasting effect; a disordered psychic or behavioral state resulting from mental or emotional stress or physical injury. From the Greek *trauma* (meaning wound).

References

Allen JG, Smith WH: Diagnosing dissociative disorders. Bull Menninger Clin 57:328–343, 1993

American Medical Association Council on Scientific Affairs: Council report: scientific status of refreshing recollection by the use of hypnosis. JAMA 253:1918–1923, 1985

American Psychiatric Association: Diagnostic and Statistical Manual of Mental Disorders, Fourth Edition. Washington, DC, American Psychiatric Association, 1994

Baker EL: The use of hypnotic dreaming in the treatment of the border-line patient: some thoughts on resistance and transitional phenomena. Int J Clin Exp Hypn 31:19–27, 1983

Bernheim H: Hypnosis and Suggestion in Psychotherapy: A Treatise on the Nature of Hypnotism (1889). Translated by Herter CA. New Hyde Park, New York, University Books, 1964

Bliss EL: Multiple personalities: a report of 14 cases with implications for schizophrenia and hysteria. Arch Gen Psychiatry 37:1388–1397, 1980

Bliss EL: Hysteria and hypnosis. J Nerv Ment Dis 172:203–206, 1984

Bliss EL: Multiple Personality, Allied Disorders and Hypnosis. New York, Oxford University Press, 1986

Bodden JL: Accessing state-bound memories in the treatment of phobias: two case studies. Am J Clin Hypn 34:24–28, 1991

Bower GH: Mood and memory. Am Psychol 36:129–148, 1981

Braun BG, Sachs RG: The development of multiple personality disorder: predisposing, precipitating, and perpetuating factors, in Childhood Antecedents of Multiple Personality. Edited by Kluft RP. Washington, DC, American Psychiatric Press, 1985, pp 37–64

Bremner JD, Southwick S, Brett E, et al: Dissociation and posttraumatic stress disorder in Vietnam combat veterans. Am J Psychiatry 149: 328–332, 1992

Bremner JD, Southwick SM, Johnson DR, et al: Childhood physical abuse and combat-related posttraumatic stress disorder in Vietnam veterans. Am J Psychiatry 150:235–239, 1993

Breuer J, Freud S: Studies on hysteria (1893–1895), in The Standard Edition of the Complete Psychological Works of Sigmund Freud, Vol 2. Translated and edited by Strachey J. London, Hogarth Press, 1955, pp 1–319

Brooks B: Familial influences in father-daughter incest. Journal of Psychiatric Treatment and Evaluation 4:117–124, 1982

Brown GR, Anderson B: Psychiatric morbidity in adult inpatients with childhood histories of sexual and physical abuse. Am J Psychiatry 148:55–61, 1991

Bryer JB, Nelson BA, Miller JB, et al: Childhood sexual and physical abuse as factors in adult psychiatric illness. Am J Psychiatry 144:1426–1430, 1987

California Legislature, AB 2669, Hypnosis of Witnesses, added to Ch 7, Div 6, of the evidence code, enacted January 1, 1985

Cardena E, Spiegel D: Dissociative reactions to the San Francisco Bay Area earthquake of 1989. Am J Psychiatry 150:474–478, 1993

Carlson EB, Putnam FW: Integrating research on dissociation and hypnotizability: are there two pathways to hypnotizability? Dissociation 2:32–38, 1989

Charcot JM: Oeuvres Completes de JM Charcot, Tome IX. Paris, Lecrosnier et Babe, 1890

Chu DA, Dill DL: Dissociative symptoms in relation to childhood physical and sexual abuse. Am J Psychiatry 147:887–892, 1990

Classen C, Koopman C, Spiegel D: Trauma and dissociation. Bull Menninger Clin 2:179–194, 1993

Coons PM, Milstein V: Psychosexual disturbances in multiple personality: characteristics, etiology, and treatment. J Clin Psychiatry 47: 106–110, 1986

Coons PM, Bowman ES, Pellow TA: Post-traumatic aspects of the treatment of victims of sexual abuse and incest. Psychiatr Clin North Am 12:325–337, 1989

Copeland DR: The application of object relations theory to the hypnotherapy of developmental arrests: the borderline patient. Int J Clin Exp Hypn 34:157–168, 1986

Copeland MD, Kitching EH: Hypnosis in mental hospital practice. Journal of Mental Science 83:316–329, 1937

Diamond BL: Inherent problems in the use of pretrial hypnosis on a prospective witness. California Law Review 68:313–349, 1980

Dywan S, Bowers KS: The use of hypnosis to enhance recall. Science 222:184–185, 1983

Erdelyi MH, Kleinbard J: Has Ebbimghaus decayed with time? the growth of recall (hypermnesia) over days. Journal of Experimental Psychology: Human Learning and Memory 4:275–289, 1978

Evans FJ, Staats JM: Suggested posthypnotic amnesia in four diagnostic groups of hospitalized psychiatric patients. Am J Clin Hypn 32:27–35, 1989

Finkelhor D: Child Sexual Abuse: New Theory and Research. New York, Free Press, 1984

Frankel FH, Orne MT: Hypnotizability and phobic behavior. Arch Gen Psychiatry 33:1259–1261, 1976

Freud A: The Ego and Mechanisms of Defense. New York, International Universities Press, 1946

Freud S: Remembering, repeating and working-through (further recommendations on the technique of psycho-analysis II) (1914), in The Standard Edition of the Complete Psychological Works of Sigmund Freud, Vol 12. Translated and edited by Strachey J. London, Hogarth Press, 1958, pp 145–156

Frischholz EJ: The relationship among dissociation, hypnosis, and child abuse in the development of multiple personality disorder, in Childhood Antecedents of Multiple Personality Disorder. Washington, DC, American Psychiatric Press, 1985, pp 99–126

Frischholz EJ, Lipman LS, Braun BG, et al: Psychopathology, hypnotizability, and dissociation. Am J Psychiatry 149:1521–1525, 1992

Gelinas D: The persisting negative effects of incest. Psychiatry 46:312–332, 1983

Gerschman J, Burrows GD, Reade P: Hypnotizability and dental phobic disorders. Int J Psychosom 34:42–47, 1987

Herman JL: Father-Daughter Incest. Cambridge, MA, Harvard University Press, 1981

Herman JL, Perry JC, van der Kolk BA: Childhood trauma in borderline personality disorder. Am J Psychiatry 146:490–495, 1989

Hilgard ER: Hypnotic Susceptibility. New York, Harcourt, Brace & World, 1965

Hilgard ER: Toward a neo-dissociation theory: multiple controls in human functioning. Perspect Biol Med 17:301–316, 1970

Hilgard ER: Divided Consciousness: Multiple Controls in Human Thoughts and Action. New York, John Wiley, 1977

Hilgard ER: The hidden observer and multiple personality. Int J Clin Exp Hypn 32:248–253, 1984

Janet P: The Major Symptoms of Hysteria. New York, Macmillan, 1920

Janet P: Psychological Healing: A Historical and Clinical Study, Vols 1 and 2. Translated by Paul E. London, George Allen & Unwin, 1925

Kardiner A, Spiegel H: War stress and neurotic illness. New York, Paul Hoeber, 1947

Keane T, Fairbank J: Survey analysis of combat-related stress disorders in Vietnam veterans. Am J Psychiatry 140:348–350, 1983

Keane TM, Wolfe J: Comorbidity in post-traumatic stress disorder: an analysis of community and clinical studies. Journal of Applied Social Psychology 20:1776–1788, 1990

Kihlstrom JF: Conscious, subconscious, unconscious: a cognitive perspective, in The Unconscious Reconsidered. Edited by Bowers KS, Meichenbaum D. New York, John Wiley, 1984, pp 149–211

Kilhstrom JF: Repression, dissociation and hypnosis, in Repression and Dissociation: Implication for Personality Theory, Psychopathology, and Health. Edited by Singer JL. Chicago, University of Chicago Press, 1990, pp 180–208

Kluft RP: Treatment of multiple personality disorder. Psychiatr Clin North Am 7:9–29,1984

Kluft RP (ed): Childhood Antecedents of Multiple Personality. Washington, DC, American Psychiatric Press, 1985

Kluft RP (ed): Incest-Related Syndromes of Adult Psychopathology. Washington, DC, American Psychiatric Press, 1990

Kluft RP: Clinical presentations of multiple personality disorder. Psychiatr Clin North Am 14:605–629, 1991

Kluft RP: The use of hypnosis with dissociative disorders. Psychiatric Medicine 10:31–46, 1992

Kluft RP: Multiple personality disorder, in Dissociative Disorders: A Clinical Review. Edited by Spiegel D. Lutherville, MD, Sidran Press, 1993

Koopman C, Classen C, Spiegel D: Predictors of posttraumatic stress symptoms among Oakland/Berkeley firestorm survivors. Am J Psychiatry 151:888–894, 1994

Kranhold C, Baumann U, Fichter M: Hypnotizability in bulimic patients and controls: a pilot study. Eur Arch Psychiatry Clin Neurosci 242: 72–76, 1992

Laurence JR, Perry C: Hypnotically created memory among highly hypnotizable subjects. Science 222:523–524, 1983

Lavoie G, Elie R: The clinical relevance of hypnotizability in psychosis: with reference to thinking processes and sample variances, in Modern Trends in Hypnosis. Edited by Waxman D, Misra P, Gibson M, et al. New York, Plenum, 1985, pp 41–66

Lavoie G, Sabourin M: Hypnosis and schizophrenia: a review of experimental and clinical studies, in Handbook of Hypnosis and Psychosomatic Medicine. Edited by Burrows GD, Dennerstein L. Amsterdam, Elsevier/North-Holland Biomedical Press, 1980, pp 377–420

Loftus EF: Leading questions and the eyewitness report. Cognitive Psychology 7:560–572, 1975

Loftus EF: The reality of repressed memories. Am Psychol 48:518–537, 1993

Loftus EF, Burns TE: Mental shock can produce retrograde amnesia. Memory and Cognition 10:318–323, 1982

Maldonado JR, Spiegel D: Treatment of posttraumatic stress disorder, in Dissociation: Clinical and Theoretical Perspectives. Edited by Lynn SJ, Rhue JW. New York, Guilford, 1994, pp 215–241

Maldonado JR, Spiegel D: Using hypnosis, in Treating Women Molested in Childhood. Edited by Classen C. San Francisco, CA, Jossey-Bass, 1995, pp 163–186

Marmar CR, Weiss DS, Schlenger WE, et al: Peritraumatic dissociation and posttraumatic stress in male Vietnam theater veterans. Am J Psychiatry 151:902–907, 1994

McConkey KM: The effects of hypnotic procedures on remembering, in Contemporary Hypnosis Research. Edited by Fromm E, Nash MR. New York, Guilford, 1992, pp 405–426

McFarlane AC: Posttraumatic morbidity of a disaster: a study of cases presenting for psychiatric treatment. J Nerv Ment Dis 174:4–13, 1986

McFarlane AC: The longitudinal course of posttraumatic morbidity: the range of outcomes and their predictors. J Nerv Ment Dis 176:30–39, 1988

Menzies RG, Clarke JC: The etiology of fear of heights and its relationship to severity and individual response patterns. Behav Res Ther 31:355–365, 1993

Morgan AH, Hilgard ER: Age differences in susceptibility to hypnosis. Int J Clin Exp Hypn 21:78–85, 1973

Murray-Jobsis J: An exploratory study of hypnotic capacity of schizophrenic and borderline patients in a clinical setting. Am J Clin Hypn 33:150–160, 1991

Nash MR, Lynn SJ: Child abuse and hypnotic ability. Imagination, Cognition and Personality 5:211–218, 1986

Nash MR, Lynn SJ, Givens DL: Adult hypnotic susceptibility, childhood punishment, and child abuse: a brief communication. Int J Clin Exp Hypn 32:6–11, 1984

Nemiah JC: Dissociative disorders, in Comprehensive Textbook of Psychiatry/IV, 4th Edition. Baltimore, MD, Williams & Wilkins, 1985, pp 942–957

Nigg JT, Silk KR, Westen D, et al: Object representations in the early memories of sexually abused borderline patients. Am J Psychiatry 148:864–869, 1991

Orne MT: The use and misuse of hypnosis in court. Int J Clin Exp Hypn 27:311–341, 1979

People v Guerra, C-41916 Supreme Court, CA, Orange Co, 1984

People v Hughes, 59 NY 2d 523, 466 NYS 2d 255, 543 NE 2d 484, 1983

People v Hurd, Supreme Court, NJ, Somerset Co, April 2, 1980

People v Schoenfeld, 168 Cal Rptr 762, 111 CA 3d 671, 1980

People v Shirley, 31 Cal 3d 18, 641 P2d 775, 1982; modified 918a, 1982

Pettinati HM: Measuring hypnotizability in psychotic patients. Int J Clin Exp Hypn 30:404–416, 1982

Pettinati HM, Kogan LG, Evans FJ, et al: Hypnotizability of psychiatric inpatients according to two different scales. Am J Psychiatry 147: 69–75, 1990

Piccione C, Hilgard ER, Zimbardo PG: On the degree of stability of measured hypnotizability over a 25-year period. J Pers Soc Psychol 56: 289–295, 1989

Pribor EF, Dinwiddie SH: 1992 Psychiatric correlates of incest in childhood. Am J Psychiatry 149:52–56, 1992

Putnam FW: Dissociation as a response to extreme trauma, in Childhood Antecedents of Multiple Personality. Edited by Kluft RP. Washington, DC, American Psychiatric Press, 1985, pp 65–79

Putnam FW: Dissociative phenomena, in American Psychiatric Press Review of Psychiatry, Vol 10. Edited by Tasman A, Goldfinger SM. Washington, DC, American Psychiatric Press, pp 145–160, 1991

Putnam FW: Using hypnosis for therapeutic abreactions. Psychiatric Medicine 10:51–65, 1992

Putnam FW: Dissociative disorders in children: behavioral profiles and problems. Child Abuse Negl 17:39–45, 1993

Putnam FW, Guroff JJ, Silberman EK, et al: The clinical phenomenology of multiple personality disorder: review of 100 recent cases. J Clin Psychiatry 47:285–293, 1986

Rodolfa ER, Kraft W, Reilley RR: Etiology and treatment of dental anxiety and phobia. Am J Clin Hypn 33:22–28, 1990

Ross CA, Norton GR, Wozney K: Multiple personality disorder: an analysis of 236 cases. Can J Psychiatry 34:413–418, 1989

Rowan AB, Foy DW, Rodriguez N, et al: Posttraumatic stress disorder in a clinical sample of adults sexually abused as children. Child Abuse Negl 18:51–61, 1994

Salzman JP, Salzman C, Wolfson AN, et al: Association between borderline personality structure and history of childhood abuse in adult volunteers. Compr Psychiatry 34:254–257, 1993

Sanders B, Giolas MH: Dissociation and childhood trauma in psychologically disturbed adolescents. Am J Psychiatry 148:50–54, 1991

Saunders EA, Arnold F: A critique of conceptual and treatment approaches to borderline psychopathology in light of findings about childhood abuse. Psychiatry 56:188–203, 1993

Scheflin AW, Shapiro JL: Trance on Trial. New York, Guilford, 1989

Smith WH: Hypnosis in the treatment of anxiety. Bull Menninger Clin 54:209–216, 1990

Solomon Z, Mikulincer M, Benbenishty R: Combat stress reaction: clinical manifestations and correlates. Military Psychology 1:35–47, 1989

Spiegel D: Vietnam grief work using hypnosis. Am J Clin Hypn 24:33–40, 1981

Spiegel D: Multiple personality as a post-traumatic stress disorder. Psychiatr Clin North Am 7:101–110, 1984

Spiegel D: Dissociating damage. Am J Clin Hypn 29:123–131, 1986

Spiegel D: The Shirley decision: the cure is worse than the disease, in Advances in Forensic Psychology and Psychiatry, Vol 2. Edited by Rieber R. Norwood, NJ, Ablex, 1987

Spiegel D: Dissociation and hypnosis in posttraumatic stress disorder. J Trauma Stress 1:17–33, 1988

Spiegel D: Hypnosis in the treatment of victims of sexual abuse. Psychiatr Clin North Am 12:295–305, 1989

Spiegel D: Hypnosis, dissociation and trauma: hidden and overt observers, in Repression and Dissociation. Edited by Singer JL. Chicago, University of Chicago Press, 1990, pp 121–142

Spiegel D: The use of hypnosis in the treatment of PTSD. Psychiatric Medicine 10:21–30, 1992

Spiegel D, Cardena E: New uses of hypnosis in the treatment of posttraumatic stress disorder. J Clin Psychiatry 51 (suppl 10):39–43, 1990

Spiegel D, Cardena E: Disintegrated experience: the dissociative disorders revisited. J Abnorm Psychol 100:366–378, 1991

Spiegel D, Fink R: Hysterical psychosis and hypnotizability. Am J Psychiatry 136:777–781, 1979

Spiegel D, Scheflin AW: Dissociated or fabricated? psychiatric aspects of repressed memory in criminal and civil cases. Int J Clin Exp Hypn 42:411–432, 1994

Spiegel D, Spiegel H: Forensic uses of hypnosis, in Handbook of Forensic Psychology. Edited by Weiner IB, Hess AK. New York, John Wiley & Sons, 1986

Spiegel D, Detrick D, Frischholz E: Hypnotizability and Psychopathology. Am J Psychiatry 139:431–437, 1982

Spiegel D, Hunt T, Dondershine HE: Dissociation and hypnotizability in posttraumatic stress disorder. Am J Psychiatry 145:301–305, 1988

Spiegel D, Frischholz EJ, Lipman LS, et al: Dissociation, hypnotizability and trauma. Paper presented at the annual meeting of the American Psychiatric Association, San Francisco, CA, May 1989

Spiegel H: The grade 5 syndrome: the highly hypnotizable person. Int J Clin Exp Hypn 22:303–319, 1974

Spiegel H: Hypnosis and evidence: help or hindrance? Ann N Y Acad Sci 347:73–85, 1980

Spiegel H, Spiegel D: Trance and Treatment: Clinical Uses of Hypnosis. New York, Basic Books, 1987

State ex rel Collins v Superior Court, 132 Ariz 180, 644 P2d 1266, 1982; supplemental opinion filed May 4, 1982

Stein JA, Golding JM, Siegel JM, et al: Long-term psychological sequelae of child sexual abuse: the Los Angeles epidemiologic catchment area study, in Lasting Effects of Child Sexual Abuse. Edited by Wyatt GE, Powell GJ. Newbury Park, CA, Sage, 1989, pp 135–154

Steingard S, Frankel FH: Dissociation and psychotic symptoms. Am J Psychiatry 142:953–955, 1985

Stern DL, Spiegel H, Nee JCM: The Hypnotic Induction Profile: normative observations, reliability, and validity. Am J Clin Hypn 21:109–132, 1979

Stone MH: Borderline syndrome: a consideration of subtypes and an overview: directions for research. Psychiatr Clin North Am 4:3–23, 1981

Stuntman RK, Bliss EL: Posttraumatic stress disorder, hypnotizability and imagery. Am J Psychiatry 142:741–743, 1985

Tellegen A: Practicing the two disciplines for relaxation and enlightenment: comment on "Role of the feedback signal in electromyograph biofeedback: the relevance of attention," by Qualls and Sheegan. J Exp Psychol Gen 110:217–226, 1981

Tellegen A, Atkinson G: Openness to absorbing and self-altering experiences (" absorption"): a trait related to hypnotic susceptibility. J Abnorm Psychol 83:268–277, 1974

Terr LC: Childhood traumas: an outline and overview. Am J Psychiatry 148:10–20, 1991

van der Kolk BA, van der Hart O: Pierre Janet and the breakdown of adaptation in psychological trauma. Am J Psychiatry 146:1530–1540, 1989

van der Kolk BA, Perry JC, Herman JL: Childhood origins of self-destructive behavior. Am J Psychiatry 148:1665–1671, 1991

Watkins JG: Hypnotherapeutic Technique: The Practice of Clinical Hypnosis, Vols 1 and 2. New York, Irvington Publishers, 1987

Weaver TL, Clum GA: Early family environments and traumatic experiences associated with borderline personality disorder. J Consult Clin Psychol 61:1068–1075, 1993

Weitzenhoffer AM, Hilgard ER: Stanford Hypnotic Susceptibility Scale-Form C. Palo Alto, CA, Consulting Psychologists Press, 1962

Westen D, Ludolph P, Misle B, et al: Physical and sexual abuse in adolescent girls with borderline personality disorder. Am J Orthopsychiatry 60:55–66, 1990

Wilkinson CB: Aftermath of a disaster: the collapse of the Hyatt Regency Hotel skywalks. Am J Psychiatry 140:1134–1139, 1983

Williams LM: Recall of childhood trauma: a prospective study of women's memories of childhood sexual abuse. J Consult Clin Psychol 62:1167–1176, 1994

Zanarini MC, Gunderson JG, Manrino MF, et al: Childhood experiences of borderline patients. Compr Psychiatry 30:18–25, 1989

Chapter 4

Dissociation and Hypnotizability: A Conceptual and Methodological Perspective on Two Distinct Concepts

Eric Vermetten, M.D., J. Douglas Bremner, M.D., and David Spiegel, M.D.

Overview

In this chapter, we describe the concepts of hypnosis and dissociation, focusing on the conceptualization of both terms, their phenomena, and their similarities and differences in measurement of hypnotizability and dissociative capacity or "dissociativity." There is a strong conceptual relationship between hypnosis and dissociation. Hypnotizability and dissociation can be conceptualized as dimensional constructs, reflecting ranges of intensity along a continuum. There is some degree of overlap between hypnotizability and dissociation. The exact degree to which there is overlap continues to be a subject of debate. Hypnosis may account for many of the findings attributed to dissociation and dissociative disorders. The viewpoint is described that dissociative processes can range along a continuum from normal dissociation to DSM-IV (American Psychiatric Association 1994) Axis I psychopathology.

Dissociation seems to account for a shift in modern psychology and psychiatry through its widespread clinical relevance and recognition by cognitive sciences. It is strongly related to consciousness, conflict/trauma, and unity of the self. Like hypnosis, dissociation can be measured by various scales, all focusing on slightly different aspects of the concepts and using different methodologies. Dissociation raises fundamental questions about the relation of the mind to the body.

Hypnotic and dissociative capacities are potentially both a liability and an asset. They could be advantageous or beneficial for the human organism in certain contexts or time frames (e.g., forgetting about or not feeling painful stimuli; being distracted from irrelevant information), but high hypnotic and dissociative capacities can be disadvantageous and harmful and can lead to various dysfunctions, pathology (e.g., amnesia, time gaps, flashbacks, conversion disorders), and severe psychopathology (e.g., dissociative identity disorder [DID]). Both hypnotizability and dissociation are related to control versus loss of control over psychological and physical functions. Physical, emotional, or sexual trauma can play a major role in the shift of this control function. Evidence is reviewed that trauma can lead to various dysfunctions that can manifest in psychological and/or bodily or somatic problems. Trauma plays a major role at least in the clinical connection between hypnotizability and dissociation. The methodology of the measurements of both hypnotizability and dissociation can serve an important purpose for a better understanding of their combined meaning in research and clinical practice.

Everyone knows what is meant by *hypnosis* and *dissociation*, even though the specific nature of these terms is difficult to describe. Hypnosis and dissociation seem to be both widely used in modern psychology and psychiatry and are at the same time rather unclear or controversial concepts.

Hypnosis and dissociation have a long history in both disciplines. Hypnosis was first used by Braid in 1843 to describe a state that he termed "neurypnology," whereas Janet wrote about dissociation in 1892 (Ellenberger 1970). Janet first used the term "desagregation mentale" to describe this process. Reviews of the literature of the last three decades shows that a robust physiological phenomenon underlies hypnosis (e.g., see Barber 1961; Spiegel and Vermetten 1994). Moreover, hypnosis has found itself a legitimate place in both medical and psychotherapeutic practice (Frankel 1987), and dissociation has been the focus of attention of a large body of research for approximately a decade (Klein and Do-

ane 1994; Lynn and Rhue 1994; Spiegel 1994). The section on dissociative identity disorders in DSM-IV shows that dissociation has
been given a place in diagnostic psychiatric practice and research.

Hypnosis Revisited

Following the decline of hypnosis after Freud, there has been a revival of interest in hypnosis since 1960. The so-called golden age of
hypnosis has been one of striking productivity, methodological
innovations, and theoretical turmoil. Traditionally, hypnosis has
been viewed as having a strong relation to suggestibility, and treatments using hypnosis have been regarded especially applicable in
cases of hysterical and neurotic complaints (Ellenberger 1970).
There is a long tradition of employing hypnotic capacity in the
treatment of these "dissociative psychoses" (Kihlstrom 1994). Early
in this century (e.g., through the work of the Dutch psychiatrist
Breukink), it was reported that hysterical psychoses were trauma
induced and certainly curable and that psychotherapy using
hypnosis was the treatment of choice. Hypnosis was used for
symptom-oriented therapy, for a comfortable and supportive mental state, and for the uncovering and integrating of traumatic
memories (van der Hart and Spiegel 1993). Hypnosis also has been
described as "artificial hysteria" (Bliss 1984). Ever since its discovery, hysteria has been linked with forgotten early traumas that
were responsible for symptoms of hysteria in patients. These amnestic traumas could in turn be revealed by hypnosis. Now that
hysteria as a diagnostic category has gone out of fashion, disorders
that previously would have been labeled hysterical are divided by
DSM-IV into or among a number of different categories: posttraumatic stress disorder (PTSD), somatoform disorder, conversion disorder, and dissociative disorder. (For a review, see Chapter 1 of this
volume.) The focus in these disorders has been on factors different
from those explaining and describing hysteria, although the psychodynamic explanation of the symptoms may be the same.

Hypnosis in the golden age has had important impact because
of the work of Barber (1969), the neodissociative position of E. R.
Hilgard (1977), and the social psychological approach of Sarbin

and Coe (1972), Spanos (1982), and Spanos and Chaves (1989). Hypnosis may be best described as consisting of three factors: absorption, dissociation, and suggestibility (Spiegel 1991). No one factor can explain the concept of hypnosis completely. In this three-factor concept, *absorption* is described as the narrowing of attention and a disposition for having episodes of single total attention that fully engage one's representational resources. *Dissociation* is described as a kind of divided or parallel access to awareness, wherein several systems may occur seemingly independently. *Suggestion* is described as a certain role behavior or the nonvolitional transformation of a suggested idea to a suggested effect. Dissociation is only one aspect of this conceptualization of hypnosis. Different researchers and therapists emphasize the different factors, dissociation, absorption, and suggestibility, in their use of hypnosis. The literature includes lively debates about state and nonstate issues regarding hypnosis and hypnotic susceptibility or hypnotizability (Barber and Wilson 1977; Coe 1973; Orne 1977). The controversy was not so much about the reality of the responses that were observed, but was about whether the state was an explanation in itself or whether it needed explanation. An ego psychology definition that describes both a "state" and a "talent" regarding hypnosis and hypnotic susceptibility is as follows:

> Hypnosis is an altered state of consciousness into which people can go if they have the talent to do so: in which they experience heightened ego receptivity (equals suggestibility) and ego activity; attention changes; more primary process thinking, more imagery; dissociative phenomena (for instance, the observing ego versus the experiencing ego); regression in the service of the ego; fading of the Generalized Reality Orientation; and stronger and quicker transference phenomena. (Fromm and Nash 1992, p. 85)

Classical phenomena of hypnosis are amnesia; catalepsy; ideomotor phenomena, such as automatic writing; posthypnotic effects with amnesia for the event; hypermnesia; age regression; and hallucinatory phenomena, with either positive or negative hallucinations. Traditionally, the state of hypnosis occurs after an induction procedure. Whether this procedure must be formal or can be informal can be and has been argued. Through research it was possible to gain substantial agreement upon the classical representative phenomena of hypnosis (E. R. Hilgard 1987).

Despite different descriptions of the conceptualization of hypnosis, its current contribution to medical and psychotherapeutic practice has never been more important. The recent renewed interest in cognitive psychology with its rediscovery of the unconscious, the influences of information-processing theories linked to computer systems, and the attractive practical uses in therapy that evolve from these perspectives has given hypnosis a strong and steady push forward in the acknowledgment of its value.

Dissociation, Neodissociation Theory, and Neural Network Models

Dissociation is ubiquitous, a priori a necessary and normal mental process. It can be viewed as being the opposite of what occurs in common life and can be viewed as the integrative function of the mind. Different stimuli (e.g., visual, acoustic, or sensory) are dissociated at root but "automatically" are formed into one piece of memory, establishing coherence and identity (Spiegel and Cardena 1991b). Dissociation seems to prohibit this integrative function and compartmentalizes different experiences. Dissociation may take the form of a physical sense (e.g., a hypnotized subject experiences one hand as being not as much a part of his or her body as the other hand). There is an involuntariness to movements, numbness, and tingling, and the hand seems to be constituted in a different relation to the rest of the body, as if two separate systems for interpreting somatic perception were occurring at the same time rather than one system incorporating similar sensations from all parts of the body (Spiegel 1990). Time distortion, negative hallucinations, and posthypnotic amnesia can be viewed as being dissociative symptoms occurring in or after hypnosis. In the dissociative process, bodily perceptions can change, as well as mental, behavioral, and emotional perceptions:

I look at my hands, which are writing this; how odd it is! Are they really concerned with what they are doing? I look at my reflection in the window, and find myself to be strange, novel. For a moment I was almost afraid of the image the window pane returned to me—of this phantom of myself. (Nemiah 1995, p. 1289)

Or,

Things don't look the way they used to. Everything I see, even the decorations on the wall of my room, seem strange to me. It's as if I were seeing everything for the first time. Everything appears unreal to me. When I go out, it seems to me that the street is not the same. It's like a city I haven't seen for a long time. Suddenly everything around me gives me the effect of having become odd. It's as though reality were deformed. (Nemiah 1995, p. 1289).

Symptoms or phenomena of more severe and potentially patho-logical dissociation are stupor, derealization, depersonalization, numbing, and amnesia for the event:

A Vietnam combat veteran who reported "I felt myself separating from myself and looking down at the person who was in combat, and feeling sorry for him" dissociated, leaving his body stuporous and numb on the battlefield. Later he had no memory for what hap-pened. (Bremner et al. 1992, p. 331)

Dissociation as a concept is supposed to describe and, through theoretical underpinning, explain symptoms of fragmentation or loss of integrative functions. It can do so by the assumptions that there are changes in the continuity of awareness and that there are altered or parallel layers of consciousness.

Of importance in the theoretical framework of dissociation has been the previously mentioned neodissociation theory of E. R. Hil-gard (1977, 1986), which expands on the concepts of hypnotic dissociation and Janet's ideas of dissociation. E. R. Hilgard empha-sized a horizontal rather than a vertical depiction of the relation between conscious and unconscious states (i.e., when two tasks are performed simultaneously, one on a conscious and one on an unconscious level, each is performed less efficiently because of the effort required for the other task and because of the effort to keep the unconscious task out of awareness). For example, when a subject's arm is made to rise in the air, the cognitive control structure for the arm has been dissociated from the main part of the central control structure. E. R. Hilgard's theory involved the coexistence in connection with the same organism of two separate streams of consciousness that are coactive and that pursue their courses not necessarily without mutual interference, but with limited mutual cognizance and a large measure of independence. His theory was not complete but served as a mapping out of the direction that a theory of hypnosis and dissociative phenomena should take.

The neodissociation theory now unwittingly seems to fit with neural network models, with subsequent connectionist viewpoints on learning and memory, and with physical evidence of the parallel distributed nature of various aspects of the functioning human brain (Parks et al. 1991). The social organization of mind contributes also to the modern assumption that memory processes are dissociated in nature (Minsky 1986; Spiegel and Cardena 1991b). Hypnotic dissociation has been described in recent models of neural networks regarding nonlinearity of long-term memorizing processes (Kuzin 1995; Li and Spiegel 1992). Together with clinical observations and research on dissociation, these neodissociation ideas seem to constitute an important shift for psychology and give dissociation a legitimate place in cognitive science because parallel distributed processing (PDP) models and neural network models have been fruitful concepts when they have been applied to simple learning and to attention, memory, language, and perceptual and motor processes (Corbetta et al. 1990; Feldman and Ballard 1982). An example of the parallel operation of two high-level information processors is the "hidden observer" phenomenon in the neodissociation theory of E. R. Hilgard (1977, 1992), in which a highly hypnotizable subject is able to produce analgesia for pain, and yet a hidden proportion of consciousness acknowledges feeling sensory pain and marks considerable discomfort. The hidden-observer theory allows for separate nonconscious parallel processing of all perception, isolated from awareness via amnesia and retrievable via a hidden observer. The narrowing of the awareness indeed affects the way in which the percepts are processed: there is reduction of cortical processing of the dissociated percept (Sigalowitz et al. 1991; Spiegel et al. 1985, 1989).

Conceptual Issues in Dissociation: Consciousness, Conflict, and Unity of the Self

Dissociation as a concept has been criticized as an oversimplification of the complexity of human behavior and human suffering (Frankel 1991). Dissociation is also described as a metaphor that can be better understood in the vocabulary of skills rather than in the vocabulary of autonomous state of mind or personality traits (Sarbin 1994; 1995). There has been, and still may be, a lively debate about differences between repression and dissociation. Both are contents of the mind and are banished from awareness, but there is no consensus yet about how and where both concepts differ (Cardena 1994; Kihlstrom 1987; Singer 1990; Spiegel 1990).

Despite the criticism, there seems to be sufficient agreement that dissociation is fundamental to cognitive function (Kihlstrom et al. 1994). The term has been used in cognitive psychology to describe differential performance in tasks presumably mediated by distinct mental processes or to explain performance in free recall completion tests (Denny and Hunt 1992; Goodglass and Budin 1988). In the field of personality and clinical psychology, dissociation is described as resembling semi-independent mental modules that are not consciously accessible, as representing an alteration in consciousness where the individual becomes disconnected or disengaged, and as a defense mechanism warding off physical or emotional pain or other alterations of consciousness. The term should not be overextended (e.g., used as a shorthand for any kind of conscious or alternate mental process or used in arguing that not all state-dependent memory is dissociative in general) (Cardena 1994). Cardena (1994) reports on different fields of study wherein dissociation is used as a descriptive or explanatory concept for apparently disparate phenomena ranging from hypnosis with perception without awareness, to forms of psychopathology, to cognitive responses to trauma and particular neurological syndromes. He proposes a model whereby dissociative phenomena are arranged along two orthogonal dimensions of normality/pathology and psychological/neurological causation. Hypnosis, together with out-of-body experiences and automatisms, is localized in this model in the lower-right quadrant, the psychological-normal cluster.

In a psychobiological model, dissociation has been described as representing a process whereby certain mental functions that are ordinarily integrated with other functions presumably operate in a more compartmentalized or automatic way, usually outside the sphere of conscious awareness or memory recall (Ludwig 1983). Dissociation is depicted in this model as having great individual and species survival value. The processes, or the consequences, of dissociation are measurable, sensible to cultural differences, and important in the mind-body relationship (Spiegel 1994). Nemiah (1993) described the broad field dissociation can cover and the impact it can have on an individual:

> The term dissociation refers to the exclusion from consciousness and the inaccessibility of voluntary recall of mental events, singly or in clusters of varying degrees of complexity, such as memories, sensations, feelings, fantasies, and attitudes. (p. 106)

Underlying the theoretical concept of dissociation and its presumed survival value, concepts concerning consciousness, conflict, mind-body relationships, and unity of the self can be found. A functional conceptualization leading to an etiological description and a discussion of how and where dissociation affects the mind-body relationship are explained separately later in this chapter. Consciousness, conflict, and unity of the self are described in relation to dissociation as follows:

1. *Consciousness.* In most of the recent literature on dissociation, when the term *consciousness* is used, the approach is phenomenological and descriptive rather than conceptual and construc-

tive. This approach is similarly used for the term *unconscious*. The unconscious in this respect is not a conceptual construction or an imaginary entity created to explain phenomenal facts, as it is in a psychoanalytical perspective. Dissociation is a description of phenomenological facts and can be viewed as a unique form of consciousness. Dissociation enables (or causes) detachment from anticipation or actual experiences of fear, pain, and helplessness (Bremner and Brett 1997; Marmar et al. 1994; Spiegel 1990, 1993; Spiegel et al. 1988). Dissociation can be viewed as the lack of connection between one piece of memory or consciousness and another (Bremner et al. 1992). PDP can be used to model the dissociative mental processes. Both the conscious/unconscious and the dissociation/integration (or dissociation/association) dichotomies are descriptive in their primary purposes, with emphasis placed on the absence or presence of awareness in the former and memory or perception in the latter.

2. *Conflict.* The defense-deficiency controversy regarding dissociation has led to lively debates (Cardena 1994; Erdelyi 1994; Gabbard 1994; Singer 1990). This controversy recalls the debate at the beginning of this century between Janet and Freud. According to Freud, dissociation was an active defense phenomenon. When the integrity of the overall system was threatened, subsystems of ideas/wishes/memories/thoughts would be forcibly repressed, dissociated, or split off. In Janet's theory, dissociation was a deficit phenomenon, an insufficiency of binding energy, caused by hereditary factors, life stresses or traumas, or an interaction among them modeled on Hughlings Jackson's hierarchy of mental functions. These processes resulted in the splitting of fragments. In Jackson's theory, dissociation had to do with a lack of integration between mental processes and especially an inaccessibility of mental contents or processes to phenomenological awareness.

Regarding the differences between dissociation and repression, Kluft (1991) states that the dissociated material maintains in the dynamic unconscious, in a series of parallel consciousnesses. Dissociation defends against traumatic experiences associated with external events, and repression defends one from forbidden internal wishes. But why dissociation is a defense against external stimuli and repression is a defense against anxiety-provoking internal stimuli has not been resolved. In dissociative amnesia, the memories are internal even though the trigger may have been caused environmentally or externally (Cardena 1994). Dissociation and repression seem to be similar, but their theoretical underpinnings differ.

The dissociation in memory is different in Freud's conversion notion. It is not that repressed memories are converted into symptoms, but in the absence of conscious recollection, the sequelae of trauma/conflict persist in procedural formats. Erdelyi (1994) tried to overcome the controversy when he proposed an alternative to Freud's conversion hypothesis, stating that repression defeats declarative memory but it does not affect procedural memory. Traumatic memory in this model preferentially involves procedural memory.

3. *Unity of the self; autobiographical memory.* Dissociated mental contents are not consciously linked with one's history or sense of the self. The state of emergency in the self triggers a defensive reorganization of consciousness, an attentional shift that excludes aspects of the self from the context of experience. The continuity of experience should not be taken for granted; the continuity of experience, memory, and identity is an accomplishment (Spiegel 1991). Self-organization exists because of reciprocity of dissociation-association, which is under continual construction. Dennett (1991) describes the self as the center of narrative gravity, stressing the need for giving verbal account of experiences to promote integrative functions. What can be forgotten and what needs to be remembered therefore must be consciously processed first, and preferably discussed, before they can be stored in memory. Creating a spatial-temporal track of both the immediate past and the ordinary continuity of experience is important. Synthesis of self-experience then takes place automatically and unconsciously. Kihlstrom (1992) discusses the difference between dissociation and automaticity. According to Kihlstrom (1992), dissociation

can delete the spatial-temporal context that is normally associated with memory for events, leading to a disruption of episodic memory and autobiographic memory. As such, dissociation is made manifest by a failure to integrate thoughts, feelings, memories, and actions into a unified sense of consciousness. Dissociation in DID is observed when cohesion of the subselves that form a unity is lost and when subselves act independently or in a contradictory manner.

Dissociative phenomena demonstrate that coherence of identity is not automatic self-evidence from which symptoms may be subtracted. Integrated identity is an accomplishment that is subject to disruption through trauma, hypnotic influences, or dysfunctions in information-processing strategies (Kihlstrom 1987; Spiegel and Cardena 1991b). We construct a sense of personal continuity by maintaining a consistent stream of memory, a kind of smoothing function in which we subsume disparate experiences under a common heading of personal integrity and identity (Spiegel 1990).

Overwhelming experiences might not be processed in an integrated manner. The information is not lost but encoded in terms of emotion and personal identity. Encoding the experience emotionally is a state-dependent and momentary reaction that protects the individual, with an automatization of cognitive and motor procedures. Encoding the experience in terms of personal identity occurs within a certain time span and has a more reflexive, self-referential nature (Kihlstrom 1987), contributing to the process of identity alteration.

A Functional Conceptualization of Dissociation

Dissociation could be conceptualized as a specific response to overwhelming stimuli. Ludwig (1983) favored individual and species survival value as being the psychobiological functions of this response. He argued that dissociation could represent the fundamental psychobiological mechanism underlying a wide variety of altered forms of consciousness. In evolutionary history, these ideas could be related to the freezing response of animals confronted with a predator or other life-endangering threat or could be related to other primitive coping styles against fearful situations. Ludwig (1983) described dissociation and the dissociative process.

The adaptive value of dissociation has led to different descriptive models of dissociative disorders. Dissociative phenomena have been described as existing on a continuum and as becoming maladaptive when they exceed limits in frequency or intensity or when they occur in contexts that are inappropriate (Putnam 1989). Only in extreme cases does dissociation give rise to a set of psychiatric syndromes known as the dissociative disorders (Putnam 1991).

Phenomena occur that are described in DID or multiple personality disorder (MPD) patients at the moment of a switch between altered states: automation of behavior, resolution of irreconcilable conflicts, escape from the constraints of reality, isolation of catastrophic experiences, cathartic discharge of feelings, submersion of the individual for group identity, analgesia, and depersonalization (Putnam 1988). Reorganization occurs in a switch process, as Putnam (1988) describes it, and changes state-related variables, such as affect, access to memories, sense of self, and cognitive and perceptual styles. The switch process is often reflected in alterations in facial expression, speech and motor activity, and interpersonal relatedness. These alterations are characterized by an apparent general polarity, with an "on-off" quality. An example is hyperarousal (flashback) alternating with detachment and numbing (derealization and depersonalization) (Spiegel 1993). Herman (1992) describes this oscillation as the dialectic of trauma.

The central and organizing paradigm for dissociation seems to be linked with a sudden activation of altered states of consciousness as a reaction to psychological trauma. These experiences induce an altered state in which memories and affects relating to the trauma are encoded. After trauma, there is often posttraumatic amnesia for these events; however, the memories and affects may manifest themselves in nonverbal forms. Amnesia in an undifferentiated form can be a manifestation of the barrier between what is and what is not integrated. In the case of psychogenic amnesia, Loewenstein (1993) differentiates two subgroups in the disorder: 1) amnesia that is primarily related to traumatization and 2) amnesia that develops in the context of overwhelming psychological conflict in an individual predisposed to dissociate.

Regarding the dissociated experience mechanism of dissociation, in which an amnesia-like barrier keeps (traumatic) experience out of consciousness, Miller and Bowers (1993) describe a different model in which a dissociated control mechanism rather than a dissociative experience explains the dissociation. Their view of dissociated control implies that suggestive communication can more or less directly activate subsystems of control and minimize the influence of executive initiative and effort. They represent an opposite position regarding the neodissociation theory of E. R. Hilgard. In their view, dissociated control is central to the nonvolitional hypnotic responding.

Some Elements Describing Hypnotic and Dissociative Processes

Some fundamental descriptions of hypnosis and dissociation are similar. They are related to what Counts (1990) described as the importance of making a distinction between different frames of reference in the process of dissociation compared with the content of dissociation. Evans (1992) proposes the same distinction between dissociation of content and dissociation of context, discussing the issue of source amnesia. The content may be an affect or a visual image that can be reported after the process of dissociation. The following three issues concerning the processes of hypnosis and dissociation should be considered:

1. *Descriptions of context and content.* The word *dissociate* is often used as a verb in clinical settings: "This patient is dissociating." Statements of this kind are often heard on clinical wards. Categorizing a patient can occur when therapists do not specify what caused the dissociation or what was dissociated. Of rele-

vance can be whether the dissociation concerned memories, sensations, feelings, fantasies, or attitudes (see definition of dissociation, Nemiah 1993). Adding information about the context and content of the dissociation could be more beneficial for the patient.

2. *Frames of reference: subjective experience versus observable behavior.* Different frames of reference can be taken into account to describe the process of dissociation. The subjective experience of perceptions, the more objective behaviors, or both may indicate the process of dissociation. While dissociating, patients may interpret their subjective experiences differently from the way they interpret them some moments later. Self-reports of patients who spoke about numbness, who felt as if they were somewhere else, or who had amnesia for a certain time frame indicate that the verb dissociate can also be used in the past tense: "The patient dissociated." Consequently, the term refers to the content of the phenomena. Dissociation is the split in the perceptual or cognitive mode; the split itself is a process. One might suggest, based on observable phenomena, that at the time of the split the patient is in hypnosis or in a trance (it can be hard to distinguish whether this really is or was the case). After hypnosis, the perceived subjective hypnotic experience can be taken into account. However, the observed phenomena in (formally) induced hypnosis are easier to distinguish because one can see what the behavior of the person is related to exactly. In the case of spontaneous trance, this observation is much more difficult. Therefore, at the time of dissociation, only the context and the observable behavior can be taken into account to describe what is happening.

3. *Involuntariness.* Involuntariness is a fundamental feature of hypnotic responding. Most individuals who successfully carry out a suggestion report that the response takes little or no effort and seems to happen by itself. Highly hypnotizable individuals experience hypnotic suggestions as involuntary, even while engaging in conflicting thoughts and imagery and attending closely to their behavior. These findings are precisely what dissociation theory would predict. If a person is given a suggestion

of arm rigidity, the person's volition seems to play no part in making the response happen, even though he or she is trying as hard as he or she can. Being physically able to bend the arm, the person must be doing something to prevent it from bending. Involuntariness goes beyond a sociocognitive theory of hypnosis (Zamansky and Ruehle 1995). A comparison between dissociation and sleeping can be made: just as someone cannot consciously start sleeping or fall asleep, one cannot consciously dissociate. It can be said that someone was sleeping for a certain moment or period, but the statement "I am sleeping right now" seems illogical. If said, it is meant in relational terms. Both dissociation and hypnosis do not have a relational meaning per se; they are personal reactions to environmental stimuli.

Hypnotizability Scales

In research and clinical practice where hypnosis is used, the importance of hypnotizability ratings is strongly stressed. These ratings are important for research purposes and predict prognosis to therapy when hypnosis is used. Different hypnotic susceptibility or hypnotizability scales have been developed, and their names (susceptibility versus hypnotizability) favor a conceptual standpoint regarding hypnosis. In the 1980s, there was vivid discussion about the style of hypnotic communication, which resulted in the conclusion that these variations in style were less important than the subject's characteristics or the subject's hypnotizability. The same could be said for preferences in using one of the scales (Spinhoven et al. 1988).

Hypnotizability is normally distributed in the general population and slowly declines with age (E. R. Hilgard 1965). A great deal of research has shown that hypnotizability is a fairly stable trait for individuals over time (J. R. Hilgard 1979; Morgan et al. 1974). Test-retest correlation of .60 over periods of 10–25 years have been shown (Piccione et al. 1989). Hypnotizability seems to peak between ages 6 and 10 years and then begins a gradual decline until death (Morgan et al. 1974). Approximately 10%–15% of the population are highly susceptible to hypnosis, 10%–15% are unresponsive, and the remaining 70%–80% are moderately susceptible to varying degrees (Perry et al. 1992). (For a review of the measurement of hypnotizability, see Perry et al. 1992). The following seven scales, in chronological order, can be considered most representative of the field of hypnotizability scales:

1. The development of the Stanford Hypnotic Susceptibility Scale, Forms A, B, and C (SHSS; Weitzenhoffer and Hilgard 1959, 1962) can be considered a milestone in the field of hypnosis research. This scale consists of 12 items of progressive difficulty. The administration of the scale takes at least 45 minutes. The scales are behaviorally oriented and scored for subjects' observable responses rather than internal experiences. Scores range from 0–12. Items include, for example, postural sway, arm rigidity, or verbal inhibition. Form C differs because items are tested in order of increasing difficulty, and newer items of greater difficulty are included (e.g., age regression, anosmia to ammonia, a negative visual hallucination). The scales were later criticized by their senior author because they lacked measures of classic suggestion and involuntariness (Weitzenhoffer 1980). Morgan and Hilgard (1978–1979) developed an analogous scale for children, the Stanford Hypnotic Clinical Scale for Children (SHCS Child). This is a short scale composed of seven items pertinent to clinical hypnosis, with items such as hand lowering, arm rigidity, visual and auditory hallucination, dream, age regression, and posthypnotic suggestion.

2. The Harvard Group Scale of Hypnotic Susceptibility (HGSHS; Shor and Orne 1962) is a group version of the SHSS. The scale was originally designed as a screening instrument for research purposes; therefore, it is less ideal for clinical purposes than the SHCS–C. In the HGSHS, the subject is asked to give a subjective estimate of what an observer would have seen as reactions on items similar to the SHSS–A and B, such as hand lowering, arm rigidity, communication inhibition, and experiencing a fly (e.g.,"You were told to become aware of the buzzing of a fly which was said to become annoying, and then you were told to shoo it away. Would you estimate that an onlooker would have

observed you make any grimacing, any movement, any out-
ward acknowledgment of an effect?"). Induction and testing
are similar to SHSS. Psychometric features (reliability and validity) are satisfactory. The scale has norms for large samples of
control subjects, as well as cross-sectional and cross-cultural
norms (Coe 1964; Lamas et al. 1989).
3. At the same time of the SHSS and the HGSHS, a Children's
Hypnotic Susceptibility Scale (CHSS) was developed by London (1962). The instructions were given depending on the age
of the group, 5–12 or 13–17 years. Items, testing, and scoring are
similar to the SHSS.
4. The Barber Suggestibility Scale (BSS; Barber 1965) did not
depend on the induction of a standardized hypnotic state. The
instructions make no mention of hypnosis. The procedure is
analogous to the SHSS, and the scale contains eight items (e.g.,
arm lowering, hallucination of thirst, body immobility). Subjects receive both objective and subjective scores on this scale,
each having a maximum score of 8.
5. The Hypnotic Induction Profile (HIP; D. Spiegel, unpublished
instrument, 1977; H. Spiegel and D. Spiegel, unpublished instrument, 1978) is different from traditional susceptibility
scales. It includes questions about the subjective experience of
dissociation and involuntariness. It was designed to be used in
a clinical setting and takes 5–10 minutes to administer. The HIP
is purported to be a measure of clinically usable hypnotizability. It measures eye roll, which is the degree to which subjects
can roll the eyes upward and keep them in this position while
closing the eyes. The induction consists of an arm levitation
with a posthypnotic suggestion, followed by questions of the
subjects' experience of trance. Differing from other scales (e.g.,
the control differential) in which subjects compare sensations
in one arm that is in an upright position with the opposite
"neutral" arm, the HIP does not rely as much on overt behavior
as the SHSS but includes a large subjective component. The induction score is a sum score. Items constituting the induction
score are dissociation, challenged arm levitation, sense of involuntariness, response to the cutoff signal, and sensory altera-

tion; there are 2 points given for each item, with scores ranging from 0 to 10. The induction score had a test-retest reliability of .76 and interrater reliability of .75. The scores for the eye roll on these items were .90 and .73–.80. There are moderate correlations with the SHSS (Frischholz et al. 1980; Orne et al. 1979). One study reports a correlation of .63 between the HIP and the SSHS among 61 highly motivated subjects (Frischholz et al. 1980).

6. Spanos et al. (1983) developed the Carleton University Responsiveness to Suggestion Scale. This scale contains seven items, of which two are ideomotor (arm levitation and arms moving apart), two challenge (catalepsy and immobility), and three cognitive suggestions (visual and auditory hallucination and amnesia). It takes 6 minutes to administer the scale. The scale can be used in a group or on an individual basis. Subjects receive objective, subjective, objective involuntariness, and voluntary cooperation scores. There is little reported research on this scale (Perry et al. 1992). Recently, a new instrument has been developed called the Phenomenology of Consciousness Inventory (Forbes and Pekala 1993). This is a self-report inventory on the experience of hypnosis. The inventory is developed to be a useful instrument in predicting hypnotizability in a less obtrusive fashion than the HGSHS.

7. Recently, a hypnotic susceptibility scale for the deaf was developed, the University of Tennessee Hypnotic Susceptibility Scale for the Deaf (UTHSS–D; Repka and Nash 1995). This is a signed videotaped version of a standard hypnotic induction with 12 standard suggestions. When this scale was administered, deaf participants were found to be less responsive to hypnosis when assessed behaviorally but equally responsive to hypnosis when assessed subjectively.

Dissociation Scales

In the last decade, several scales used to measure dissociation have been developed. The following list of 13 scales is not a thorough one; these are the most recent and, to different extents, well-developed ones. Most of these scales focus on depersonalization-derealization and other classical hypnotic phenomena as they occur in daily life. The first report of a scale measuring dissociation dates back to 1985 and is based on DSM-III-R criteria (Steinberg 1985).

1. The Structured Clinical Interview for DSM-IV Dissociative Disorders (SCID-D; Steinberg 1993) is a semistructured diagnostic interview for assessing five core dissociative symptoms: amnesia, depersonalization, derealization, identity confusion, and identity alteration. It assesses presence, severity, and phenomenology of these five symptoms. It is modeled on the format of the Structured Clinical Interview for DSM-III-R (SCID), developed by Spitzer et al. (1987). Each question is open-ended to allow the subject to use his or her own descriptions. The SCID-D contains no direct questions about trauma; it does contain questions about dissociative defenses that enabled the subject to survive traumatic experiences. The SCID-D has shown good reliability and validity (Steinberg 1994). The interview takes 30 minutes to 1 hour. The questions are asked in a way that the subject can describe the frequency of the suggested dissociative symptom (e.g., "Have you ever felt as if there were large gaps in your memory?" or "Have you ever felt as if there is a struggle inside of you?"). Amnesia often shows highest differences between patients and control subjects (Bremner et al. 1993d). The mini-SCID-D is an abbreviated version of the SCID-D. The miniscale is also based on DSM criteria for dissociative disorders. This scale seems to be more focused on experiences of dissociation per se and is less saturated with normal experiences of absorption and imaginative involvement (Steinberg et al. 1990).

2. Dissociation can also be measured by using the Dissociative Experiences Scale (DES; Bernstein and Putnam 1986), a self-report screening instrument containing a number of items tapping disturbances of awareness, memory, and identity, including depersonalization and derealization. The percentage of time

that the subject experiences a symptom is marked on a visual analogue scale. The sum of scores is divided by the number of items in the list. The scale takes about 10 minutes to complete and yields item and total scores ranging from 0 to 100. A score of 25 indicates that the subject reports dissociative symptoms 25% of the time. Kihlstrom et al. (1994) summarizes seven research studies indicating discriminant validity for the DES as a measure of dissociation. This scale is configured so that it assumes dissociation to be a normal experience; all items are added to determine a total score, and there is no cutoff point on each separate item that makes a distinction between normal and pathological experiences. According to the developers of the scale, reliability testing showed that the scale had good test-retest and good split-half reliability. Item-scale score correlations were all significant, indicating good internal consistency and construct validity. In a factor analysis of the DES, three underlying dimensions repeatedly emerged: absorption and imaginative involvement, amnesia and other activities of dissociated states, and depersonalization/derealization (Ross et al. 1991). Other analyses show that similar but more factors emerged: fantasy and absorption; different types of amnesia, including segment amnesia (inability to remember some aspect of one's life), critical events amnesia (inability to remember important life events), and in situ amnesia (in which one awakes to the current situation); depersonalization; different selves; and denial of dissociation (M. J. Angiulo and J. F. Kihlstrom: "Dissociative Experiences in a College Population," 1993; Ray et al. 1992; W. J. Ray, M. Faith, and J. Mathieu: "Factor Structure of the Dissociative Experience Scale: A College Age Population Study," 1992). Fischer and Elnitsky (1990) found disturbances in cognition control to be the most replicable and reliable factor for the DES. The DES has proved to be a reliable measure. The predictive capacity of the DES, with a cutoff score of 30 in a large (n = 1934) multicenter study, showed a sensitivity rate of 74% and a specificity rate of 80% (Carlson et al. 1993). A Child Dissociative Checklist (Putnam et al. 1993) (see item 4) has been developed and an Adolescent DES (DES-A) is being developed

by the same authors of the DES. No data have yet been published on the latter scale.

3. The Dissociative Disorders Interview Schedule (DDIS; Ross et
al. 1989a) is a structured interview for diagnosing dissociative
disorders. This questionnaire consists of 131 questions and
items, divided into 16 sections, that help to develop a fuller
clinical picture and differentiation between schizoaffective disorder, borderline personality disorder, and atypical dissociation. The subject is asked to respond yes, no, or unsure on all
questions. This interview includes all symptoms of somatization, in addition to a variety of dissociative symptom clusters; it
gathers information about physical and sexual abuse and docu-
ments prior psychiatric treatment. The interview can be administered in 30–45 minutes.

4. After Hornstein and Putnam (1992) investigated the phenomenology of child and adolescent dissociative disorders and concluded that there was good construct validity for assessing
dissociative disorders in childhood, a Child Dissociative Checklist (CDC; Putnam et al. 1993) was developed. Until this scale
was developed, no measures of dissociation existed for children younger than ages 12–14 years. This scale is a 20-item
observer-report measure of dissociative behaviors exhibited by
children. The CDC includes questions about amnesia, alterations in identity, hallucinations, spontaneous trance phenomena, rapid shifts in demeanor, access to information, skills,
knowledge, habits, and age-appropriate behavior. The CDC
had a 1-year test-retest reliability of .69 in 73 subjects, including
healthy control girls and sexually abused girls. The CDC had
high discriminant validity among four test samples, including
healthy control girls, sexually abused girls, boys and girls with
dissociative disorder not otherwise specified, and boys and
girls with MPD. The CDC is intended to be used as a clinical
screening instrument and as a research measure; it is not designed to be used as a diagnostic instrument.

5. The Clinician-Administered Dissociative States Scale (CADSS;
Bremner et al., in press) is a clinical scale for measuring dissociation in clinical observations at specific times. It is used to as-

sess symptoms of amnesia, depersonalization, and derealization. After assessing 23 items in an interview, the observer scores the behavior of the subject at the time of the interview through a series of 5 questions, including "Does the subject appear to be separated or detached from what is going on, as if not part of the experience or not responding in a way that you would expect?" The observed phenomena are not induced. Psychometric assessment of the CADSS showed convergent validity with other measures of dissociation and high levels of interrater and test-retest reliability (Bremner et al., in press).[1]

6. The Perceptual Alteration Scale (PAS; S. Sanders 1986) contains items tapping normal states of absorption and imaginative involvement. A factor analysis study in 507 undergraduate students showed disturbances in affect-control to be the most reliable dimension of two scales measuring dissociation (Fischer and Elnitsky 1990). This scale has not been tested in clinical populations and therefore has no clinical reliability or validity.

7. No data on the Questionnaire of Experiences of Dissociation (QED; Riley 1988) are available yet, except the initial report data on reliability and validity. Like the PAS, this scale contains questions about absorption and imaginative involvement.

8. Briere and Runtz (1990) have developed a dissociative subscale that complements the Hopkins Symptom Checklist—90 (HSCL-90; Derogatis et al. 1974), a self-report measuring general psychopathology with nine subscales. This subscale is sensitive to a history of trauma and to elevations on DES and DDIS dissociative symptom clusters.

9. The Dissociation Questionnaire (DIS-Q; Vanderlinden et al. 1993) is a diagnostic screening scale that contains 63 items, assessing 4 factors: identity confusion and fragmentation, loss of

---

[1]The CADSS is available on the World Wide Web at the following address: http://info.med.yale.edu/psych/org/ypi/trauma/cadss.txt

control, amnesia, and increased concentration. Subjects report how much each item relates to their situation. A maximum score of 5 points is given for each item, and the total score is divided by the amount of items. A cutoff score of 2.5 for the total scale is suggested; cutoff scores for separate factors are being developed. This self-report method is useful; a comparison study with the DES shows a correlation of $r = 0.85$ in a study by Vanderlinden et al. (1991) and $r = 0.87$ in a study by Sainton et al. (1993).

10. The Stanford Acute Stress Reaction Questionnaire (SASRQ) is a self-report measure. Respondents indicate the frequency with which they experience a variety of dissociative and anxiety symptoms during or after a stressful event. Versions of this measure have been used in studies assessing acute reactions to an earthquake (Cardena and Spiegel 1993), to an execution (Freinkel et al. 1994), and to a firestorm (Koopman et al. 1994). Internal consistency using Cronbach's alpha has been found to be high overall (.93) and also high for particular symptom subscales (.72–.88; C. Classen, unpublished data, May 1996). The concurrent validity of this measure is supported by the strong correlations obtained between overall SASRQ symptom scores and scores on the subscales of the Impact of Events Scale (IES; Horowitz et al. 1979) ($r = .83$, $P < .0001$ for intrusion; $r = .59$, $P < .001$ for avoidance) and between the SASRQ symptom subscale scores and the IES intrusion ($r = .57–.89$, $P < .001$) and avoidance ($r = .44–.54$, $P < .01–.001$) subscales.

11. The Dissociative Experience Questionnaire (DEQ; Marmar et al. 1994) is a scale ranging from 0 to 13, and it consists of 13 questions. The score on the DEQ is determined by the total number of positive responses to 13 questions about dissociative states. The scale measures dissociative states during trauma. Subjects are asked to relate their most traumatic event (e.g., combat, childhood), and the DEQ is used to assess dissociative states at that time.

12. The a dissociative subscale for the Minnesota Multiphasic Personality Inventory–2 (MMPI–2; Hathaway and McKinley 1989) was developed by (Waelde et al. 1995). When using the DES to

discriminate high and low dissociation (cutoff score of 30) in a group of 211 Vietnam veterans, investigators found that 16 items of the MMPI–2 discriminated significantly ($P < .001$) between the dissociation groups when generalized psychopathology was statistically controlled. The scale correlated significantly with the DES and DEQ and had good internal consistency.

13. The Somatic Dissociation Questionnaire (E. R. Nijenhuis et al.: "Somatic Dissociation Questionnaire," unpublished document, 1996) is being developed and focuses on bodily experiences to assess dissociative symptoms.

Similarities and Differences in Measurements of Hypnotizability and Dissociation

Our understanding of hypnosis and dissociation is in part shaped by the scales we use to measure the phenomena of these concepts. We know that hypnosis and dissociation are not identical phenomena. As stated earlier in this chapter, their historical definitions and contemporary measurements are not the same. From the overview of the scales, it also can be observed that the first hypnotizability scale was developed in 1959, whereas the first dissociation scale was developed more than 25 years later. In these years a shift in attention has occurred from hypnotizability to dissociation research. In the last 10 years, more scales measuring dissociation have been developed than are known for hypnotizability. The development of this range of diagnostic tools has gone along with the increasing prevalence of dissociative disorders diagnoses. If dissociation was a clear cut phenomenon, like length, or temperature, only one scale would be sufficient. Of course, this view is rather naive, but every dissociation scale seems to focus on a somewhat different aspect of the complex construct of dissociation serving a research goal or fitting into a broader theory.

Consistent with this assumption, intercorrelations are not high enough ($r = 0.6–0.7$) to use different hypnotizability scales as interchangeable measures (Frischholz et al. 1992a). There is no hypnotizability scale that excludes dissociation from its measurement; moreover, there is no dissociation subscale in hypnotizability scales. Dissociation is an element that cannot be measured separately, presumably because in hypnosis there is always an interactive component allowing suggestibility to sneak in as a confounding factor. Overall, hypnosis seems to serve as a broader concept than dissociation does. Several authors have noted a (clinical) relationship between hypnotizability and dissociation, showing that patients with a dissociative disorder have higher hypnotizability scores than other groups and showing correlations between dissociation and hypnotizability in PTSD patients (Frischholz 1985; Frischholz et al. 1992a; Spiegel et al. 1988).

Carlson and Putnam (1989) consider the scales that are used to measure hypnotizability and those that measure dissociation to be developed from different concepts; therefore, the scales should not be equated. Carlson (1994) concludes that the ability to experience hypnotic phenomena and the tendency to dissociate on a day-to-day basis are related but distinct constructs. She describes unpublished research by Perry who selected three groups of subjects according to their level of hypnotizability (low, medium, and high). He found the mean scores for the levels of dissociativity to be 10.3, 18.5, and 30.8, respectively, indicating that higher levels of hypnotizability are related to higher DES scores (Carlson 1994). The statistical relationship between measures of hypnotizability and dissociation was performed in a study of 311 undergraduates by using DES (total score) and HGSHS (summary score), showing significant correlations of .12 ($P < .05$), and by using DES (total score) with subjects' self-ratings of hypnotizability, showing correlations of .13 ($P < .05$) (Frischholz et al. 1992a). These correlations, however, are of low magnitude, and the findings suggest that individual differences in the frequency of self-reported dissociative experiences are not strongly related to individual differences in hypnotizability in student populations.

Hypnosis and dissociation scales include items from different domains. Hypnotizability scales measure alterations in motor, sensory, and cognitive functions, whereas the dissociation scales measure alterations in memory, awareness, identity, cognitive functions, and perceptions. In hypnotizability scales, hypnosis is mostly experienced after a formal induction procedure. Hypnosis occurs within a specific time frame and can be considered a micro-level experience. It lasts as long as the measurement takes, or less. In an experimental or clinical situation, except for self-hypnosis, the hypnotic experience is observed by an observer or therapist; in most dissociation measurements, dissociation is experienced out-side of the clinical setting, in the life of the subjects, during or following sequential time frames. The amount, frequency, or in-tensity of dissociation is later reported in questionnaires or inter-views. Hypnosis can occur after induction, in an experimental or clinical setting, and is therefore controlled. Dissociation occurs more or less spontaneously, after a trigger that is or is not recog-nized, and it occurs nonvolitionally. Dissociation scales rely on self-reported phenomena, reflecting a subject's memory, affect, behavior, perception, knowledge, or attitude. In most of the scales, the dissociative symptoms are reported, not observed, at least not during measurement. The CADSS and the CDC are the only ques-tionnaires in which dissociation can be measured and dissociative phenomena observed during the interview. Dissociation therefore relies mostly on self-observation. Hypnosis, on the other hand, is mostly measured after and by inducing and evaluating the phe-nomena (e.g., arm levitation, catalepsy, hallucination, or anesthe-sia). Hypnotizability can be measured in a group or an individual. Only in the HIP is dissociation measured by a (motor) control dif-ferential between an elevated and a nonelevated arm. Dissociation is measured in a hypnotic context. Table 4–1 summarizes the most prominent differences in the hypnotizability and dissociation scales.

The Role of Absorption in Dissociation and Hypnotizability

The dissociative compartmentalization of experience is accom-plished through a complementary focusing of attention. Hypnotic and dissociative phenomena may be understood as clarifying ex-

Table 4–1.   Differences in hypnotizability scales versus dissociation
scales

Hypnotizability scales	Dissociation scales
Induced hypnosis	Not induced
Suggested experience	Spontaneous and involuntary experience
Phenomena at the time of trance	Phenomena on day-to-day basis
Subjective estimate or observable behavioral characteristics	Self-reports, written question-naires, or interviews (post-dissociation)
Individual or in group	Individual
Microlevel experience, one time frame	Macrolevel experience, sequential time frame
Measures hypnotizability	Measures dissociativity

tremes of human attentional processes (Spiegel et al. 1988). Absorption is described as a tendency to become fully involved in an imaginative or ideational experience. Individuals prone to this type of cognition are more highly hypnotizable than those who never fully engage in such experiences. The Tellegen Absorption Scale (TAS; Tellegen and Atkinson 1974) is a measure of involvement in various imaginative activities suggestive of passive and effortless rather than active attention. This scale was developed through factor analysis and consists of true/false items on the following subscales: dissociation, openness to experience, devotion-trust, autonomy-criticality, reality absorption, and fantasy absorption. There is some similarity with the fantasy-prone personalities as described by Barber and Wilson (1977) and later by Lynn and Rhue (1994). Correlational studies of hypnotizability have used the TAS, showing correlations usually at .40 (Roche and McConkey 1990). Two separate focused attentional abilities can be discriminated: 1) moderately focused attention, resembling ambient attention; and 2) extremely focused attention and disattention, related to hypnotizability. The first is the ability to attend moderately so that noise in the environment is no longer disruptive but may be attended and the second is the ability to attend so fully to a task that noise and irrelevant stimuli in the environment are apparently not even noticed and provide no distraction (Crawford 1969).

Using the HGSHS, Glisky and Kihlstrom (1993) investigated the relationship among hypnotizability and absorption, "intellectance" (or intelligence), and liberalism, all of which are different kinds of what they described as "openness," in 651 subjects. They found modest relationships among the three dimensions of openness, and only absorption was significantly related to hypnotizability. They concluded that by adding intellectance and liberalism to absorption, the prediction of hypnotizability could not be enhanced. Absorption and hypnosis share a kind of imaginative involvement that is not necessarily part of other kinds of openness, such as intellectance and liberalism (Glisky and Kihlstrom 1993). Absorption or imagery abilities are generally related to hypnotizability, but they do not appear to be necessary in all cases, and they only explain a relatively small proportion of the variance in research. Frischholz et al. (1987) found correlation scores ranging from .33 to .53 between HIP scores and absorption scores by using the TAS in three groups: smokers ($n = 226$), phobia patients ($n = 95$), and chronic pain patients ($n = 65$).

A few items of the TAS describe experiences of dissociation (e.g., item 13: I sometimes step outside my usual self and experience an entirely different state of being; item 22: If I wish, I can imagine that my body is so heavy that I could not move it if I wanted to). These items refer to an altered sense of reality and the self. As the focus on the attentional object becomes magnified, and other aspects recede from awareness, this can create feelings of distortion and unreality of the individual. This description is certainly like the experience of dissociation. However, lessening of reality testing in dissociation is not invariably part of the absorption experience. If so, it would seem that all of those who were capable of absorption would also be capable of entering a hypnotic state. This seems not to be the case. Although absorption experiences are related to feelings of unreality and dissociation, they are not the same. Both absorption and dissociation can be seen as complementary and essential aspects of hypnosis. The capacity for absorption allows the individual to become fully engaged in the hypnotic suggestion, and the capacity for dissociation allows the individual temporarily to suspend or disengage from or to other levels of awareness, finally resulting in a different processing of information.

Highly hypnotizable individuals have the capacity to become involved in internal stimuli and thus become more distanced or dissociated from their environment. However, these individuals also have the capacity to become absorbed in external stimuli. The object of attentional variables can differ, but they do have the ability to engage and be immersed in their imagination and perception.

A Continuum Perspective of Hypnotizability and Dissociation

A person might inherit or develop a dissociative capacity in early life. This dissociative capacity seems to differ from the capacity that underlies the ability to enter trance: it involves the ability to segregate and idiosyncratically encode experience into separate psychological or psychobiological processes, with associated alterations in identity. Among nonclinical populations, extreme distress may significantly increase the prevalence and severity of transient dissociative phenomena and anxiety (e.g., the experience of witnessing an execution was associated with the development of dissociative symptoms in several journalists [Freinkel et al. 1994]). These phenomena provide further evidence of the role that dissociation plays in the response to inescapable stress or trauma and are of considerable clinical and theoretical importance in view of the lifetime prevalence of traumatic experiences in the general population (Breslau and Davis 1992).

Dissociation can be seen as one extreme on a continuum of awareness and can describe a rather wide range of clinical phenomena. This continuum of awareness ranges from full awareness to suppression, denial, repression, and dissociation. Braun (1988) developed a model for understanding the phenomena of dissociation by dividing dissociation into behavior, affect, sensation, and

knowledge changes of general awareness. These four phenomenological processes function in parallel on a time continuum
(Braun 1988). The model seemed conceptually well thought out
but was rather hard to operationalize in research and clinical
practice.

Dissociation also can be seen as a continuum ranging from minor or normative forms to major or pathological forms (Bernstein
and Putnam 1986). Evidence for the continuum of dissociation
comes from studies of the distribution of hypnotizability in both
healthy control subjects and psychiatric populations and studies
of the distribution of dissociation using the DES (Bernstein and
Putnam 1986). The continuum of dissociation ranges from a normal to a dissociative episode, dissociative disorder, posttraumatic
disorder, atypical disorder, atypical personality disorder, and finally DID, where intensity/severity and frequency or the experienced phenomena are cumulative or scaled along the same axis.
Although it has been proposed that PTSD is on the continuum of
dissociative disorders (Braun 1988), it is not categorized as a dissociative disorder in DSM-IV, although some good evidence of
dissociative symptoms has been found in patients with PTSD
(Bremner et al. 1992, 1993d; Koopman et al. 1994; Spiegel et al.
1988). In DSM-IV, a dissociative symptom is described as a disruption in the usually integrated functions of consciousness, memory,
identity, or perception of the environment. The dissociative disorders seem not to be characterized by a single set of symptoms that
qualitatively differentiate to make the diagnosis, but rather by
quantitative differences in the frequency, extent, or intensity of
dissociative symptoms displayed by individuals (Kihlstrom et al.
1994).

When the DES was developed, Bernstein and Putnam (1986)
presumed the number and frequency of dissociative experiences
to lie along a continuum. This continuum was their first hypothesis tested in developing the DES, and it proved to be of major
significance in the design of the scale. Most definitions of dissociation are concerned with distinguishing normal from abnormal or
pathological dissociative experiences. The definition of what
should be considered pathological changed over time since the

early dissociation theory of Janet. Nemiah (1995) considered pathological dissociative reactions to be characterized by a disruption in the individual's sense of identity and by disturbances of memory. There has been a debate about the threshold or cutoff between normal and pathological dissociation. For the DES, there is no consensus. Some report a score higher than 15–20 to be pathological (Ross et al. 1991), whereas some are in favor a higher score of 30 (Carlson et al. 1993). A cutoff score may overestimate the risk of pathological dissociation in the population at large. Kihlstrom (1994) reports on a sample collected at the University of Arizona in which 10% of subjects exceeded a cutoff score of 20 on the DES and 6% exceeded a cutoff score of 30. He recommends the need for a normative study of dissociative experiences in a sample that is representative of the population at large.

The setting of somewhat arbitrary thresholds of severity is intended to define more clinically relevant and homogeneous groupings but creates a gap between severe and milder cases on what may actually be a continuum of severity. These problems might be circumvented by using continuum measures of dimensions in research studies. Accordingly, it can be useful to approach dissociation as a dimensional construct in which pathological cases exist on a continuum with subclinical levels of dissociation and levels leading to dissociative disorders with failure of integration. Two dimensional constructs can be described: state-dependent emotional disturbances on one end and personality alteration on the other.

A continuum in hypnotizability has been evidenced in previous research on hypnotizability scales. Various normative data were collected in past decades when different hypnotizability scales were used. Routine hypnotizability assessment could be useful in differential diagnosis of patients with psychopathological disorders. Frischholz et al. (1992b, 1992c) used hypnotizability measurement in different patient populations. Dissociative disorder patients in this study had significantly higher hypnotizability scores, on the SHSS and the HIP, than groups of patients with schizophrenia, mood disorders, and anxiety disorders and healthy college students. Patients with a dissociative disorder were observed to have significantly higher hypnotizability scores on various measures compared with healthy control subjects or other clinical groups. Dissociative disorder patients initially also recalled significantly fewer items when the posthypnotic amnesia suggestion was in effect and reversed significantly more items when the suggestion was canceled. It can be concluded that routine hypnotizability assessment may be useful in the differential diagnosis of patients with dissociative disorders (Frischholz et al. 1992b, 1992c). Hypnotizability also can serve as a predictor of outcome in treatment. Hypnotizability and living with a significant other predicted the 2-year maintenance of treatment response on smoking abstinence following a single-session intervention with self-hypnosis (Spiegel et al. 1993).

Compared with hypnosis research, dissociation is a relatively new concept in research. One of the central differences seems to be that in hypnotizability research, subjects are brought to or guided in the dissociated or altered state of consciousness, whereas in dissociation research, subjects report from a sort of metaperspective about feelings and memories in these altered dissociated states.

Mind-Body Relations: Hypnosis and Dissociation

> Parts of the body that previously experienced physical disease of trauma seem to be especially vulnerable to reactivation of that response with hypnosis. High hypnotizable individuals are likely to use their intensified mind/body relatedness unwittingly as a means of experiencing and expressing conflict. (Spiegel 1994)

Research in previous decades has provided considerable evidence for the importance of suggestion and hypnotic ability in the healing or amelioration of various somatic disorders (Bowers and Kelly 1979). The facts of hypnotic influence sometimes exceed the capacity of science to understand them. How would one account for the well-witnessed success in Mason's case (1952; 1955), which describes suggested healing of a severe congenital skin disease one limb at a time? Different placebo-controlled studies have reported reduced pain and anxiety during painful procedures (Zelt-zer and LeBaron 1982), treatment of nausea and vomiting in chemotherapy (Zeltzer et al. 1984), treatment of irritable bowel disease (Whorwell et al. 1984, 1987), and effects on smoking cessation (Spiegel et al. 1993; Williams and Hall 1988) when hypnosis is used as treatment. These results confronted many people with the relationship between words and healing or between mind and body and have led to the question, How does information received and processed at a semantic level become transduced into information at a somatic level?

The work of Barber (1961), Bowers and Kelly (1979), Frankel (1987), and Spiegel and Vermetten (1994) has shown that hypnosis and subsequent dissociative states have unusual effects on the body. These states could be viewed as vehicles for increased control over neurophysiological and peripheral somatic functions. The literature suggests that highly hypnotizable individuals and those with dissociative symptoms are capable of an unusual degree of psychological control over various somatic functions or conversely demonstrate a loss of control over these various functions. Highly hypnotizable subjects may dissociate without provocation of trauma and suffer more dissociative symptoms when they sustain traumatic experiences. Dissociation enables one to detach from painful or acute traumatic situations but is complicated by a failure to integrate. It therefore can be seen as beneficial for the moment but harmful in the long run.

The somatoform disorders could be viewed as an involuntary unconscious use of dissociative defenses. These defenses could be understood as conversion symptoms—disturbances of sensory or motor function that follow the patient's model of illness rather than neuroanatomical pathways. These symptoms can be conceptualized as dissociative phenomena and are related to hypnotizability (Wickramasekera 1995). In a sample of patients with somatoform disorders ($n = 83$), the hypnotizability was not normally distributed. The patients' score for hypnotizability on the HGSHS was significantly higher ($P < .001$) than that of control subjects ($n = 78$). Both low- and high-scoring patients had a larger percentage of somatic symptoms than psychological symptoms, whereas somatic and psychological symptoms were more evenly distributed among control subjects.

There is an intensified relationship with the body in both extremes of high- and low-hypnotizable persons. Highly hypnotizable individuals tend to become intensely absorbed in noxious sensations and tend to develop dissociative (in this case somatoform) disorders. Low-hypnotizable individuals have an inability to block out noxious sensations with normal levels of concentration and absorption (Kirmayer et al. 1994) and may be prone to react with cognitions of control rather than cognitions of loss of control. It is known that individuals with low hypnotizability lack words for feelings (Frankel et al. 1977). Threat perception in individuals with low hypnotizability may be absent from verbal report or consciousness but may be present in measures of sympathetic activation or motor behavior. They are hypothesized to "know the words but miss the music." They develop primarily somatic symptoms and do not react with psychological symptoms such as dissociative experiences. Highly hypnotizable individuals may spontaneously enter the hypnotic mode of information processing and experience "involuntary" changes in perception, memory, and mood that can amplify perception of fear and pain; they are prone to "surplus pattern recognition," seeing meaning in events that seem randomly distributed or meaningless to low-hypnotizable persons; and they are at risk for threat-related disorders because they are prone to "surplus empathy," in which they involuntarily absorb the pain or negative affect of others (Wickramasekara 1995). These notions relate to the long-standing clinical impression of an association between conversion, hysteria, and high hypnotizability. It may take less severe stress or trauma to trigger a conversion symptom or other dissociative symptom in individuals who are highly hypnotizable. Highly hypnotizable individuals seem to be vulnerable to conversion symptoms or conversion disorder, suggesting that hypnotic states may be mobilized spontaneously or may produce pseudosomatic conversion symptoms (Bliss 1984; Nemiah 1993). For example, in a review of special characteristics of highly hypnotizable persons, Wilson and Barber (1981, 1983) observed that 60% of their study sample of highly hypnotizable subjects had experienced pseudocyesis, with symptoms that included amenorrhea, breast changes, and abdominal enlargement. These subjects also experienced dramatic physical symptoms stimulated by stress. Patients with PTSD show similar dissociative symptoms as those of dissociative disorder patients (Bremner et al. 1992, 1993d; Hyer et al. 1993). Earlier findings show higher hypnotizability in patients with PTSD compared with patients who have a general anxiety disorder (Spiegel et al. 1988).

Analogous to the way we can regard dissociation as a dimensional construct in which pathological cases exist on a continuum with subclinical levels of dissociation, Kirmayer et al. (1994) propose the same for somatization. For somatization, the focus is on three dimensional constructs: 1) the tendency to experience and report functional symptoms, 2) the tendency to worry or to be convinced that one is sick, and 3) the tendency for some individuals with depression or anxiety to present clinically with predominantly somatic symptoms (Kirmayer et al. 1994). This analogy suggests that dissociation may be elicited by, and may in turn represent, an adaptation to somatic distress. In addition to the social learning processes of modeling and reinforcement, there is growing evidence that childhood traumatic experiences affect body perceptions that may be associated with medically unexplained somatic symptoms in adulthood. In a group of 14 psychiatric inpatients with dissociative disorders measured with the DDIS (Ross et al. 1989a), more gastrointestinal symptoms, pain symptoms, cardiopulmonary symptoms, and conversion symptoms were reported compared with a matched inpatient group with few dissociative symptoms (Saxe et al. 1994). Somatization is a serious problem for patients with dissociative disorders. These patients have more somatic symptoms, are more likely to have a somatization disorder, and use more medical services than patients who do not dissociate. Women with chronic pelvic pain, in a study by Walker et al.(1992), were more likely to use dissociation as a coping mechanism, to show current psychological distress, to see themselves as medically disabled, to experience social decrements in function, and to amplify physical symptoms. In Walker et al.'s (1992) study, women with a history of childhood abuse had higher scores on measures of psychological distress, somatization, and dissociation. Pseudoseizures and their relationship to dissociation need further exploration. There is good evidence that pseudoseizures originate from dissociated personalities or ego-states, are expressions of dissociated memories of child abuse, and can be triggered by recent stresses or traumas (Alper 1994; Bowman 1993; Loewenstein and Putnam 1988). Spiegel (1991) suggests that there is a dissociative syndrome associated with certain kinds of temporal lobe epilepsy that is phenomenologically similar to classical dissociative disorders but that is historically distinct. Gainer (1993) describes how hypnosis can be useful in treating dissociated traumatic memories in a case of reflex sympathetic dystrophy. Prospective longitudinal studies are needed to relate these findings adequately to the hypotheses.

Patients with extreme dissociative disorders, such as DID, grossly show these unusual somatic symptoms (Ross 1994). Ross describes somatic disorders involving genitourinary functioning to be natural consequences of sexual abuse. Siemens and Ross (1991) also have shown that disorders of the gastrointestinal tract, such as irritable bowel syndrome, are associated with a history of trauma. Psychosomatic symptoms from all body symptoms often can be considered dissociative and related to chronic severe childhood trauma (Ross et al. 1989b). Certain somatic disorders also have been found to be associated with higher scores on the DES. These disorders include the luteal phase of premenstrual syndrome and bulimia (Carlson 1994). Ross (1994) reports anecdotal observations like fast wound healing and suggests that lower doses of narcotics could be required in terminal malignancies for those who have higher DES scores. He reports higher rates of delirium tremens and postoperative psychosis in subjects who have high scores on the DES. These observations give rise to a link between trauma, dissociation, somatization, and pathophysiology.

In a study in psychologically disturbed adolescents, B. Sanders and Giolas (1991) tested their hypothesis that dissociation is positively correlated with stress or early experiences of abuse. They found support for the view that dissociation represents a reaction to early negative experience. In their view, MPD can be placed at the extreme end of a continuum of dissociative sequelae of child-hood trauma. B. Sanders and Giolas (1991) stress the importance of trying to identify psychiatric patients with prominent dissociative characteristics or symptoms and attempting to correlate this phe-nomenology with negative earlier experiences. Although in chil-dren the dissociative symptomatology may be subtle, the effects in adults all relate to the problem of embodiment, which varies from DID to eating disorders, somatization disorder, self-mutilation, suicide, and suicide attempts (McElroy 1994; Roesler and McKen-zie 1994; Young 1992). The central problem in disorders where dissociation is involved is not the barrier of amnesia, but the dis-ruption in integration of self across highly discrete states of con-sciousness (Putnam 1991), leading to segregation and lack of cohesion of normal embodiment processes (van der Kolk 1994).

Controlled Versus Noncontrolled Dissociation: The Role of Trauma

A great deal of the current literature on dissociation connects the phenomena of dissociation etiologically with trauma, including combat-related trauma, childhood physical or sexual abuse, civilian violence such as rape, and natural disasters such as earthquakes, floods, and fires. Although there is a strong relationship with these categories of trauma, dissociation seems not invariably linked to trauma itself. It occurs with the existence of two or more incompati-ble mental contents that exclude one another from consciousness (Spiegel 1990). The person is unable to think about two or more contents in connection with one another. The perception of some-thing traumatic can be or can have incompatible mental content.

Recent literature shows that individuals who respond to trau-mas or overwhelming events by using dissociation develop long-term changes in psycho- and neurobiological systems (Bremner et al. 1993c; Charney et al. 1993; Koopman et al. 1994; Krystal et al. 1995; Southwick et al. 1994). One initial study has found evidence for alterations in dopaminergic, serotonergic, and opioid systems associated with the clinical expression of dissociation (Demitrack et al. 1993). Dissociative symptoms are important elements of the long-term psychopathological response to trauma (Spiegel et al. 1988). Long-term changes in neurobiological and neurochemical systems may in turn result in dissociative responses to subsequent events, increased general dissociative symptoms, and increased risk for stress-related psychiatric disorders (Bremner et al. 1995). These dissociative disorders can be understood as more extreme and unconscious eruptions of normal dissociative phenomena, often elicited in the face of traumatic stress (Carlson 1994; Spiegel 1993).

Essential in the pathophysiology of a dissociative disorder or DID is the capacity to dissociate (Braun and Sachs 1985; Putnam 1985). Hypnosis has been thought of as a controlled dissociation, and dissociation in turn has been thought of as a form of spontaneous self-hypnosis. Hypnosis, in this respect, is a valuable tool in the treatment of dissociative disorders: what was originally invoked in the individual by traumatic experiences can be beneficially influenced in treatment by controlled hypnotic interventions. Kluft (1982) and Putnam (1989) stress that, although hypnosis can simulate phenomena of different dissociative reactions or disorders, there is no evidence that the profound disturbances in identity, consciousness, and memory as found in dissociative disorders can be caused by hypnosis.

It has been hypothesized that persons with DID tend to be highly hypnotizable, presumably because of their extensive use of hypnosis-like dissociative strategies in coping with (early) life trauma. Hypnotizable individuals are supposed to have a propensity to dissociate defensively under stress. First data do not seem to support this notion. In a matched control study among 54 sexually abused girls, ages 6–15 years, no significant differences were found in hypnotizability between abused subjects and control subjects (Putnam et al. 1995). There were significant differences in clinical dissociation initially and on 1-year retest between the groups. The highly hypnotizable subjects in the abused group were significantly more dissociative on the CDC than poorly hypnotizable subjects in the abuse group. Higher levels of clinical dissociation were associated with abuse by multiple perpetrators and copresence of physical abuse independent of sexual abuse. Putnam et al. (1995) discriminate a subgroup in abused children, described as having "double dissociation." This description means that these subjects show both high clinical dissociation and high hypnotizability. Double dissociation in traumatized children may subsequently be a marker for a dissociative disorder.

Dissociation ends when congruity among dissociated components of experience (behavior, affect, sensation, thought) is established (Braun 1988). Common in a broad array of psychotherapeutic techniques is the intent to orient the patient back to current sensory experience with a strong emphasis on learning control (Allen 1993; Braun 1988; Spiegel 1993).

Summary: Perspective on the Measurement of Two Distinct Constructs

Measuring hypnotizability where hypnosis is introduced as a controlled and structured dissociation could serve the goals of the therapist who measures the susceptibility level and the patient who seeks a strategy to modify control. Hypnotizability is described as a measurable concept with long-term stability and reproducibility within the individual. Various scales have been developed in the past 30 years for the measurement of both hypnotizability and dissociation, and recent research on the impact of trauma sheds new light on the relationship between hypnotizability and dissociation. Although most research on hypnotizability was done in the 1970s and early 1980s, a new perspective on the relationship between hypnosis and dissociation can evolve. The 1980s provided a body of literature on correlations between scales, reliability studies, and developments of new scales; however; research now focuses more on dissociation and dissociative disorders and its measurement. Hypnosis may account for many of the findings attributed to dissociation and dissociative disorders; the methodology of the measurements and the additional expertise from previous research could serve a valuable purpose.

Dissociation seems to account for a shift in modern psychology and psychiatry through its widespread clinical relevance and recognition by cognitive sciences. It is strongly related to consciousness, conflict/trauma, and unity of the self. Dissociation can be assessed by questionnaires in which the intensity of dissociation or capacity to dissociate can be measured. We favored describing dissociation as a dimensional construct where pathological cases exist on a continuum with subclinical levels of dissociation. The contribution of hypnosis as a descriptive or explanatory variable in dissociation has not yet gained consensus. Although dissociation can be regarded as one aspect of the broader concept of hypnosis, the operation of both constructs is different. Dissociation raises fundamental questions about the relationship between mind and body. It can be concluded that there is a strong conceptual relationship between hypnosis and dissociation. A troublesome relationship derives from measuring differences between the hypnotizability and dissociativity scales.

Dissociation and dissociative disorders reflect an emphasis by psychiatric nosology on turning the concept and the disorders into discrete entities. Hypnosis and dissociation have a long history, share historical analogies, and are widely used concepts in research and clinical practice, but both concepts leave us with some fundamental questions. Despite a widespread stable acceptance in academic and clinical settings, hypnosis and hypnotizability leave unanswered questions about the concept of hypnosis, the variety of scales used to measure hypnotizability, and the contributing factors to hypnois. Dissociation and the dissociative disorders leave us with even more unanswered questions. Recent theories might need to change in response to new data. At least in the clinical connection between hypnotizability and dissociation, trauma plays a major role. A combination of the methodologies used for measuring hypnosis and dissociation can lead to a better understanding of their combined meaning in research and clinical practice.

References

Allen JG: Dissociative processes: theoretical underpinnings of a working model for clinician and patient. Bull Menninger Clin 57:287–308, 1993

Alper K: Nonepileptic seizures. Neurol Clin 12:153–173, 1994

American Psychiatric Association: Diagnostic and Statistical Manual of Mental Disorders, 4th Edition. Washington, DC, American Psychiatric Association, 1994

Barber TX: Physiological effects of "hypnosis." Psychol Bull 58:390–419, 1961

Barber TX: Measuring "hypnotic like" suggestibility with and without "hypnotic induction": psychometric properties, norms, and variables influencing response to the Barber Suggestibility Scale (BSS). Psychol Rep (monogr suppl) 16:809–844, 1965

Barber TX: Hypnosis: A Scientific Approach. New York, Van Nostrand Reinhold, 1969

Barber TX, Wilson SC: Hypnosis, suggestions, and altered states of consciousness: experimental evaluation of the new cognitive behavioral theory and the traditional trance state theory of "hypnosis." Ann N Y Acad Sci 296:34–47, 1977

Bernstein EM, Putnam FW: Development, reliability and validity of a dissociation scale. J Nerv Ment Dis 174:727–735, 1986

Bliss EL: Hysteria and hypnosis. J Nerv Ment Dis 172:203–206, 1984

Bowers KS, Kelly P: Stress, disease, psychotherapy and hypnosis. J Abnorm Psychol 88:490–505, 1979

Bowman ES: Etiology and clinical course of pseudoseizures: relationship to trauma, depression and dissociation. Psychosomatics 34:333–342, 1993

Braun BG: The BASK model of dissociation. Dissociation 1:4–23, 1988

Braun BG: Dissociative disorders as sequelae to incest, in Incest-Related Syndromes of Adult Psychopathology. Edited by Kluft RP. Washington, DC, American Psychiatric Press, 1990, pp 227–247

Braun BG, Sachs RG: The development of multiple personality disorder: predisposing, precipitating, and perpetuating factors, in Childhood Antecedents of Multiple Personality. Edited by Kluft RP. Washington, DC, American Psychiatric Press, 1985, pp 37–64

Bremner JD, Brett E: Increased dissociative states and long-term psychopathology in posttraumatic stress disorder. Journal of Traumatic Stress 10:37–49, 1997

Bremner JD, Southwick S, Brett E, et al: Dissociation and posttraumatic stress disorder in Vietnam combat veterans. Am J Psychiatry 149:328–333, 1992

Bremner JD, Scott TM, Delaney RC, et al: Deficits in short-term memory in posttraumatic stress disorder. Am J Psychiatry 150:1015–1019, 1993a

Bremner JD, Davis M, Southwick SM, et al: Neurobiology of posttraumatic stress disorder, in American Psychiatric Press Review of Psychiatry, Vol 12. Edited by Oldham JM, Riba MB, Tasman A. Washington, DC, American Psychiatric Press, 1993b, pp 183–205

Bremner JD, Steinberg M, Southwick SM, et al: Use of Structured Clinical Interview for DSM-IV Dissociative Disorders for systematic assessment of dissociative symptoms in posttraumatic stress disorder. Am J Psychiatry 150:1011–1014, 1993c

Bremner JD, Krystal JH, Southwick SM, et al: Functional neuroanatomical correlates of the effects of stress on memory. J Trauma Stress 8:527–555, 1995

Bremner JD, Mazure CM, Putnam FW, et al: Measurement of dissociative states with the Clinician-Administered Dissociative States Scale (CADSS). Journal of Traumatic Stress, in press

Breslau N, Davis GC: Posttraumatic stress disorder in an urban population of young adults: risk factors for chronicity. Am J Psychiatry 149: 671–675, 1992

Briere J, Runtz M: Augmenting Hopkins SCL scales to measure dissociative symptoms: data from two nonclinical samples. J Pers Assess 55: 376–379, 1990

Cardena E: The domain of dissociation, in Dissociation: Clinical and Theoretical Perspectives. Edited by Lynn SJ, Rhue JW. New York, Guilford, 1994, pp 15–32

Cardena E, Spiegel D: Dissociative reactions to the San Francisco Bay area earthquake. Am J Psychiatry 150: 474–478, 1993

Carlson EB: Studying the interaction between physical and psychological states with the Dissociative Experiences Scale, in Dissociation: Culture, Mind, and Body. Edited by Spiegel D. Washington, DC, American Psychiatric Press, 1994, pp 41–58

Carlson EB, Putnam FW: Integrating research on dissociation and hypnotizability: are there two pathways to hypnotizability? Dissociation 2:32–38, 1989

Carlson EB, Putnam FW, Ross CA, et al: Validity of the Dissociative Experiences Scale in screening for multiple personality disorder: a multicenter study. Am J Psychiatry 150:1030–1036, 1993

Charney DS, Deutch AY, Krystal JH, et al: Psychobiologic mechanisms of posttraumatic stress disorder. Arch Gen Psychiatry 50:294–299, 1993

Coe WC: Further norms on the Harvard Group Scale of Hypnotic Susceptibility, Form A. Int J Clin Exp Hypn 12:184–190, 1964

Coe WC: Experimental designs and the state-nonstate issue in hypnosis. Am J Clin Hypn 16:118–128, 1973

Corbetta M, Miezin FM, Dobmeyer S, et al: Attention modulation of neural processing of shape, color, and velocity in humans. Science 248: 1556–1559, 1990

Counts RM: The concept of dissociation. J Am Acad Psychoanal 18: 460–479, 1990

Crawford HJ: Brain dynamics and hypnosis: attentional and disattentional processes. Int J Clin Exp Hypn 42:204–232, 1994

Demitrack MA, Putnam FW, Rubinow DR, et al: Relation of dissociative phenomena of cerebrospinal fluid monoamine metabolites and beta-endorphin in patients with eating disorders: a pilot study. Psychiatry Res 49:1–10, 1993

Dennett D: Consciousness Explained. Boston, Little, Brown, 1991

Denny EB, Hunt RR: Affective valence and memory in depression: dissociation of recall and fragment completion. J Abnorm Psychol 101: 575–580, 1992

Derogatis LR, Lipman RS, Rickels K, et al: The Hopkins Symptom Checklist—90 (HSCL-90): a self-report symptom inventory. Behav Sci 19: 1–15, 1974

Ellenberger HF: The Discovery of the Unconscious. New York, Basic Books, 1970

Erdelyi MH: Dissociation, defense, and the unconscious, in Dissociation: Culture, Mind, and Body. Edited by Spiegel D. Washington, DC, American Psychiatric Press, 1994, pp 3–20

Evans F: Posthypnotic amnesia: dissociation of content and context, in Hypnosis and Memory. Edited by Pettinati HM. New York, Guilford, 1992, pp 157–192

Feldman JA, Ballard DA: Connectionist models and their properties. Cognitive Science 6:205–254, 1982

Fischer DG, Elnitsky S: A factor analytic study of two scales measuring dissociation. American Journal of Clinical Hypnotherapy 32:200–206, 1990

Forbes EJ, Pekala RJ: Predicting hypnotic susceptibility via a phenomenological approach. Psychol Rep 73:1251–1256, 1993

Frankel FH: Significant developments in medical hypnosis during the past 25 years. Int J Clin Exp Hypn 35:231–247, 1987

Frankel FH: Hypnotizability and dissociation. Am J Psychiatry 147: 823–839, 1991

Frankel FH, Apfel-Savitz R, Nemiah JC, et al: The relationship between hypnotizability and alexithymia. Psychother Psychosom 8:172–178, 1977

Freinkel A, Koopman C, Spiegel D: Dissociative symptoms in media eye-witnesses of an execution. Am J Psychiatry 151:1335–1339, 1994

Frischholz EJ: The Relationship among dissociation, hypnosis and child abuse in the development of multiple personality, in Childhood Antecedents of Multiple Personality. Edited by Kluft RP. Washington, DC, American Psychiatric Press, 1985, pp 99–126

Frischholz EJ, Tyron WW, Vellios AT, et al: The relationship between the Hypnotic Induction Profile and the Stanford Hypnotic Susceptibility Scale, Form C: a replication. Am J Clin Hypn 22:185–196, 1980

Frischholz EJ, Spiegel D, Trentalange MJ, et al: The Hypnotic Induction Profile and absorption. Am J Clin Hypn 30:87–93, 1987

Frischholz EJ, Braun BG, Sachs RG, et al: Construct validity of the Dissociative Experiences Scale, II: its relationship to hypnotizability. Am J Clin Hypn 35:145–152, 1992a

Frischholz EJ, Lipman LS, Braun BG, et al: Psychopathology, hypnotizability and dissociation. Am J Psychiatry 149:1521–1525, 1992b

Frischholz EJ, Braun BG, Lipman LS, et al: Suggested posthypnotic amnesia in psychiatric patients and normals. Am J Clin Hypn 35:29–39, 1992c

Fromm E, Nash MR (eds): Contemporary Hypnosis Research. New York, Guilford, 1992

Gabbard GO: Psychodynamic Psychiatry in Clinical Practice, the DSM-IV Edition. Washington, DC, American Psychiatric Press, 1994

Gainer M: Somatization of dissociated traumatic memories in a case of reflex sympathetic dystrophy. Am J Clin Hypn 36:124–131, 1993

Ganaway GK: Hypnosis, childhood trauma and dissociative identity disorder: towards an integrative theory. Int J Clin Exp Hypn 43:127–144, 1995

Glisky M, Kihlstrom JF: Hypnotizability and facets of openness. Int J Clin Exp Hypn 41:112–123, 1993

Goodglass H, Budin C: Category and modality specific dissociations in word comprehension and concurrent phonological dyslexia. Neuropsychologia 26:67–78, 1988

Hathaway SR, McKinley JC: Minnesota Multiphasic Personality Inventory–2. Minneapolis, MN, University of Minnesota, 1989

Herman JL: Trauma and Recovery. New York, Basic Books, 1992

Hilgard ER: Hypnotic Susceptibility. New York, Harcourt, Brace & World, 1965

Hilgard ER: Divided Consciousness: Multiple Controls in Human Thought and Action. New York, Wiley, 1977

Hilgard ER: Divided Consciousness: Multiple Controls in Human Thought and Action, Expanded Edition. New York, Wiley, 1986

Hilgard ER: Research advances in hypnosis: issues and methods. Int J Clin Exp Hypn 35:248–264, 1987

Hilgard ER: Dissociation and theories of hypnosis, in Contemporary Hypnosis Research. Edited by Fromm E, Nash MR. New York, Guilford, 1992, pp 69–101

Hilgard JR: Personality and Hypnosis: A Study of Imaginative Involvement, Revised Edition. Chicago, University of Chicago Press, 1979

Hornstein NL, Putnam FW: Clinical phenomenology of child and adolescent dissociative disorders. J American Acad Child Adolesc Psychiatry 31:1077–1085, 1992

Horowitz MJ, Wilner NR, Alvarez W: Impact of Events Scale: a measure of subjective distress. Psychosomatic Medicine 41:208–218, 1979

Hyer LA, Albrecht JW, Boudewyns PA, et al: Dissociative experiences of Vietnam veterans with chronic posttraumatic stress disorder. Psychol Rep 73:519–530, 1993

Jaschke V, Spiegel D: A case of probable dissociative disorder. Bull Menninger Clin 56:246–260, 1992

Kihlstrom JF: The cognitive unconscious. Science 37:1445–1452, 1987

Kihlstrom JF: Hypnosis: a sesquicentennial essay. Int J Clin Exp Hypn 40:219–227, 1992

Kihlstrom JF: One hundred years of hysteria, in Dissociation: Clinical and Theoretical Perspectives. Edited by Lynn SJ, Rhue JW. New York, Guilford, 1994, pp 365–394

Kihlstrom JF, Glisky ML, Angiulo MJ: Dissociative tendencies and dissociative disorders. J Abnorm Psychol 103:117–124, 1994

Kirmayer LJ, Robbins JM, Paris J: Somatoform disorders: personality and the social matrix of somatic distress. J Abnorm Psychol 103:125–136, 1994

Klein RM, Doane BK (eds): Psychological Concepts and Dissociative Disorders. Hillsdale, NJ, Lawrence Erlbaum, 1994

Kluft RP: Varieties of hypnotic interventions in the treatment of multiple personality. Am J Clin Hypn 24:230–240, 1982

Kluft RP: Multiple personality, in American Psychiatric Press Review of Psychiatry, Vol 10. Edited by Tasman A, Goldfinger SM. Washington, DC, American Psychiatric Press, 1991, pp 161–188

Koopman C, Classen C, Spiegel D: Predictors of posttraumatic stress symptoms among survivors of the Oakland/Berkeley, California, firestorm. Am J Psychiatry 151:888–894, 1994

Krystal JH, Bennett A, Bremner JD, et al: Toward a cognitive neuroscience of dissociation and altered memory functions in post-traumatic stress disorder, in Neurobiological and Clinical Consequences of Stress: From Normal Adaptation to Post Traumatic Stress Disorder. Edited by Friedman MJ, Charney DS, Deutch AY. Philadelphia, JB Lippincott, 1995, pp 239–271

Kuzin IA: Hypnosis modelling in neural networks. Bull Math Biol 57:1–20, 1995

Lamas JR, del Valle-Inclan F, Blanco MJ, et al: Spanish norms for the Harvard Group Scale of Hypnotic Susceptibility, Form A. Int J Clin Exp Hypn 37:264–273, 1989

Loewenstein RJ: Dissociation, development and the psychobiology of trauma. J Am Acad Psychoanal 21:581–603, 1993

Loewenstein RJ, Putnam F: A comparison study of dissociative symptoms in patients with complex partial seizures, MPD, and PTSD. Dissociation 1:17–23, 1988

London P: The Children's Hypnotic Susceptibility Scale. Palo Alto, CA, Consulting Psychologists Press, 1962

Ludwig AM: The psychobiological functions of dissociation. Am J Clin Hypn 26:93–99, 1983

Lynn SJ, Rhue JW (eds): Dissociation: Clinical and Theoretical Perspectives. New York, Guilford, 1994

Marmar CR, Weiss DS, Schlenger DS, et al: Peritraumatic dissociation and posttraumatic stress in male Vietnam theater veterans. Am J Psychiatry 151:902–907, 1994

Mason AA: A case of congenital ichthyosiform erythrodermia treated by hypnosis. BMJ 2:422–423, 1952

Mason AA: Ichthyosis and hypnosis. BMJ 2:57, 1955

McElroy LP: Early indicators of pathological dissociation in sexually abused children. Child Abuse Negl 16:833–846, 1994

Miller M, Bowers K: Hypnotic analgesia: dissociated experience or dissociated control? J Abnorm Psychol 102:29–38, 1993

Minsky M: The Society of Mind. New York, Simon & Schuster, 1986

Morgan AH, Hilgard JR: The Stanford Hypnotic Clinical Scale for Children. Am J Clin Hypn 21:148–155, 1979

Morgan AH, Johnson DL, Hilgard ER: The stability of hypnotic susceptibility: a longitudinal study. Int J Clin Exp Hypn 21:78–85, 1974

Nemiah JC: Dissociation, conversion and somatization, in Dissociative Disorders: A Clinical Review. Edited by Spiegel D. Lutherville, MD, Sidran Press, pp 104–117, 1993

Nemiah JC: Dissociative disorders (hysterical neurosis, dissociative type), in Comprehensive Textbook of Psychiatry/VI, 6th Edition, Vol 1. Edited by Kaplan HI, Sadock BJ. Baltimore, MD, Williams & Wilkins, 1995, pp 1281–1293

Orne MT: The construct of hypnosis: implications of the definition for research and practice. Ann N Y Acad Sci 296:14–33, 1977

Orne MT, Hilgard ER, Spiegel H, et al: The relation between the Hypnotic Induction Profile and the Stanford Hypnotic Susceptibility Scales, Forms A and C. Int J Clin Exp Hypn 27:85–102, 1979

Parks RW, Long DL, Levine DS, et al: Parallel distributed processing and neural networks: origins, methodology and cognitive functions. Int J Neurosci 60:195–214, 1991

Perry C, Nadon R, Button J: The measurement of hypnotic ability, in Contemporary Hypnosis Research. Edited by Fromm E, Nash MR. New York, Guilford, 1992, pp 459–491

Piccione C, Hilgard ER, Zimbardo PG: On the degree of stability of measured hypnotizability over a 25-year period. J Pers Soc Psychol 56:289–295, 1989

Putnam FW: Dissociation as a response to extreme trauma, in Childhood Antecedents of Multiple Personality. Edited by Kluft RP. Washington, DC, American Psychiatric Press, 1985, pp 65–97

Putnam FW: The switch process in multiple personality disorder and other state-change disorders. Dissociation 1:24–32, 1988

Putnam FW: Diagnosis and Treatment of Multiple Personality Disorder. New York, Guilford, 1989

Putnam FW: Dissociative phenomena, in American Psychiatric Press Review of Psychiatry, Vol 10. Edited by Tasman A, Goldfinger SM. Washington, DC, American Psychiatric Press, pp 145–160, 1991

Putnam FW, Helmers K, Trickett PK: Development, reliability, and validity of a Child Dissociation Scale. Child Abuse Negl 17:731–741, 1993

Putnam FW, Helmers K, Horowitz LA, et al: Hypnotizability and dissociativity in sexually abused girls. Child Abuse Negl 19:645–655, 1995

Ray WJ, June K, Turaj K, et al: Dissociative experiences in a college age population: a factor analytic study of two dissociation scales. Personality and Individual Differences 13:417–424, 1992

Repka RJ, Nash MR: Hypnotic responsivity of the deaf: the development of the University of Tennessee Hypnotic Susceptibility Scale for the Deaf. Int J Clin Exp Hypn 43:316–313, 1995

Riley KC: Measurement of dissociation. J Nerv Ment Dis 176:449–450, 1988

Roche SM, McConkey KM: Absorption, nature, assessment, and correlates. J Pers Soc Psychol 59:91–101, 1990

Roesler TA, McKenzie N: Effects of childhood trauma on psychological functioning in adults sexually abused as children. J Nerv Ment Dis 182:145–150, 1994

Ross CA: Dissociation and physical illness, in Dissociation: Culture, Mind, and Body. Edited by Spiegel D. Washington, DC, American Psychiatric Press, 1994, pp 171–184

Ross CA, Heber S, Norton GR: The Dissociative Disorders Interview Schedule: a structured interview. Dissociation 2:169–189, 1989a

Ross CA, Heber S, Norton GR: Somatic symptoms in multiple personality disorder. Psychosomatics 30:154–160, 1989b

Ross CA, Joshi S, Currie R: Dissociative experiences in the general population: a factor analysis. Hospital and Community Psychiatry 42:297–301 , 1991

Sainton K, Ellason J, Mayran L, et al: Reliability of the new form of the Dissociative Experiences Scale (DES) and the Dissociation Questionnaire (DIS-Q) (abstract), in Dissociative Disorders 1993: Proceedings of the Tenth International Conference on Multiple Personality/Dissociative States. Edited by Braun BG, Parks JP. Chicago, Rush-Presbyterian-St. Luke's Medical Center, 1993, p 125

Sanders B, Giolas MH: Dissociation and childhood trauma in psychologically disturbed adolescents. Am J Psychiatry 148:50–54, 1991

Sanders S: The perceptual alteration scale: a scale measuring dissociation. Am J Clin Hypn 29:95–102, 1986

Sarbin TR, Coe WC: Hypnosis: A Social Psychological Analysis of Influence Communication. New York, Holt, Rinehart & Winston, 1972

Sarbin TR: Dissociation: state, trait or skill? Contemporary Hypnosis 11:47–54, 1994

Sarbin TR: On the belief that one body may be host to two or more personalities. Int J Clin Exp Hypn 43:163–183, 1995

Saxe GN, Chinman G, Berkowitz R, et al: Somatization in patients with dissociative disorder. Am J Psychiatry 151:1329–1334, 1994

Shor RE, Orne EC: Harvard Group Scale of Hypnotic Susceptibility. Palo Alto, CA, Consulting Psychologists Press, 1962

Siemens JG, Ross CA: Childhood sexual abuse and somatic symptoms in patients with gastrointestinal disorders (abstract), in Proceedings of the Eighth International Conference on Multiple Personality/Dissociative States. Edited by Braun BG, Carlson EB. Chicago, Rush-Presbyterian-St. Luke's Medical Center, 1991, p 86

Sigalowitz SJ, Dywan J, Ismailos L: Electrocortical evidence that hypnotically induced hallucinations are experienced. Paper presented at the Society for Clinical and Experimental Hypnosis symposium, "Dissociations in Conscious Experience: Electrophysical and Behavioral Evidence," New Orleans, LA, October 9–13, 1991

Singer JL (ed): Repression and Dissociation: Implication for Personality Theory, Psychopathology, and Health. Chicago, University of Chicago Press, 1990

Southwick SM, Bremner JD, Krystal JH, et al: Psychobiologic research in post-traumatic stress disorder. Psychiatr Clin North Am 17:251–264, 1994

Spanos NP: Hypnotic behavior: a cognitive, social psychological perspective. Research Communications in Psychology, Psychiatry and Behavior 7:199–213, 1982

Spanos NP, Chaves JF (eds): Hypnosis: The Cognitive-Behavioral Perspective. Buffalo, NY, Prometheus Books, 1989

Spanos NP, Radtke HL, Hodgins DC, et al: The Carleton University Responsiveness to Suggestion Scale: stability, reliability, and relationships with expectancy and "hypnotic experiences." Psychol Rep 53:555–563, 1983

Spiegel D: Dissociation, double binds and posttraumatic stress in multiple personality disorder, in Treatment of Multiple Personality Disorder. Edited by Braun BG. Washington, DC, American Psychiatric Press, 1986, pp 61–77

Spiegel D: Hypnosis, dissociation and trauma: hidden and overt observers, in Repression and Dissociation. Edited by Singer JL. Chicago, University of Chicago Press, 1990, pp 121–142

Spiegel D: Neurophysiological correlates in patients of hypnosis and dissociation. J Neuropsychiatry Clin Neurosci 3:440–445, 1991

Spiegel D: Dissociation and trauma, in Dissociative Disorders: A Clinical Review. Lutherville, MD, Sidran Press, 1993, pp 117–131

Spiegel D (ed): Dissociation: Culture, Mind, and Body. Washington, DC, American Psychiatric Press, 1994

Spiegel D, Cardena E: The disintegrated experience: the dissociative disorders revisited. J Abnorm Psychol 100:366–387, 1991b

Spiegel D, Vermetten E: Physiological correlates of hypnosis and dissociation, in Dissociation: Culture, Mind, and Body. Edited by Spiegel D. Washington, DC, American Psychiatric Press, 1994, pp 185–209

Spiegel D, Cutcomb S, Ren C, et al: Hypnotic hallucination alters evoked potentials. J Abnorm Psychol 94:249–255, 1985

Spiegel D, Hunt T, Dondershine HE: Dissociation and hypnotizability in posttraumatic stress disorder. Am J Psychiatry 145:301–305, 1988

Spiegel D, Bierre P, Rootenberg J: Hypnotic alteration of somatosensory perception. Am J Psychiatry 146:749–754, 1989

Spiegel D, Frischholz EJ, Fleiss JL, et al: Predictors of smoking abstinence following a single-session restructuring intervention with self-hypnosis. Am J Psychiatry 150:1090–1097, 1993

Spinhoven PH, Baak D, Van Dyck R, et al: The effectiveness of an authoritative versus permissive style of hypnotic communication. Int J Clin Exp Hypn 36:182–191, 1988

Spitzer RL, Williams JB, Gibbon M: Structured Clinical Interview for DSM-III-R (SCID). New York, New York State Psychiatric Institute, Biometrics Research Department, 1987

Steinberg M: Structured Clinical Interview for DSM-IV Dissociative Disorders (SCID-D). Washington, DC, American Psychiatric Press, 1993

Steinberg M: Systematizing dissociation: symptomatology and diagnostic assessment, in Dissociation: Culture, Mind, and Body. Edited by Spiegel D. Washington, DC, American Psychiatric Press, 1994, pp 59–88

Steinberg M, Rounsaville B, Ciccetti DV: The Structured Clinical Interview for DSM-III-R Dissociative Disorders: preliminary report on a new diagnostic instrument. Am J Psychiatry 147:77–83, 1990

Tellegen A, Atkinson G: Openness to absorbing and self-altering experiences (" absorption"), a trait related to hypnotic susceptibility. J Abnorm Psychol 83:286–277, 1974

van der Hart O, Spiegel D: Hypnotic assessment and treatment of trauma-induced psychoses: the early psychotherapy of H. Breukink and modern views. Int J Clin Exp Hypn 41:191–209, 1993

Vanderlinden J, Van Dyck R, Vandereyken MD: Dissociative experiences in the general population in the Netherlands and Belgium: a study with the Dissociative Questionnaire (DIS-Q). Dissociation 4:180–184, 1991

Vanderlinden J, Van Dyck R, Vandereyken W, et al: The Dissociation Questionnaire: development and characteristics of a new self-reporting questionnaire. Child Psychology and Psychotherapy 1: 21–27, 1993

Waelde LC, Fairbank JA, Uddo M, et al: Empirical development of an MMPI-2 subscale for assessing dissociative symptomatology in post-traumatic stress disorder. Paper and abstract presented at the International Society of Traumatic Stress Studies, Boston, November 1995

Walker E, Katon WJ, Neraas K, et al: Dissociation in women with chronic pelvis pain. Am J Psychiatry 149:534–537, 1992

Weitzenhoffer AM: Hypnotic susceptibility revisited. Am J Clin Hypn 22:130–146, 1980

Weitzenhoffer AM, Hilgard ER: Stanford Hypnotic Susceptibility Scale: Forms A and B. Palo Alto, CA, Consulting Psychologists Press, 1959

Weitzenhoffer AM, Hilgard ER: Stanford Hypnotic Susceptibility Scale: Form C. Palo Alto, CA, Consulting Psychologists Press, 1962

Wickramasekera IE: Somatization: concepts, data and predictions from the high risk model of threat perception. J Nerv Ment Dis 183:15–23, 1995

Williams JM, Hall DW: Use of single session hypnosis for smoking cessation. Addict Behav 13:205–208, 1988

Whorwell PJ, Prior A, Faragher EB: Controlled trial of hypnotherapy in the treatment of severe refractory irritable bowel syndrome. Lancet 12:1232–1234, 1984

Whorwell PJ, Prior A, Colgan SM: Hypnotherapy in severe irritable bowel syndrome: further experience. Gut 28:423–425, 1987

Wilson SC, Barber TX: Vivid fantasy and hallucinatory abilities in the life histories of excellent hypnotic subjects (" somnabules"): preliminary report with female subjects, in Imagery, Vol 2: Concepts, Results and Applications. Edited by Klinger E. New York, Plenum, 1981, pp 133–149

Wilson SC, Barber TX : The fantasy prone personality: implication for understanding imagery, hypnosis, and parapsychological phenomena, in Imagery: Current Theory, Research and Application. Edited by Sheikh AA. New York, Wiley, 1983, pp 340–387

Young L: Sexual abuse and the problem of embodiment. Child Abuse Negl 16:89–100, 1992

Zamansky HS, Ruehle BL: Making hypnosis happen: the involuntariness of the hypnotic experience. Int J Clin Exp Hypn 18:386–398, 1995

Zeltzer L, LeBaron S: Hypnosis and nonhypnotic techniques for reduction of pain and anxiety during painful procedures in children and adolescents with cancer. J Pediatr 101:1032–1035, 1982

Zeltzer L, Lebaron S, Zeltzer PM: The effectiveness of behavioral intervention for reduction of nausea and vomiting in children and adolescents receiving chemotherapy. J Clin Oncol 6:83–90, 1984

Chapter 5

Trauma, Dissociation, and Somatization

Gary Rodin, M.D., Janet de Groot, M.D., and
Harold Spivak, M.D.

In this chapter, we address the association among trauma, dissociation, and somatization. *Dissociation* has been defined as a psychological process by which information—incoming, stored, or outgoing—is deflected from integration with its usual or expected associations (West 1967). It is also regarded as a coping mechanism by which individuals attempt to remove themselves from an emotional experience that is too intense or distressing (Spiegel and Cardena 1991). The predominant use of this coping mechanism is sometimes considered pathological. In DSM-IV (American Psychiatric Association 1994), disruption in the usual integration of functions such as consciousness, memory, identity, and perception of the environment, when associated with impairment in social, occupational, or other areas of functioning, is considered an essential feature of the so-called dissociative disorders (American Psychiatric Association 1994). What is not specifically emphasized in the DSM-IV definition is that dissociation may represent an attempt to manage overwhelming emotional experience. Furthermore, none of these definitions takes into account the possibility that dissociation reflects a relative failure in the development of the capacity for affect integration. Although impaired affect integration may be present in a variety of pathological and nonpathological conditions, it is the hallmark of the dissociative disorders.

The discussion of the relationship between antecedent trauma and dissociation will be broadened in this chapter to include not only discrete gross events but also "microscopic," repetitive emotional injury. Most of the psychiatric literature linking dissociation with trauma has focused on gross trauma, particularly physical and sexual abuse. However, repetitive subtle trauma, specifically parental failures in attunement and responsiveness to the emotional experience of the child, may have profound effects on the child's capacity to organize affects and perceptions (Emde 1983; Stern 1985; Stolorow et al. 1987). Indeed, parental understanding and responsiveness to the child's emotional experience may be vital in the development of the child's capacity for affect integration. Furthermore, family environments that inflict or permit gross trauma are also likely to be disruptive or inattentive to a wide range of a child's other developmental needs.

Somatization refers to the tendency to experience distress in terms of physical symptoms, bodily preoccupation, and/or illness-related worry (Barsky and Klerman 1983) and/or to experience oneself predominantly in physical terms (Rodin 1991). It reflects a disturbance in affect integration to the extent that the psychological and physical aspects of experience are not integrated. In these terms, somatization also reflects a disturbance in the sense of self. The belief that somatization might be associated with both antecedent trauma and the defense mechanism of dissociation is not new. In fact, Janet (1920) hypothesized that memories of traumatic experiences that are stored apart from conscious awareness may contribute to dissociation and somatization in the form of hysteria. Freud (1893/1962) similarly suggested a link between defensive operations and the subsequent development of somatic symptoms. He postulated that unacceptable thoughts and feelings were transformed into somatic symptoms through the mechanism of conversion. However, this emphasis on the defensive function of somatization did not take into account the direct, experiential nature of many somatic symptoms (Rodin 1991). Furthermore, somatization, like dissociation, may reflect a failure to develop the capacity to integrate emotion into the ongoing flow of subjective experience. This failure most often arises in the context of relative parental unavailability to validate the child's emotional experience and to assist with its integration and modulation.

Some of the recent literature documenting the association between dissociation and trauma in selected somatizing conditions is briefly noted in this chapter. This relationship between dissociation and somatization is addressed not only because sexual and physical abuse have been associated with both phenomena, but also because both may reflect disturbances in the organization and integration of subjective experience. The psychological mechanisms by which dissociation and somatization may be linked to each other and to antecedent trauma are considered. Finally, some of the implications for psychotherapeutic treatment are addressed.

Trauma, Dissociation, and Somatization: Evidence for an Association

Somatization may be found in the general population; in the so-called somatoform disorders; in conditions such as anorexia nervosa or bulimia nervosa, in which bodily preoccupation is a predominant feature; in factitious disorders, in which illness is simulated or induced; and in a variety of other psychiatric disorders, such as depression and schizophrenia (Rodin 1984). The biological, social, and psychological determinants of somatization are beyond the scope of this chapter; however, the significance of dissociation and trauma in the somatizing conditions is reviewed.

Somatoform Disorders

The somatoform disorders include conditions such as somatization disorder, conversion disorder, pain disorder, hypochondriasis, and body dysmorphic disorder. All of these conditions are associated with physical symptoms that are not fully explained by a medical condition and with impairment in social, occupational, or other areas of functioning (American Psychiatric Association 1994). Somatization disorder refers to a chronic, severe, somatizing condition, with symptoms occurring over a number of years, beginning before age 30, and involving multiple organ systems. Some studies of this condition have demonstrated a strong association with a prior history of trauma and dissociative symptoms. For example, Pribor et al. (1993) found that more than 90% of women with somatization disorder reported a history of emotional, physical, or sexual abuse and 80% reported some type of sexual abuse. Saxe et al. (1994) found that the majority of psychiatric inpatients with somatization disorder also met diagnostic criteria for dissociative disorder and that the degree of dissociation correlated with the degree of somatization. Other reports have suggested a possible association between sexual trauma and subsequent functional somatic symptoms, including irritable bowel and chronic pelvic pain (Drossman et al. 1990; Felitti 1991; Walker and Stenchever 1993). Furthermore, Walker et al. (1992) reported that women with chronic pelvic pain were more likely than those in a control group to use dissociation as a coping mechanism.

A number of recent studies suggest that a history of trauma and a propensity toward dissociation may be found in patients with somatoform disorders and related conditions. However, it has not been demonstrated that either trauma or dissociation are linked more specifically to the somatoform disorders than to other psychiatric conditions.

Eating Disorders

Anorexia nervosa and bulimia nervosa are conditions that occur predominantly in women in late adolescence and early adulthood (Fairburn and Beglin 1991). These disorders are associated with bodily preoccupation, undue influence of body weight and shape on self-evaluation, and a variety of extreme weight loss behaviors (American Psychiatric Association 1994). Many of the behavioral manifestations of these conditions, such as bingeing, self-starvation, self-induced vomiting, laxative abuse, and extreme exercise, are intended to heighten somatic experience.

Dissociation and other disturbances in the processing of emotions have been documented in patients with eating disorders. For example, systematic studies have shown that diminished emotional awareness, referred to as alexithymia when present in an extreme form, has been observed in patients with eating disorders (de Groot et al. 1995; Schmidt et al. 1993). In addition, initial case reports documenting the association between dissociation and eating disorders (Chandarana and Malla 1989; Sands 1991; Torem 1990) have been confirmed by systematic research (Berger et al. 1994). Demitrack et al. (1990) found significantly higher scores on the Dissociative Experiences Scale (Bernstein and Putnam 1986) in patients with eating disorders compared with age-matched control subjects. Vanderlinden et al. (1993) also found that both trauma and dissociative experiences were significantly more common in patients with eating disorders than in control subjects and that the degree of dissociation was related to the seriousness of previous trauma. Torem and Curdue (1988) found that more than 80% of patients with multiple personality disorder had pathological eating behaviors as presenting symptoms. Although the significance of the relationship between eating disorders and dissociation is not well established, it seems likely that dissociation as a prominent mechanism, and/or the presence of an eating disorder, often reflects or is associated with a disturbance in the processing and management of emotional experience.

Uncontrolled studies of patients with eating disorders have demonstrated widely varying rates of sexual abuse, ranging from 7%–100% (Bulik et al. 1989; Lacey 1990; Oppenheimer et al. 1985; Root and Fallon 1988; Sloan and Leichner 1986). Miller et al. (1993) found that a history of both sexual abuse and dissociative experiences was more common in bulimic women than in a control group. However, a recent cross-cultural study involving students with a diagnosis of bulimia nervosa from Austria, Brazil, and the United States indicated that a history of sexual abuse in these individuals was no more common than in the general population (Pope et al. 1994). Indeed, a history of childhood sexual abuse has been reported by up to 54% of women in the general population (Peters et al. 1986; Russell 1983). A community-based study that specifically elicited a history of sexual abuse involving physical contact found that it was more common among women with bulimia nervosa than among those without this disorder (Welch and Fairburn 1994). However, in this study, the rate of reporting sexual abuse in both a community and clinical sample of women with bulimia nervosa was not greater than in those with other psychiatric disorders. These findings suggest that the trauma of sexual abuse may not be specifically linked to eating disorders and is, at most, a nonspecific risk factor for psychiatric morbidity.

Although there may not be a specific association between eating disorders and sexual abuse, the latter may be a marker for more severe psychopathology among those with eating disorders. In this regard, we found that patients with eating disorders who reported sexual abuse tended to demonstrate more psychopathology than women with eating disorders who did not report such a history (de Groot et al. 1992). Similarly, Herzog et al. (1993) found that women with eating disorders who reported childhood sexual abuse had higher scores on the Dissociative Experiences Scale (Bernstein and Putnam 1986) than those who did not. Others have suggested that combinations of sexual, physical, and psychological abuse, rather than sexual abuse alone, are more common in women with bulimia nervosa than in control subjects (Rorty et al. 1994). Chronically abusive or traumatic family environments may lead to disturbances in personality and may lead to specific syndromes, such as eating disorders. Borderline personality disorder, for example, has been shown to be independently associated with both sexual abuse (Brown and Anderson 1991; Ogata et al. 1990) and eating disorders (Gartner et al. 1989; Wonderlich and Swift 1990). In fact, borderline personality disorder has been diagnosed in up to 46% of patients with bulimia nervosa or anorexia nervosa (Gartner et al. 1989; Johnson et al. 1989; Pope and Hudson 1989; Wonderlich and Swift 1990).

Some researchers have suggested that disturbed family dynamics may account for the link between sexual abuse and eating disorders (Abramson and Lucido 1991; de Groot et al. 1992; Pribor and Dinwoodie 1992). Kinzl et al. (1994) reported that disturbances in the family dynamics of female college students were even more strongly associated with eating disorders than was a history of sexual abuse. It has been hypothesized that both mothers (Leibowitz 1991; Sands 1989) and fathers (Bemporad et al. 1992) of patients with eating disorders have tended to use their daughters to mirror their own needs and have failed to validate adequately the emotional experiences of their children. This parental failure, when associated with other risk factors, may contribute to the subsequent development of anorexia nervosa and bulimia nervosa. However, the specificity or universality of such observations is not known.

Unresponsiveness to the emotional life of a child, and specifically to "child-initiated cues" (Bruch 1982), is considered by some to be the critical traumatic factor in the genesis of the emotional disturbances associated with eating disorders. When emotional states have been too intense or traumatic or when parents have failed to provide sufficient calmness and have failed to accept and respond to the child's emotional life, the child's capacity for affect integration may be adversely affected (Stolorow et al. 1987). Trauma of this kind leads to difficulty in being able to identify, trust, and integrate emotional experience. de Groot et al. (1995) found that women with bulimia nervosa tend to have greater disturbances in emotional awareness than control women, even after the remission of current eating disorder symptoms.

Factitious Disorders

Factitious disorders are conditions in which emotional distress is manifested by intentionally producing or feigning physical signs or symptoms (American Psychiatric Association 1994). There are no systematic studies of either dissociation or trauma in patients with chronic factitious disorder. However, there is some evidence to suggest that many of these patients suffer from disturbances in the sense of reality and in the sense of self (Spivak et al. 1994). Consistent with this finding, a diagnosis of borderline personality disorder has been made in up to 30% of patients with factitious disorder (Sutherland and Rodin 1990).

There has been much speculation about the psychological basis for factitious disorders (Spivak et al. 1994). Classical psychoanalytic theory emphasized the role of conflict and retroflexed anger. More recent speculations have focused on psychological defects and disturbances in the subjective experience of patients with factitious disorder. Physical illness may be induced or simulated by individuals with factitious disorder to concretize and validate their subjective sense of suffering and their need for assistance.

Assistance is sought in a medical environment that is structured and therefore safe and in which the responsiveness of others is organized around physical interventions. Physical responsiveness and interventions may be valued because they are experienced as more tangible, meaningful, and real than are psychological interventions.

Chronic fabrication of illness, in which the illness experience becomes central to the individual's identity, may occur in response to a fundamental defect in the sense of self (Spivak et al. 1994). The simulation or adoption of illness may provide a sense of identity and organization for individuals in whom it is otherwise lacking. Paradoxically, "medical imposture" may heighten the sense of reality because physical symptoms, diseases, and interventions are experienced as more valid or real, even when fabricated or falsely induced, than are other aspects of emotional experience (Greenacre 1958). Although Western culture generally attaches legitimacy to distress that is medically based (Good 1994), medical imposture may occur only with individuals who have great difficulty regarding their own subjective experience or sense of identity as valid or real. Indeed, an individual's sense of reality may need to be impaired to permit fabrication of illness without evoking the subjective experience of lying. Dissociative mechanisms may contribute to fabrication or imposture without the subjective experience of lying by suspending reality testing in these patients (Spivak et al. 1994).

Trauma, Dissociation, and Somatization: How Are They Linked?

Some evidence has been cited thus far to support the presence of an association among trauma, dissociation, and somatization. What accounts for this link needs to be explained. It is possible that these phenomena are related because all are associated with or represent disturbances in the nature and processing of emotional experience. The psychiatric literature on dissociation has tended to focus on the effects of gross trauma in producing intense and intolerable emotional states that are deflected or warded off by this coping mechanism (Putnam 1989). However, the premorbid and subsequent capacity to experience, tolerate, and trust emotional experience and the emotional availability of significant others may be equally important in determining the effects of trauma. Environments that not only provoke intense emotionality but also fail to assist with affect integration and modulation may be most likely to contribute to dissociation, somatization, and other disturbances in the sense of self.

Developing the capacity for affect integration depends, at least in part, on the extent to which caregivers have been attuned and responsive to a child's subjective experience. Optimally, caregivers help the child to identify and verbalize affects, which are initially experienced in predominantly somatic terms. In this way, the child learns to distinguish somatic from psychological experience and comes to comprehend that intense and contradictory affects can arise from a unified self (Stolorow et al. 1987). This integration of affective experience into conscious awareness facilitates the progressive articulation of self-experience (de Groot and Rodin 1994). When affective states are not recognized by caregivers or are perceived as threatening, they may be defensively walled off and/or experienced as invalid or poorly differentiated. The relative absence of a parental relationship that facilitates the integration of affects also may lead to disturbances in the sense of self and the tendency to somatize. The tendency to exclude or dismiss affective states inevitably interferes with psychological development because affects are so central to the organization of self-experience (Demos 1987; Emde 1983; Stern 1985) and because the mutual sharing of affective states helps to establish an inner sense of emotional relatedness (Stern 1985).

The literature on dissociation has emphasized gross trauma as the critical pathogenic factor in the development of pathological dissociation. However, developmental theorists also have pointed to the traumatic effect of parent-child interactions that do not assist or that interfere with the child's emerging capacity to regulate affects (Demos 1987; Stern 1985). Achieving the capacity to experience affective states in an integrated fashion depends, in part, on caregivers who are attuned to the child's emotional life. The relative failure of parents to respond to a child's emotional experience may contribute to the child's tendency to be emotionally unaware and/or to deflect feeling states from awareness. The latter is a central characteristic of dissociation. A recent study confirmed that there may be a relationship between diminished emotional awareness, also referred to as alexithymia, and the tendency to dissociate (Berenbaum and James 1994). Dissociation presumably operates in this situation to protect the individual from feeling overwhelmed by disturbing and poorly differentiated feeling states. However, when chronic and predominant, this coping mechanism may also interfere with the individual's capacity to experience emotions and to regard them as real. A disturbance in the sense of reality is also a typical feature of dissociative states.

Somatization, like dissociation, may be associated with a tendency to feel overwhelmed by affective states that are intense and poorly differentiated. Somatic symptoms may represent an attempt to organize and concretize inner chaotic affective states (Goodsitt 1983) or to rely upon bodily experiences, which are regarded as more real or more authentic (Spivak et al. 1994). Some individuals can regard their suffering as real only when it can be experienced or communicated in physical terms (Spivak et al. 1994).

Treatment

Patients with somatization and/or dissociation may benefit from treatment that is supportive or directive (Sharpe et al. 1992), including techniques intended to reduce the intensity of emotional experience (e.g., relaxation therapy) and to correct cognitive distortions related to physical and/or emotional well-being. In patients who have anorexia nervosa and bulimia nervosa, structured treatments also have been shown to be effective in the short term (Fairburn et al. 1993), although long-term morbidity persists (Steinhausen and Glanville 1983; Windauer et al. 1993).

Traditional psychoanalytic approaches that rely on verbal interpretations of unconscious conflict are often ineffective in patients with somatizing conditions (de Groot and Rodin 1994). When psychotherapeutic interpretations are not based on the data of subjective experience, treatment may actually interfere with the capacity of patients to identify and trust their inner world. This risk is great for patients with somatization disorder or other patients who already have difficulty identifying feeling states or who are at risk of compliantly accepting explanations provided by therapists or others in positions of authority (Bruch 1982). Treatments directed toward identifying and validating emotional experience have been recommended for patients with eating disorders, although empirical studies of effectiveness have not yet been reported.

Patients with dissociative disorders may experience emotional states as intense, unreal, and poorly integrated with other aspects of their intrapsychic or interpersonal world. The goal of treatment may be to help such individuals become better able to modulate the intensity of their emotional experience and to integrate it with other aspects of experience. Some of these issues are described in the case example.

Case Example

A 35-year-old woman had chronic symptoms of depression and fatigue that met criteria for the diagnoses of dysthymic disorder, recurrent major depression, and chronic fatigue. Her symptoms of fatigue, which were medically unexplained, were often triggered by upper respiratory infections and were associated with a variety of somatic symptoms, including incapacitating weakness and muscular pain. She complained of difficulties in relationships, which tended to be either superficial or else intense but compartmentalized. She believed that her depressive symptoms and fatigue were unrelated, and she reported disturbing thoughts that seemed to arise spontaneously and to be disconnected from her conscious concerns. She often wondered whether her feelings were real and reported periodically banging her head against a wall or taking pills to calm herself when she felt overwhelmed by intense and painful feeling states.

This patient's history was significant in that it was characterized by chronic emotional isolation. She regarded her parents as caring but unable to be attuned to her inner experience. As a child, she often felt terrified but unable to communicate her fears. She tended to experience emotions intensely and to respond adversely to a wide range of emotional and physical stimuli. There was no history of gross trauma. She reported a wide range of somatic symptoms over the preceding decade, including migraine headache, fatigue, muscle pain, and sleep disturbance. She tended to be overly conscientious in her work and in her responsibilities to others and subsequently felt overburdened and exhausted.

This patient demonstrated a tendency toward both dissociation and somatization. Her history was devoid of gross trauma but was striking in terms of the chronic sense of perceived misattunement and empathic failure. She began weekly expressive therapy focused on her symptoms of depression, problems in relationships, and difficulty tolerating and sharing her feelings. In the first phase of treatment, she was preoccupied with the fear that her perspective would not be valued or understood. She was usually unable to describe her feelings during the sessions but would often report intense and distressing feelings of injury afterward. It was necessary for the therapist to avoid theoretical speculation, to "de-center" from his own experience, and to remain immersed in the patient's subjective experience. Nonverbal cues from the patient were often the most reliable guide to understanding her experience. At times, she felt that she was understood, but still wondered whether the therapist actually "knew" her. She often described feeling "not here" and being unable to identify feelings triggered in the sessions. Most problematic for both patient and therapist was her profound feelings of hopelessness about the future. In particular, she felt pessimistic about establishing a relationship in which her deeper feelings and broader interests could be understood and shared.

We have recommended that treatment in many patients with somatization disorder should focus, at least initially, on identifying felt emotional experience, particularly that which emerges in treatment sessions (de Groot and Rodin 1994). This approach must be used cautiously, particularly with patients who are prone to be flooded by intense or undifferentiated affective states. It is usually most successful to focus on small moments of the patients' experiences rather than on more global phenomena. With patients who tend to somatize and to feel detached from affect, particular attention should be paid to felt experience and to the sense of reality. Often, feelings that are intensely experienced are nevertheless regarded as unreal or "imagined."

With those who have difficulty experiencing affect, there is always the danger of therapy becoming an intellectual exercise. It requires a shift for therapists, accustomed to focusing on psychological symptoms, to begin listening with interest to the bodily complaints and concerns of their patients. Therapists who place particular value on the verbal articulation of psychological experience may unwittingly lead patients with somatization disorder to communicate in experience-distant psychological language rather than in the language of more deeply felt bodily experience. Such pressure may be counterproductive because the most authentic aspects of self-experience may be manifested in the bodily realm.

The presence of a helping relationship and the structure of the therapeutic situation provide relief to many patients. A posture of "sustained empathic enquiry" (Stolorow et al. 1987) by therapists may further facilitate the identification and articulation of patients' subjective experiences. Patients with somatization disorder who have difficulty identifying their feelings or experiencing the therapeutic relationship as sustaining may require more engagement by their therapists. Over time, the progressive elaboration of emotional experience may lead to an increased capacity of patients to experience themselves in psychological terms, to distinguish the psychological from the physical aspects of self experience, and to tolerate and integrate feeling states.

Conclusion

Somatization and dissociation both may reflect disturbances in the integration of subjective experience. Somatization involves a relative inability to differentiate the psychological and physical aspects of experience or to experience oneself in psychological terms. Dissociation involves the failure to experience diverse aspects of subjective experience in an integrated form. Dissociation may become prominent and chronic when gross trauma has triggered affective states that are overwhelming and painful. Both somatization and dissociation may be more likely to occur when there has been chronic empathic failure and emotional misattunement in relationships with caregivers during important developmental periods. Psychotherapeutic treatment may involve assistance with identifying, integrating, and articulating intense and diverse affective states. This process may gradually lead to greater organization and consolidation of self experience and may reduce the need to compartmentalize and ward off emotional experience.

References

Abramson EE, Lucido GM: Brief report: childhood sexual experience and bulimia. Addict Behav 16:529–532, 1991

American Psychiatric Association: Diagnostic and Statistical Manual of Mental Disorders, 4th Edition. Washington, DC, American Psychiatric Association, 1994

Barsky AJ, Klerman GL: Overview: Hypochondriasis, bodily complaints, and somatic styles. Am J Psychiatry 140:273–283, 1983

Bemporad J, Beresin E, Ratey J, et al: A psychoanalytic study of eating disorders, I: a developmental profile of 67 index cases. J Am Acad Psychoanal 20:509–531, 1992

Berenbaum H, James T: Correlates and retrospectively reported antecedents of alexithymia. Psychosom Med 56:353–359, 1994

Berger D, Saito S, Ono Y, et al: Dissociation and child abuse histories on an eating disorder cohort in Japan. Acta Psychiatr Scand 90:274–280, 1994

Bernstein EM, Putnam FW: Development, reliability and validity of a dissociation scale. J Nerv Ment Dis 174:727–735, 1986

Brown GR, Anderson B: Psychiatric morbidity in adult inpatients with childhood histories of sexual and physical abuse. Am J Psychiatry 148:55–61, 1991

Bruch H: Anorexia nervosa: therapy and theory. Am J Psychiatry 39:1531–1538, 1982

Bulik CM, Sullivan PF, Rorty M: Childhood sexual abuse in women with bulimia. J Clin Psychiatry 50:460–464, 1989

Chandarana P, Malla A: Bulimia and dissociative states: a case report. Can J Psychiatry 34:137–139, 1989 de Groot JM, Rodin G: Eating disorders, female psychology, and the self. J Am Acad Psychoanal 22:299–317, 1994

de Groot J, Kennedy S, Rodin G, et al: Correlates of sexual abuse in women with anorexia nervosa and bulimia nervosa. Can J Psychiatry 37:516–518, 1992

de Groot J, Rodin G, Olmsted M: Alexithymia, depression and treatment outcome in bulimia nervosa. Compr Psychiatry 36:53–60, 1995

Demitrack MA, Putnam FW, Brewerton TD, et al: Relation of clinical variables to dissociative phenomena in eating disorders. Am J Psychiatry 147:1184–1188, 1990

Demos EV: Affect and the development of the self: a new frontier, in Frontiers in Self Psychology. Edited by Goldberg A. Hillsdale, NJ, Analytic Press, pp 27–53, 1987

Drossman DA, Leserman J, Nachman G, et al: Sexual and physical abuse in women with functional or organic gastrointestinal disorders. Ann Intern Med 113:828–833, 1990

Emde RN: The prepresentational self and its affective core. Psychoanal Study Child 38:165–192, 1983

Fairburn CG, Beglin SJ: Studies of the epidemiology of bulimia nervosa. Am J Psychiatry 147:401–408, 1991

Fairburn CG, Jones R, Peveler RC, et al: Psychotherapy and bulimia nervosa: longer-term effects of interpersonal psychotherapy, behavior therapy, and cognitive behavior therapy. Arch Gen Psychiatry 50:419–428, 1993

Felitti VJ: Long-term medical consequences of incest, rape and molestation. South Med J 84:328–331, 1991

Freud S: On the physical mechanism of hysterical phenomena: preliminary communication (1893), in The Standard Edition of the Complete Psychological Works of Sigmund Freud, Vol 3. Translated and edited by Strachey J. London, Hogarth Press, 1962, pp 224–314

Gartner AF, Marcus RN, Halmi K, et al: DSM-III-R personality disorders in patients with eating disorders. Am J Psychiatry 146:1585–1591, 1989

Good BJ: How medicine constructs its objects, in Medicine, Rationality, and Experience: An Anthropological Perspective. Edited by Good BJ. Cambridge, England, Cambridge University Press, 1994, pp 65–87

Goodsitt A: Self-regulatory disturbances in eating disorders. Int J Eat Disord 2:51–60, 1983

Greenacre P: The impostor. Psychoanal Q 27:359–382, 1958

Herzog DB, Staley JE, Carmody S, et al: Childhood sexual abuse in ano-
    rexia nervosa and bulimia nervosa: a pilot study. J Am Acad Child
    Adolesc Psychiatry 32:962–966, 1993
Janet P: The Major Symptoms of Hysteria. New York, Macmillan, 1920
Johnson C, Tobin D, Enright A: Prevalence and clinical characteristics of
    borderline patients in an eating-disordered population. J Clin Psy-
    chiatry 50:9–15, 1989
Kinzl JF, Traweger C, Guenther V, et al: Family background and sexual
    abuse associated with eating disorders. Am J Psychiatry 151:
    1127–1131, 1994
Lacey JH: Incest, incestuous fantasy and indecency: a clinical catchment
    area study of normal-weight bulimic women. Br J Psychiatry 157:
    399–403, 1990
Leibowitz EB: Bulimia: A self psychological study, in Psychoanalytic Ap-
    proaches to Addiction. Edited by Smaldino A. New York, Brunner/
    Mazel, 1991, pp 96–122
Miller DA, McCluskey-Fawcett K, Irving LM: The relationship between
    childhood sexual abuse and subsequent onset of bulimia nervosa.
    Child Abuse Negl 17:305–314, 1993
Ogata SN, Silk KR, Goodrich S, et al: Childhood sexual and physical
    abuse in adult patients with borderline personality disorder. Am J
    Psychiatry 147:1008–1013, 1990
Oppenheimer R, Howells K, Palmer RL et al: Adverse sexual experience
    in childhood and clinical eating disorders: a preliminary description. J
    Psychosom Res 19:357–361, 1985
Peters SD, Wyatt GE, Finkelhor D: Prevalence, in A Sourcebook on Child
    Sexual Abuse. Edited by Finkelhor D. and Associates. Beverly Hills,
    CA, Sage, 1986, pp 15–59
Pope HG, Hudson JI: Are eating disorders associated with borderline
    personality disorder? a critical review. Int J Eat Disord 8:1–9, 1989
Pope HG, Mangweth B, Negrao AB, et al: Childhood sexual abuse and
    bulimia nervosa: a comparison of American, Austrian and Brazilian
    women. Am J Psychiatry 151:732–737, 1994
Pribor EF, Dinwoodie SH: Psychiatric correlates of incest in childhood.
    Am J Psychiatry 149:52–56, 1992
Pribor EF, Yutzy SH, Dean JT et al: Briquet's syndrome, dissociation, and
    abuse. Am J Psychiatry 150:1507–1511, 1993
Putnam FW: Diagnosis and Treatment of Multiple Personality Disorder.
    New York, Guilford, 1989

Rodin GM: Somatization and the self. Am J Psychother 38:257–263, 1984

Rodin GM: Somatization: a perspective from self psychology. J Am Acad Psychoanal 19:367–384, 1991

Root MPP, Fallon P: The incidence of victimization experiences in a bulimic sample. International Journal of Violence 3:161–173, 1988

Rorty M, Yager J, Rossotto E: Childhood sexual, physical and psychological abuse in bulimia nervosa. Am J Psychiatry 151:1122–1126, 1994

Russell DE: The incidence and prevalence of intrafamilial and extrafamilial sexual abuse of female children. Child Abuse Negl 18:133–246, 1983

Sands SH: Eating disorders and female development: a self-psychological perspective, in Dimensions of Self Experience: Progress in Self Psychology, Vol 5. Edited by Goldberg A. Hillsdale, NJ, Analytic Press, 1989, pp 75–103

Sands SH: Bulimia, dissociation and empathy: a self-psychological view, in Psychodynamic Treatment of Anorexia Nervosa and Bulimia. Edited by Johnson C. New York, Guilford, 1991, pp 34–50

Saxe GN, Chinman G, Berkowitz R, et al: Somatization in patients with dissociative disorders. Am J Psychiatry 151:1329–1334, 1994

Schmidt U, Jiwany A, Treasure J: A controlled study of alexithymia in eating disorders. Compr Psychiatry 34:54–58, 1993

Sharpe M, Peveler R, Mayou R: The psychological treatment of patients with functional somatic symptoms: a practical guide. J Psychosom Res 36:525–529, 1992

Sloan G, Leichner P: Is there a relationship between sexual abuse or incest and eating disorders? Can J Psychiatry 31:656–660, 1986

Spiegel D, Cardena E: Disintegrated experience: the dissociative disorders revisited. J Abnorm Psychol 100:366–378, 1991

Spivak H, Rodin G, Sutherland A: The psychology of factitious disorders: a reconsideration. Psychosomatics 35:25–34, 1994

Steinhausen HC, Glanville K: A long-term follow-up of adolescent anorexia nervosa. Acta Psychiatr Scand 68:1–10, 1983

Stern D: The Interpersonal World of the Infant: A View from Psychoanalysis and Developmental Psychology. New York, Basic Books, 1985

Stolorow RD, Brandchaft B, Atwood GE: Psychoanalytic Treatment: An Intersubjective Approach. Hillsdale, NJ, Analytic Press, 1987

Sutherland AJ, Rodin GM: Factitious disorders in a general hospital setting: clinical features and a review of the literature. Psychosomatics 31:392–399, 1990

Torem MS: Covert multiple personality underlying eating disorders. Am
    J Psychother 44:357–368, 1990

Torem MS, Curdue W: PTSD presenting as an eating disorder. Stress
    Medicine 4:139–142, 1988

Vanderlinden J, Vandereycken W, Van Dyck R, et al: Dissociative experi-
    ence and trauma in eating disorders. Int J Eat Disord 13:187–193, 1993

Walker EA, Stenchever MA: Sexual victimization and chronic pelvic pain
    (review). Obstet Gynecol Clin North Am 20:795–807, 1993

Walker EA, Katon WJ, Neraas K, et al: Dissociation in women with
    chronic pelvic pain. Am J Psychiatry 149:534–537, 1992

Welch SL, Fairburn CG: Sexual abuse and bulimia nervosa: three inte-
    grated case control comparisons. Am J Psychiatry 151:402–407, 1994

West LJ: Dissociative reaction, in Comprehensive Textbook of Psychiatry.
    Edited by Freedman AM, Kaplan HI. Baltimore, MD, Williams &
    Wilkins, 1967, p 885

Windauer U, Lennerts W, Talbot P, et al: How well are "cured" anorexia
    nervosa patients? an investigation of 16 weight-recovered anorexic
    patients. Br J Psychiatry 163:195–200, 1993

Wonderlich SA, Swift WJ: Borderline versus other personality disorders
    in the eating disorders: clinical description. Int J Eat Disord 9:629–638,
    1990

Chapter 6

Dissociative Symptomatology in Adult Patients With Histories of Childhood Physical and Sexual Abuse

James A. Chu, M.D.

The abuse and maltreatment of children—some of the most vulnerable members of our society—continues at near epidemic proportions. In the United States in 1990, 2.7 million cases of suspected child maltreatment were reported to child protective agencies, and in nearly half of the cases, child maltreatment was substantiated (National Research Council 1993). These figures may represent a substantial underestimate of prevalence as intrafamilial abuse often occurs in great secrecy and often goes unreported to child protective agencies. While not all, and perhaps not even most, of these children will develop serious psychiatric difficulties, a substantial number are likely to suffer lasting effects.

Over the past decade, we have begun to understand some of the psychological and psychiatric effects of childhood abuse. Clinical investigations have suggested that early abuse may be associated with numerous psychological and psychiatric difficulties, including depression, anxiety, impaired self-esteem, poor social functioning, self-destructive behavior, impaired personality development, alcohol and drug abuse, eating disorders, somatization, and various physiological changes (Bagley and Ramsey 1986; Barksy et al. 1994; Bryer et al. 1987; Courtois 1979; Finkelhor 1984; Gelinas 1983; Goldman et al. 1992; Hall et al. 1986; Herman 1981; Herman and van der Kolk 1987; Herman et al. 1986, 1989; Loewenstein 1990; Ludolph et al. 1990; Morrison 1989; National Victim

Center and Crime Victims Research and Treatment Center 1992; Ogata et al. 1990; Pribor and Dinwiddie 1992; Pribor et al. 1993; Russell 1986; Shapiro 1987; Summit 1983; Swanson and Biaggo 1985; van der Kolk 1987; van der Kolk et al. 1991; Welch and Fairburn 1994; Zanarini et al. 1987). Although many of these associated difficulties are based on clinical observations and preliminary studies, there appears to be considerable morbidity associated with certain kinds of early traumatization. In recent years, clinicians and investigators have focused on posttraumatic and dissociative symptoms that appear to be etiologically related to childhood traumatization (Bernstein and Putnam 1986; Braun 1990; Chu 1991; Chu and Dill 1990; Coons et al. 1990; Donaldson and Gardner 1985; Kirby et al. 1993; Putnam 1985; Putnam et al. 1986; Ross et al. 1991; Saxe et al. 1993; Ulman and Brothers 1988; van der Kolk and Kadish 1987). Dissociative symptoms, including depersonalization, derealization, dissociative amnesia, fragmentation of identity, and posttraumatic reexperiencing phenomena (e.g., "flashbacks" of traumatic events), are frequent clinical findings in disorders that derive from childhood abuse. In this chapter, I present several studies of dissociative symptoms in psychiatric patients and describe some of the common clinical presentations of patients with dissociative symptomatology.

Dissociative Symptoms in Relation to Childhood Abuse

Until the mid-1980s, childhood trauma was not generally acknowledged as a major cause of adult psychiatric psychopathology. It is only in the past few years that clinicians have begun to ask routinely about histories of childhood abuse and about posttraumatic and dissociative symptomatology. Dissociative symptoms resulting from traumatic experiences appear to be particularly prominent because they offer a psychological defense against overwhelming stimuli. Painful events can be made less intense through dissociative alterations in perceptions (depersonalization and derealization); can be made unconscious (dissociative amnesia); can be

fragmented into separate cognitive, affective, and somatic components (various forms of posttraumatic stress disorder [PTSD]); or
even can be disowned (dissociative identity disorder). However,
repressed and dissociated experiences do not remain dormant.
As noted both by classic psychoanalytic theorists (e.g., Freud
1920/1955; Janet 1907) and by modern investigators of PTSD (e.g.,
Chu 1991; Putnam 1985; van der Kolk and Kadish 1987), repressed
and dissociated experiences are reexperienced in the form of
dreams and nightmares, flashbacks, and flooding of feelings and
sensations related to the original experiences. Thus, many patients
who have used dissociation to cope with traumatic experiences
have a constellation of symptoms that include both dissociative
defenses and reexperiencing phenomena. In our studies, both of
these clusters of symptoms are defined as dissociative experiences.

The recognition of dissocia-
tive symptoms and trauma-related disorders in general psychiatric populations was relatively rare. In 1988, we began a survey of
women psychiatric inpatients to determine the prevalence of histories of abuse, dissociative symptoms, and any correlation between histories of abuse and dissociation (Chu and Dill 1990). The
target group for this initial study included all adult women con-
secutively admitted to a large private psychiatric hospital. One
hundred fifty-six women were asked to participate and 103 (66%)
agreed to participate; 18 of the 156 women (12%) were judged not
competent to give informed consent to participate, and 35 (22%)
refused. Of the 103 participants, data for 5 were incomplete, leaving 98 subjects.

The subjects' mean age was 34 years. Nearly all (93) were white.
Fifty-one had never been married, 25 were married, and 22 were
separated, divorced, or widowed. Forty-four were employed. Subjects completed three self-report instruments: the Symptom
Checklist-90—Revised (SCL-90-R; Derogatis 1983), the Dissociative Experiences Scale (DES; Bernstein and Putnam 1986), and a
Life Experiences Questionnaire (Bryer et al. 1987) that includes
questions about childhood trauma. Estimates of the prevalence of
abuse were based on responses to the Life Experiences Questionnaire, which includes questions about being "hit really hard,

kicked, punched, stabbed, or thrown down" and being "pressured against your will into forced contact with the sexual parts of your body or his/her body." A stringent definition of sexual abuse was used requiring genital contact. Estimates of the prevalence of dissociative symptoms were based on comparisons of the subjects' symptom levels with previously established levels in posttraumatic and dissociative disorders (Bernstein and Putnam 1986). To further define correlates of dissociation, the 24 subjects who reported high levels of dissociation were compared to a randomly selected group of 24 subjects with low levels of dissociation. Finally, to test whether histories of abuse predicted adult symptoms, DES scores, SCL-90-R global severity scores, and SCL-90-R subscale scores were submitted to individual two-by-two analyses of variance.

Nearly two-thirds (63%) of the subjects reported some kind of abuse before age 16 years. Approximately half (51%) reported physical abuse, more than a third (36%) reported sexual abuse, and approximately one-quarter (23%) reported both kinds of abuse. Subjects could be in more than one group (e.g., the physical abuse group included those with only physical abuse plus those with both physical and sexual abuse). These data are comparable to those of a similar study by Bryer et al. (1987) when data from our study are corrected for the less stringent criteria that Bryer et al. used for sexual abuse (including sexualized touching/kissing) (see Table 6–1).

Of the 50 subjects reporting childhood physical abuse, the majority (92%, $n = 46$) named family members as perpetrators. With regard to subsequent victimization, our data suggest that if subjects were physically abused as children that they were more likely to be physically abused as adults, with an odds ratio of more than 17 to 1. Of the 35 subjects who reported childhood sexual abuse, most (77%, $n = 27$) were abused by family members. The majority reported multiple incidents. Twenty-eight (80%) reported that the earliest incident occurred before puberty. Childhood sexual abuse more than doubled the risk of subsequent adult sexual abuse, with an odds ratio of more than 2 to 1.

Subjects reported a high rate of dissociative symptoms on the

Table 6–1. Prevalence of childhood abuse in female psychiatric inpatients

	Chu and Dill (1990) study		
	Genital contact criteria for sexual abuse	Bryer et al. (1987) criteria for sexual abuse	Bryer et al. (1987) study
Abuse before age 16 years			
Physical abuse	51%	51%	38%
Sexual abuse	36%	47%	44%
Physical and sexual abuse	24%	31%	23%

DES. Eighty-one (83%) reported a level in excess of 4.4, the median for healthy adults as found by Bernstein and Putnam (1986). Nearly one-quarter of the sample (24%, $n = 24$) had symptom scores above the level established for PTSD, and six (6%) had scores higher than the median for multiple personality disorder (MPD) (see Table 6–2).

Although the DES is not considered a diagnostic tool, these findings are remarkable, congruent with findings from a study by Ross et al. (1991). Using a structured diagnostic interview, Ross et al. (1991) studied a general psychiatric inpatient population of both men and women and found that approximately 21% had an atypical dissociative disorder and approximately 5% had MPD.

Childhood abuse was clearly related to a higher level of adult dissociative symptoms, as shown in Table 6–3. Results showed a main effect for physical abuse, sexual abuse, and a significant interaction effect. DES scores were highest in subjects who reported experiences of both physical and sexual abuse in childhood.

Childhood abuse by family members was clearly related to a higher level of dissociative symptoms in adulthood (see Table 6–4). Extrafamilial abuse was relatively infrequent in this sample and was not clearly related to adult dissociative symptoms. Intrafamilial abuse implies boundary violations, interpersonal betrayals, and lack of care and nurturance, possibly leading to increased

Table 6–2.   Dissociative Experiences Scale (DES) scores in female
                 psychiatric inpatients

	n	%
Subjects scoring at or above the median scores for		
Control subjects (4.38)	81	83
Agoraphobia (7.38)	71	72
Schizophrenia (20.63)	32	33
Posttraumatic stress disorder (31.3)	24	24
Multiple personality disorder (57.1)	6	6

Table 6–3.   Dissociative Experiences Scale (DES) scores by category of
                 abuse in female psychiatric inpatients

	n	DES scores
Subjects with no abuse	36	11.04
Subjects with physical abuse	50	22.34[a]
Subjects with sexual abuse	35	25.76[a]
Subjects with physical and sexual abuse	23	34.11[a]

Note.   DES = Dissociative Experiences Scale.
[a]Significant at $P < .01$.

isolation of the victims. Our results also showed that only 3 of the
35 subjects (9%) who were sexually abused ever told anyone about
it around the time of occurrence. It is perhaps the absence of external family support that leads to the increased development of internal dissociative defenses.

Childhood abuse experiences were variably related to general
psychiatric symptoms in adulthood, as shown in Table 6–5. On
comparison of SCL-90-R scores of abused versus nonabused
subjects, there were significant main effects only for physical
abuse on the global severity index and the subscales for interpersonal sensitivity, anxiety, hostility, paranoid ideation, and
psychoticism.

This study demonstrated a high level of childhood abuse in psychiatric inpatients and high levels of dissociative symptoms. In

Table 6–4. Dissociative Experiences Scale (DES) scores by category of abuse and perpetrators in female psychiatric inpatients

	n	**DES scores**
Physically abused subjects (*N* = 50)		
Perpetrators were family members	46	19.20[a]
Perpetrators were not family members	4	17.05
Sexually abused subjects (*N* = 35)		
Perpetrators were family members	27	23.04[b]
Perpetrators were not family members	8	11.52

Note.   DES = Dissociative Experiences Scale.
[a]Significant at $P < .01$; [b]significant at $P < .001$.

Table 6–5. SCL-90-R Scale scores by category of abuse in female psychiatric inpatients

SCL-90-R scale	No abuse (*n* = 36)	Physical abuse only (*n* = 27)	Sexual abuse only (*n* = 12)	Physical and sexual abuse (*n* = 23)
Somatization	62	65	63	67
Obsessive-compulsive	68	71	66	73
Interpersonal sensitivity	70	72[a]	67	75
Depression	70	72	69	75
Anxiety	68	72[a]	71	76
Hostility	63	71[a]	74	72
Phobic anxiety	67	67	63	70
Paranoid ideation	63	70[a]	64	71
Psychoticism	72	79[a]	68	81
Global severity index	69	73[a]	69	79

SCL-90-R = Symptom Checklist-90—Revised.
[a]Significantly higher than scores of subjects not physically abused ($P < .005$).

further review of the clinical records of the 24 subjects with DES scores above the median for PTSD, we found little documentation of dissociative symptoms and few diagnoses of PTSD and dissociative disorders. Although the DES is not a diagnostic instrument, the absence of clinical documentation nevertheless suggested that dissociative symptoms were being overlooked. Simple questions about depersonalization, derealization, dissociative amnesia, flashbacks, and switches in ego-states would likely have substantially increased PTSD or dissociative disorder diagnoses among the 24 subjects.

This study also suggested that although there is a clear correlation between childhood abuse and high levels of dissociative symptoms, there is little clear correlation between abuse and other general psychiatric symptoms. This finding helps to explain the common clinical situation in which dissociative symptoms are not recognized and there is confusion about diagnosis. In fact, a comparison of the clinical records of the subjects with high DES scores and a matched group of subjects with lower scores showed that those with high levels of dissociation had significantly more diagnoses and more previous hospitalizations, and they had received more somatic treatments (e.g., medications and electroconvulsive therapy).

The correlation between childhood abuse experiences and elevated dissociative symptoms strongly suggests that dissociative experiences are linked to childhood trauma. Our findings also suggested that severity of abuse is related to the level of dissociative experiences. Subjects who had experienced both physical and sexual abuse had high DES scores, but those who had only a single kind of abuse had much lower scores. The scores of subjects who were abused by family members were also high. Our findings showed, unfortunately, that both combined abuse and intrafamilial abuse were common in the backgrounds of our subjects. Overall, our findings should encourage clinicians to inquire about dissociative experiences and abuse histories. In the presence of high levels of dissociative symptoms, clinicians should include PTSD and dissociative disorders in the differential diagnoses and consider possible traumatic etiologies.

Correlates of Dissociative Symptomatology

What aspects of childhood abuse may lead to more lasting and damaging effects? Our findings supported our clinical observations that higher levels of dissociation in adulthood are related to the combination of childhood physical and sexual abuse. Other studies by Saunders and Giolas (1991) and Saunders et al. (1989) showed a significant correlation between frequency and severity of subjects' past stressful experiences and higher levels of current dissociative experiences. Terr's (1991) work in examining the effects of trauma on children also suggests that high frequency of abuse increases the severity of dissociative symptoms. Terr (1991) hypothesizes that dissociation is learned by the abused child, whose attempt to mentally escape the overwhelming experience begins as a conscious effort at blocking out the abuse. However, with repetition, dissociation becomes an automatic and uncontrollable response to abuse or a stimulus associated with abuse.

In addition to the growing evidence of the role of severity and frequency of abuse in the development of dissociative symptoms, it appears that the age at which trauma occurs also may be an important factor. Herman and Schatzhow (1987) and Briere and Conte (1993) have shown that patients with incest histories were more likely to report amnesia for their sexual abuse if it had occurred prior to adolescence. Dissociation appears to occur more readily and normatively in childhood and to decrease with age. Therefore, children subjected to abusive experiences may be more likely to use and retain dissociative defenses.

Our second study (Kirby et al. 1993) investigating the nature of dissociation examined the relationship between dissociative symptomatology and several different parameters of the abuse experience. It was hypothesized that greater severity or noxiousness of abuse, greater chronicity, and earlier age at onset would result in increased use of dissociative defenses and that each of these factors would be correlated with increased dissociative symptomatology in adulthood.

Subjects were recruited from three units of a private psychiatric hospital. Of 114 patients approached, 24 refused to participate and

11 failed to complete the questionnaire. Sixty-eight (60%) completed the questionnaire. Sixty-four of the 68 reported a history of physical and/or sexual abuse and were subjects for this study. The high prevalence of childhood abuse in this subject sample resulted from recruiting the majority of the subjects (81%) from a unit specializing in the treatment of posttraumatic disorders. The remainder were recruited from units treating affective disorders (16%) and psychotic disorders (3%). The subjects' mean age was 35 years, and 88% were white. Nineteen percent were married, 28% were divorced or separated, and 50% were never married. Thirty-six percent were employed full- or part-time, and 34% were disabled. Subjects completed the Life Experiences Questionnaire (Bryer et al. 1987) and the DES (Bernstein and Putnam 1986) in addition to other measures. Subjects' responses to the Life Experiences Questionnaire were analyzed for severity of sexual abuse, frequency of physical and sexual abuse, and age at onset of physical and sexual abuse. Subjects' self-reports of sexual abuse were assigned a degree of severity according to criteria described by Russell (1986). Frequency and age at onset were determined by subjects' self-report. Two group comparisons were used to test the hypothesis that more severe abuse and greater frequency of abuse would be associated with greater dissociative symptoms. Spearman correlations were used to test the hypothesis that age at onset of abuse would be inversely correlated with higher DES scores.

Ninety-five percent of the subjects ($n = 61$) had at some time in their lives been "pressured against [their] will" into sexual contact. Eighty-three percent ($n = 53$) had experienced physical contact that involved "being hit really hard, kicked, punched, burned, stabbed, or thrown down." Seventy-eight percent ($n = 50$) had experienced both kinds of abuse.

Of 59 subjects with a history of sexual abuse and complete data regarding severity, the majority, 49 (83%) had experienced penetration or attempted penetration (most severe). Six (10%) had experienced genital fondling without attempted penetration (severe), and four (7%) had experienced abuse without genital contact (least severe). DES scores for the least severe and severe groups were pooled for comparison against the most severe group. Table 6–6 shows that subjects in the most severe group ex-hibited a higher degree of dissociation than subjects in the less se-vere group.

Of 45 patients with a history of physical abuse and complete data, more than half reported being first abused before age 5 years and nearly three-quarters before age 11 years. We found it remarkable, even with this rather specialized patient population, that most of our sample first experienced physical abuse as very young children and nearly all experienced physical abuse before adolescence (see Table 6–7). Earlier age at onset of physical abuse was correlated with higher levels of dissociative symptomatology ($P < .05$).

Similarly striking data were obtained concerning childhood sex-ual abuse. Of 56 patients with a history of sexual abuse and com-plete data, more than half were first abused before age 5 years and most before age 11years (see Table 6–7). Again, most of our sub-jects experienced abuse in early childhood and before adoles-cence. Earlier age at onset of sexual abuse was highly correlated with higher levels of dissociative symptomatology ($P < .001$).

Although subjects were asked to quantify episodes of abuse, many recorded "countless," "all my life," or "every day." These re-sponses were interpreted to mean a number greater than 10. Of the 43 subjects with a history of physical abuse and complete data, more than three-quarters reported chronic abuse. Subjects with more chronic physical abuse had a higher level of dissociative symptoms than subjects with fewer experiences (see Table 6–8).

Table 6–6.   Dissociative Experiences Scale (DES) scores by severity of abuse

	n	%	DES scores
Subjects with less severe sexual abuse (sexual fondling or abuse without genital contact)	10	17	16
Subjects with more severe sexual abuse (attempted or completed intercourse)	49	83	33[a]

Note.   DES = Dissociative Experiences Scale.
[a]Significant at $P < .05$.

Table 6–7. Age at onset of childhood abuse

	n	%
Physical abuse		
Onset before age 5 years	26	58
Onset between ages 6 and 10 years	7	16
Onset between ages 11 and 15 years	3	7
Onset between ages 16 and 38 years	9	20
Sexual abuse		
Onset before age 5 years	33	59
Onset between ages 6 and 10 years	7	13
Onset between ages 11 and 15 years	13	23
Onset between ages 16 and 21 years	3	5

Similarly, of the 42 subjects with a history of sexual abuse and complete data, most reported chronic abuse. Subjects with more chronic sexual abuse also had a higher level of dissociative symptoms than subjects who were less frequently abused (see Table 6–8). Although there was a clear trend toward more dissociative experiences with more chronic sexual abuse, the difference did not reach statistical significance because of the small number of subjects abused infrequently.

The results of this study have good face validity. More severe and noxious abuse, early age at onset, and chronic abuse all contribute to the degree of traumatization and greater dissociation. Our data also support the notion that there may be a childhood window of vulnerability to the development of significant dissociative defenses that may persist into adulthood if these defenses are used regularly. Our conclusions are limited by the subject pool that was largely recruited from a specialized population being treated for trauma-based disorders and by the high degree of intercorrelation among the variables tested (e.g., early age at onset with chronicity of abuse). Nevertheless, it appears likely that all these factors exert some influence on the degree to which dissociative symptoms are developed in response to early traumatic experiences.

Table 6–8.   Chronicity of childhood abuse and Dissociative
Experiences Scale (DES) scores

	n	%	DES scores
Physical abuse			
Less than 10 experiences	9	21	7
More than 10 experiences	34	79	32[a]
("countless," "all my life," "every day")			
Sexual abuse			
Less than 10 experiences	8	19	6
More than 10 experiences	34	81	30[b]
(" countless," "all my life," "every day")			

*Note.*DES = Dissociative Experiences Scale.
[a]$P < .01$. [b]$P = .262$ (not significant).

Controversy Concerning Dissociative Amnesia

The idea that overwhelming experiences can be "forgotten" and then later recalled has its origins in major schools of thinking concerning intrapsychic experience. Many adult patients report extensive amnesia for childhood events. To some patients, much of their childhood is foggy. Others can recount the events of their past but feel as though it happened to someone else. Many patients describe a "Swiss-cheese memory," with gaps in the recall of their early experiences, or even complete amnesia for most events over months or years. In clinical settings, this level of dissociative amnesia may be highly significant, and many patients with this kind of amnesia eventually report recovered memories of extensive childhood abuse. Our studies (Chu and Dill 1990; Kirby et al. 1993) and others (Briere and Conte 1993; Herman and Schatzhow 1987) suggest that dissociative amnesia is particularly associated with chronicity of abuse, early age at onset, and severity of abuse. In fact, a reanalysis of the data from our second study showed that the association between dissociation and each of these parameters of abuse was driven primarily by a strong correlation of each of the parameters with the amnesia subscale of the DES (Carlson and Putnam

1988). any clinicians and investigators accept recovered memories of childhood abuse as essentially valid reports of repressed or dissociated early experiences. For some patients, clinical work with recovered memories has been a vehicle to resolution of psychiatric symptomatology and has led to an enhanced understanding of the traumatic etiologies of their difficulties. Recently, however, a number of investigators (Loftus 1993; Ofshe 1992; Ofshe and Singer 1994; Pope and Hudson 1995) have questioned the validity of recovered memory and have argued that such memories can be false and that many clinicians may be colluding in the creation of pseudomemories. In particular, a heated debate has emerged in recent years regarding the role of therapists in retrieving dissociated memories of childhood abuse.

Some investigators (Crabtree 1992; Kolb 1987; van der Kolk and Ducey 1989; van der Kolk and van der Hart 1991) have suggested that traumatic memories are stored separately from ordinary narrative memory and are less subject to ongoing modification in response to new experiences. In contrast to narrative memories that are integrative, malleable, and fitted into the individual's personal cognitive schemas, traumatic memories are said to be inflexible, nonnarrative, automatic, triggered, and disconnected from ordinary experience. This nonintegration may be the basis for dissociated remembering through behavioral reenactment, somatic sensation, or intrusive images that are disconnected from explicit memory of events. Because the memories are unassimilated, they retain their original force—" unremembered and therefore unforgettable" (van der Kolk and van der Hart 1991). Whereas ordinary narrative memory is dynamic and both changes and degrades over time, traumatic memory may be less changeable and has been described as "indelible" (LeDoux 1992).

Studies in the field of cognitive psychology have shown that memories can be remarkably subject to change and distortion. Investigators have studied the nature of memory in stressful (although not truly traumatic) experiences, including testing college students under demanding conditions (Eriksen 1952, 1953; Tudor and Holmes 1973) and exposing subjects to shocking photographic material (Christianson and Loftus 1987; Kramer et al.

1991). Subjects are often remarkably inaccurate in recounting details of their experience (Christianson and Loftus 1987, 1991; Holmes 1990; Kramer et al. 1991). However, details of the experiences that are central to the individual seem to be accurately retained. The role of suggestion in the malleability of memory also has been well established in laboratory studies (Loftus 1979; Loftus et al. 1989; Schooler et al. 1986; Schumaker 1991). In some protocols, subjects are shown pictures, slides, or videotapes of an event and are then asked to recall the event. When subjects are given cues or suggestions regarding the event, they often make errors concerning peripheral details of the events. Despite evidence that memory content can be influenced by suggestion, emotional arousal, and personal meaning, the bulk of memory research actually supports the accuracy of remembered events that are known to have occurred. However, there is also evidence that persons can have memory for events that did *not* occur. One well-known personal pseudomemory was described by Piaget (1962), the well-known Swiss theorist of cognitive development in childhood. During his childhood, Piaget had clear visual memory of someone trying to kidnap him from his pram when he was age 2. The memory also involved his nanny's chasing away the potential abductor and then going home and telling the family. Years later, when Piaget was 15, the nanny returned to the Piaget family and confessed that the incident had never occurred. Her motive had been to enhance her position in the household, but she subsequently had suffered guilt about the fabrication and about a reward that she had received.

Piaget's experience suggests that after being told about certain past events by a trusted individual, persons may create pseudomemories of events that never actually occurred. The "memories" may seem valid, and persons may not recall the true source of the information (so-called source amnesia). An experiment by Loftus and Coan further demonstrated that this phenomenon can readily occur. In the experimental protocol, an older brother attempted to instill a memory of an episode that had never occurred in the subject, his younger brother. He told his brother a story about the younger brother being lost in a shopping mall some years previously. Over the next several days, the younger brother began to have fragmentary memories of this "event." By the end of 2 weeks, he had a vivid memory of being lost, complete with essential details of what he had been told and with additional elaborations. Even after being informed about the experiment, the younger brother still had trouble believing that the incident had not occurred (E. F. Loftus and Coan, unpublished study, 1993).

The now well-known case of Paul Ingram has added evidence concerning the creation of pseudomemory. As described by Ofshe (1992) and Loftus (1993), Ingram, a law enforcement officer, was accused of abusing his daughter and other children and participating in satanic cult activities, including ritual sexual abuse and murder. At first he denied everything, but after interrogation and pressure from a psychologist and other advisers, Ingram began to have vivid memories of his involvement in the alleged abuse. Ofshe, an expert witness, attempted to test Ingram's suggestibility. He told Ingram that he had been accused of forcing his son and daughter to have sex together, an event that both his children had agreed had *not* occurred. Ingram initially had no memory of this "event," but after being urged to think about the scene, he began to vividly recall it and eventually confessed to the alleged activities. This apparent pseudomemory does not necessarily invalidate Ingram's other recollections. However, the case does raise issues concerning the effect on memory of questioning, suggestion, and interrogation in both legal and clinical settings.

Clinical research has generally supported the concepts of dissociative amnesia and recovered memory. Clinical investigators have found a relatively high rate of self-reported amnesia for childhood sexual abuse with subsequent recovery of memory (19%–62%) in subjects with self-reported histories of such abuse (Briere and Conte 1993; Herman and Schatzhow 1987; Loftus et al. 1994; Williams 1994). Moreover, these studies suggest that a higher incidence of amnesia is correlated with early onset of abuse, chronicity of abuse, and severity of abuse (e.g., violence, multiple perpetrators, physical injury, fear of death). Terr's investigations (1985, 1988, 1991) with traumatized children also have demonstrated that there are different effects depending on the chronicity of abuse. Children who have experienced limited, circumscribed trauma have hypermnesia—" clear, detailed accounts of their experiences [that make] one conclude that these memories stay alive in a very special way" (Terr 1991, p.14). In contrast, chronically traumatized children demonstrate extensive amnesia: "They may forget whole segments of childhood—from birth to age 9, for instance" (Terr 1991, p.16). Furthermore, she notes that this kind of chronic traumatization profoundly shifts characterological development resulting in "relative indifference to pain, lack of empathy, failure to define or acknowledge feelings, and absolute avoidance of psychological intimacy" (Terr 1991, p. 16). Thus, these chronically traumatized patients are most likely to have amnesia for their abuse, and given the level of denial and dissociative defenses they use, the accuracy of recovered memory in these patients may be most vulnerable to distortions and errors in recall.

Implications for Clinical Practice

Our studies and others document a high prevalence of dissociative symptoms in clinical populations—levels that may approach more commonly recognized psychiatric symptoms such as depression and anxiety. Although our studies included inpatients as subjects, there are indications that outpatient populations have similarly high levels of dissociation (Surrey et al. 1990). Clinicians need to be aware of the presence of dissociative symptoms and to develop the skills to observe and detect them. Simple questions can be used to elicit reports of depersonalization (e.g., "Do you ever feel as though your body is distorted or unreal?" or "Have you ever felt as though you are outside of your body observing yourself?") and derealization (e.g., "Do you ever see the world around you as distorted, foggy, or unreal?"). Dissociative amnesia can be detected by both direct questions (e.g., "How is your memory for current and past events?") and indirect questions (e.g., "Have you ever found evidence that you said or did something that you do not recall doing?").

Clinicians also should observe state changes that are not attributable to mood disorders or chemical dependency. For example, repeatedly observed abrupt changes of affect or behavior may signal the presence of shifts in dissociative states. Direct questions may be used to elicit evidence of state changes or shifts into prolonged dissociative states (e.g., "Do you ever feel or behave in ways that are very alien to you?" or "Do you sometimes find yourself becoming internally preoccupied for long periods of time without being aware of the passage of time?"). Careful evaluation of responses to these questions may reveal dissociative symptoms.

Dissociative reexperiencing of phenomena may take many forms. Flashbacks of past traumatic experiences are the clearest form of reexperiencing, but it is more common for adults with childhood abuse and delayed-onset posttraumatic responses to have partial reexperiencing phenomena. For example, intense waves of dysphoric affect, impulsive behavior, and/or painful somatic feelings may be experienced even in the absence of clear verbal or visual memory of traumatic events (Chu 1991). These clinical presentations may be confusing for both patients and clinicians because patients may be experiencing severe symptoms without any clear idea of their relationship to past events. These clinical observations are supported by research suggesting that there are different types of memory processes, such as explicit memory (including conscious visual and verbal memory) and implicit memory (including nonconscious behavioral learning, priming, and conditioned responses), that operate independently of each other (Graf and Schacter 1985; Schacter 1992). To the extent that affective, behavioral, and somatic memory are forms of implicit memory, they may be experienced quite differently and separately from explicit visual and verbal memory.

Dissociative symptoms also must be differentiated from symptoms of other disorders. For example, the auditory hallucinations (usually perceived as coming from inside the head) that are common in severe dissociative disorders may be communications between fragmented parts of the self and not necessarily evidence of a thought disorder. The dysphoria found in posttraumatic and dissociative states can be confused with primary major depression, and dissociative state changes and posttraumatic somatic overactivation can be similar to the affective lability of mood disorders.

Finally, clinicians must wrestle with the issues concerning dissociative amnesia. Clinicians must use caution in inquiring about histories of childhood abuse. There is little evidence that direct questioning about abuse per se results in false memories of abuse. However, research concerning the use of suggestion and certain kinds of interrogation has shown that memory content can be affected by interactions with others and that pseudomemory can be induced. Therefore, clinicians must be careful not to inquire about possible abuse in a way that even subtly suggests a particular kind of response.

Critics of the concept of recovered memory note that most clinical studies are based on self-report, which may be considerably altered, distorted, or even newly created or fabricated (Loftus 1993; Pope and Hudson 1995). One clinical study in the literature presents some independent corroboration of abuse memories (Herman and Schatzhow 1987), and numerous current studies are being done to examine what can be known about the validity of recovered memory. In the context of this continuing controversy, mental health professionals must be meticulous in their clinical practice. Clinicians must understand that fantasies about abuse, suspicions of or partly formed ideas about abuse, and dreams about abuse are not the same as the actuality of abuse. Especially when memories are fragmentary, clinicians must support the psychological validity of the memories but avoid coming to premature conclusions when there is insufficient evidence to support the occurrence of abuse. Similarly, when recovered memory begins to replace amnesia, clinicians must remain open to the possibility of real abuse but also must encourage patients to reconstruct their personal histories in a way that is thoughtful and rational and consistent with what is known about the past and current symptomatology.

The results of our studies and others in the literature are beginning to document the etiological relationship between childhood trauma and dissociation, which until recently has been supported only by anecdotal clinical observations. If the difficulties by patients with histories of abuse are directly related to the abuse experiences, it seems clear that definitive treatment cannot occur without acknowledging these experiences. Although many clinicians urge caution concerning extensive exploration of traumatic memories early in treatment, it seems important at least to acknowledge trauma early in the treatment of abuse survivors. Acknowledging the reality of the abuse can profoundly shift the attitudes of both patients and clinicians. In almost all instances, patients who have been abused continue to feel guilty, damaged, and defective. Clinicians treating such patients, if unaware that traumatic etiologies of the current disturbance exist, may collude with the patients in these beliefs about themselves. Treating professionals frustrated by their inability to understand their patients' complex clinical presentation and failure to respond to standard treatment protocols may come to view such patients as difficult and untreatable. Acknowledging the reality of the abuse casts a new light on such situations: clinicians are then able to sympathize with their patients' efforts to cope with overwhelming circumstances and to help patients understand their impact. This shift in attitude is essential for treating such patients and makes the often difficult task more tolerable and productive for both clinicians and patients.

References

Bagley C, Ramsey R: Sexual abuse in childhood: psychosocial outcomes and implications for social work. Social Work Practice in Human Sexuality 4:33–47, 1986

Barksy AJ, Wool C, Barnett MC, et al: Histories of childhood trauma in adult hypochondriacal patients. Am J Psychiatry 151:397–401, 1994

Bernstein EM, Putnam FW: Development, reliability, and validity of a dissociation scale. J Nerv Ment Dis 174:727–734, 1986

Braun BG: Dissociative disorders as sequelae to incest, in Incest-Related Syndromes of Adult Psychopathology. Edited by Kluft RP. Washington, DC, American Psychiatric Press, 1990, pp 227–246

Briere J, Conte J: Self-reported amnesia for abuse in adults molested as children. J Trauma Stress 6:21–32, 1993

Bryer JB, Nelson BA, Miller JB, et al: Childhood sexual and physical abuse as factors in adult psychiatric illness. Am J Psychiatry 144:1426–1430, 1987

Carlson EB, Putnam FW: Further validation of the Dissociative Experiences Scale. Paper presented at the annual meeting of the American Psychological Association, 1988

Christianson S-Å, Loftus E: Memory for traumatic events. Applied Cognitive Psychology 1:225–239, 1987

Christianson S-Å, Loftus E: Remembering emotional events: the fate of detailed information. Memory and Cognition 5:81–108, 1991

Chu JA: The repetition compulsion revisited: reliving dissociated trauma. Psychotherapy 28:327–332, 1991

Chu JA, Dill DL: Dissociative symptoms in relation to childhood physical and sexual abuse. Am J Psychiatry 147:887–892, 1990

Coons PM, Cole C, Pellow T, et al: Symptoms of posttraumatic stress and dissociation in women victims of abuse, in Incest-Related Syndromes of Adult Psychopathology. Edited by Kluft RP. Washington, DC, American Psychiatric Press, 1990, pp 205–225

Courtois C: The incest experience and its aftermath. Victimology 4: 337–347, 1979

Crabtree A: Dissociation and memory: a two hundred year perspective. Dissociation 5:150–154, 1992

Derogatis LR: SCL-90-R: Administration, Scoring, and Procedures Manual II. Towson, MD, Clinical Psychometric Research, 1983

Donaldson MA, Gardner R: Diagnosis and treatment of traumatic stress among women after childhood incest, in Trauma and Its Wake. Edited by Figley C. New York, Brunner/Mazel, 1985, pp 356–377

Eriksen C: Defense against ego threat in memory and perception. Journal of Abnormal and Social Psychology 3:253–256, 1952

Eriksen C: Individual differences in defensive forgetting. Journal of Experimental Psychology 44:442–443, 1953

Finkelhor D: Child sexual abuse: new theory and research. New York, Free Press, 1984

Freud S: Beyond the pleasure principle (1920), in The Standard Edition of the Complete Psychological Works of Sigmund Freud, Vol 18. Translated and edited by Strachey J. London, Hogarth Press, 1955, pp 1–64

Gelinas DJ: The persisting negative effects of incest. Psychiatry 46: 312–332, 1983

Goldman SJ, D'Angelo EJ, DeMaso DR, et al: Physical and sexual abuse among children with borderline personality disorder. Am J Psychiatry 149:1723–1726, 1992

Graf P, Schacter DL: Implicit and explicit memory for new associations in normal and amnesic subjects. J Exp Psychol Learn Mem Cogn 11: 501–518, 1985

Hall RCW, Tice L, Beresford TP, et al: Sexual abuse in patients with anorexia and bulimia. Psychosomatics 30:73–79, 1986

Herman JL: Father-daughter incest. Cambridge, MA, Harvard University Press, 1981

Herman JL, Schatzhow E: Recovery and verification of memories of childhood sexual trauma. Psychoanalytic Psychology 4:1–14, 1987

Herman JL, van der Kolk BA: Traumatic antecedents of borderline personality disorder, in Psychological Trauma. Edited by van der Kolk BA. Washington, DC, American Psychiatric Press, 1987, pp 111–127

Herman JL, Russell D, Trocki K: Long-term effects of incestuous abuse in childhood. Am J Psychiatry 143:1293–1296, 1986

Herman JL, Perry JC, van der Kolk BA: Childhood trauma in borderline personality disorder. Am J Psychiatry 146:490–495, 1989

Holmes DS: Evidence for repression: an examination of 60 years of research, in Repression and Dissociation: Implication for Personality Theory, Psychopathology, and Health. Edited by Singer JL. Chicago, University of Chicago Press, 1990, pp 85–102

Janet P: The Major Symptoms of Hysteria. New York, Macmillan, 1907

Kirby JS, Chu JA, Dill DL: Severity, frequency, and age of onset of physical and sexual abuse as factors in the development of dissociative symptoms. Compr Psychiatry 34:258–263, 1993

Kolb LC: A neuropsychological hypothesis explaining posttraumatic stress disorders. Am J Psychiatry 144:989–995, 1987

Kramer TH, Buckhout R, Fox P, et al: Effects of stress on recall. Applied Cognitive Psychology 5:483–488, 1991

LeDoux JE: Emotion as memory: anatomical systems underlying indelible neural traces, in The Handbook of Emotion and Memory. Edited by Christianson S-Å. Hillsdale, NJ, Lawrence Erlbaum, 1992, pp 289–297

Loewenstein RJ: Somatoform disorders in victims of child abuse, in Incest-Related Syndromes of Adult Psychopathology. Edited by Kluft RP. Washington, DC, American Psychiatric Press, 1990, pp 75–112

Loftus EF: Reacting to blatantly contradictory information. Memory and Cognition 7:368–374, 1979

Loftus EF: The reality of repressed memories. Am Psychol 48:518–537, 1993

Loftus EF, Korf NL, Schooler JW: Misguided memories: sincere distortions of reality, in Credibility Assessment. Edited by Yuille JC. Norwell, MA, Kluwer Academic, 1989, pp 155–173

Loftus EF, Polonsky S, Fullilove MT: Memories of childhood sexual abuse. Psychology of Women Quarterly 18:64–84, 1994

Ludolph PS, Westen D, Misle B, et al: The borderline diagnosis in adolescents: symptoms and developmental history. Am J Psychiatry 147:470–476, 1990

Morrison J: Childhood sexual histories of women with somatization disorder. Am J Psychiatry 146:239–241, 1989

National Research Council, Commission on Behavioral and Social Sciences and Education, Panel on Research on Child Abuse and Neglect: Understanding Child Abuse and Neglect. Washington, DC, U.S. Government Printing Office, 1993

National Victim Center and Crime Victims Research and Treatment Center: Rape in America: a report to the nation. Arlington, VA, National Victim Center, 1992

Ofshe RJ: Inadvertent hypnosis during interrogation: false confession due to dissociative state, misidentified multiple personality and the satanic cult hypothesis. Int J Clin Exp Hypn 40:125–126, 1992

Ofshe RJ, Singer MT: Recovered-memory therapy and robust repression: influence and pseudomemories. Int J Clin Exp Hypn 42:391–410, 1994

Ogata SN, Silk KR, Goodrich S, et al: Childhood sexual and physical abuse in adult patients with borderline personality disorder. Am J Psychiatry 147:1008–1013, 1990

Piaget J: Plays, Dreams and Imitation in Childhood. New York, Norton, 1962

Pope HG, Hudson JI: Can memories of child sexual abuse be repressed? Psychol Med 25:121–126, 1995

Pribor EF, Dinwiddie SH: Psychiatric correlates of incest in childhood. Am J Psychiatry 149:53–56, 1992

Pribor EF, Yutzy SH, Dean T, et al: Briquet's syndrome, dissociation, and abuse. Am J Psychiatry 150:1507–1511, 1993

Putnam FW: Dissociation as a response to extreme trauma, in Childhood Antecedents of Multiple Personality. Edited by Kluft RP. Washington, DC, American Psychiatric Press, 1985, pp 65–97

Putnam FW, Guroff JJ, Silberman EK, et al: The clinical phenomenology of multiple personality disorder: a review of 100 cases. J Clin Psychiatry 47:258–293, 1986

Ross CA, Anderson G, Fleisher WP, et al: The frequency of multiple personality disorder among psychiatric inpatients. Am J Psychiatry 148:1717–1720, 1991

Russell DEH: The Secret Trauma: Incest in the Lives of Girls and Women. New York, Basic Books, 1986

Saunders B, Giolas MH: Dissociation and childhood trauma in psychologically disturbed adolescents. Am J Psychiatry 148:50–54, 1991

Saunders B, McRoberts G, Tollefson C: Childhood stress and dissociation in a college population. Dissociation 2:17–23, 1989

Saxe GN, van der Kolk BA, Berkowitz R, et al: Dissociative disorders in psychiatric inpatients. Am J Psychiatry 150:1037–1042, 1993

Schacter DL: Priming and multiple memory systems: perceptual mechanisms of implicit memory. Journal of Cognitive Neurosciences 4:244–256, 1992

Schooler J, Gerhard E, Loftus E: Qualities of the unreal. J Exp Psychol Learn Mem Cogn 12:171–181, 1986

Schumaker JF (ed): Human Suggestibility: Advances in Theory, Research, and Application. New York, Routledge, 1991

Shapiro S: Self-mutilation and self-blame in incest victims. Am J Psychother 41:46–54, 1987

Summit R: The child sexual abuse accommodation syndrome. Child Abuse Negl 7:177–193, 1983

Surrey J, Swett C, Michaels A, et al: Reported history of physical and sexual abuse and severity of symptomatology in women psychiatric outpatients. Am J Orthopsychiatry 60:412–417, 1990

Swanson L, Biaggo MK: Therapeutic perspectives on father-daughter incest. Am J Psychiatry 142:667–674, 1985

Terr L: Remembered images of psychic trauma. Psychoanal Study Child 40:493–533, 1985

Terr L: What happens to memories of early childhood trauma? J Am Acad Child Adolesc Psychiatry 27:96–104, 1988

Terr L: Childhood traumas: an outline and overview. Am J Psychiatry 148:10–20, 1991

Tudor TG, Holmes DS: Differential recall of successes and failures. Journal of Research in Personality 7:208–224, 1973

Ulman RB, Brothers D: The Shattered Self. Hillsdale, NJ, Analytic Press, 1988

van der Kolk BA (ed): Psychological Trauma. Washington, DC, American Psychiatric Press, 1987

van der Kolk BA, Ducey CP: The psychological processing of traumatic experience: Rorschach patterns in PTSD. J Trauma Stress 2:259–274, 1989

van der Kolk BA, Kadish W: Amnesia, dissociation and the return of the repressed, in Psychological Trauma. Edited by van der Kolk BA. Washington, DC, American Psychiatric Press, 1987, pp 173–190

van der Kolk BA, van der Hart O: The intrusive past: the flexibility of memory and the engraving of trauma. American Imago 48:425–454, 1991

van der Kolk BA, Perry JC, Herman JL: Childhood origins of self-destructive behavior. Am J Psychiatry 148:1665–1671, 1991

Welch SL, Fairburn CG: Histories of childhood trauma in bulimia nervosa: three integrated case controls. Am J Psychiatry 151:402–407, 1994

Williams LM: Recall of childhood trauma: a prospective study of women's memories of child sexual abuse. J Consult Clin Psychol 62:1167–1176, 1994

Zanarini MC, Gunderson JG, Marino MF: Childhood experiences of borderline patients. Compr Psychiatry 30:18–25, 1987

Chapter 7

Relationships Between Traumatic Experiences and Symptoms of Posttraumatic Stress, Dissociation, and Amnesia

Eve B. Carlson, Ph.D., Judith Armstrong, Ph.D., Richard Loewenstein, M.D., and David Roth, Ph.D.

E mpirical studies have begun to explore the relationships be-tween traumatic experiences and later symptoms of posttrau-matic stress, dissociation, and amnesia. In an ongoing study, we are collecting data from psychiatric inpatients relating to these vari-ables with particular attention to childhood experiences of abuse. In this chapter, we describe our understanding of the relationships between traumatic experiences and these later symptoms, and we briefly review the relevant literature. We then describe and discuss some preliminary results from our study.

When people have traumatic experiences, they show a range of psychological and physiological responses that include hypera-rousal, avoidance, aggression, and depression. We see these as broad categories that include different specific symptoms. For ex-ample, hyperarousal includes symptoms of anxiety, posttraumatic stress disorder (PTSD), and some somatic symptoms. Avoidance can take the form of behavioral avoidance, emotional avoidance, or cognitive avoidance. Emotional and cognitive avoidance also might be conceptualized as dissociation because, for trauma pa-tients, the function of dissociation may be to allow patients to avoid disturbing trauma-related emotions and cognitions. Aggres-sion would include aggressive behaviors, emotions, and thoughts directed toward oneself or toward others. Depression would include symptoms of depressed behaviors, emotions, and thoughts.

Because all of these symptoms can occur in response to trauma, we consider all of them to be possible posttraumatic stress symptoms. In this chapter, we use the term *posttraumatic stress disorder* to refer to the smaller set of posttraumatic stress symptoms that constitute DSM-III-R (American Psychiatric Association 1987) and DSM-IV (American Psychiatric Association 1994) diagnostic criteria for PTSD. Of the various responses to trauma studied to date, it appears that PTSD symptoms and dissociative symptoms are the most prominent in terms of their capacity to differentiate between persons who have had traumatic experiences and those who have not. Furthermore, these two types of symptoms seem to be the most strongly related to aspects of the traumatic experiences. For these reasons, we focus on PTSD symptoms and dissociative symptoms in this chapter.

PTSD symptoms are one facet of hyperarousal symptoms experienced following trauma. We conceptualize hyperarousal symptoms to be part of a preparatory response of the body and the mind to a generalized expectancy of danger. In other words, when trauma patients are reminded of a traumatic experience, they anticipate a loss of control over their own safety. Because of this expectation, the body and mind are put on "red alert," and these individuals experience symptoms of physiological arousal, including anxiety, somatic symptoms (as a result of chronic hyperarousal), and PTSD symptoms such as startle response, sleep problems, and autonomic arousal. They also will experience cognitive hyperarousal in the form of PTSD symptoms such as hypervigilance, intrusive thoughts, and nightmares. This conceptualization of the causal connection between trauma-related stimuli and hyperarousal symptoms is supported by findings of two studies in which combat veterans with PTSD showed hyperarousal in response to trauma cues (Orr et al. 1993; Pitman et al. 1990). We believe that this same causal relationship between trauma and hyperarousal applies to traumatic abuse experiences.

PTSD symptoms are clearly related to traumatic experiences, and countless studies have documented this relationship across a wide range of types of trauma. Research on child abuse trauma has revealed a similar pattern between trauma and PTSD symptoms. High levels of PTSD symptoms have been found in persons with histories of childhood abuse (Albach and Everaerd 1992; Coons et al. 1990; Kiser et al. 1991; Roesler and McKenzie 1994; D. Wolfe et al. 1994; V. V. Wolfe et al. 1989). At least one study has found higher levels of PTSD symptoms in samples of abused individuals than in nonabused control subjects (Briere 1988).

Behavioral, emotional, and cognitive avoidance of trauma-related stimuli are all commonly observed in trauma patients. These symptoms all seem to be natural responses to the aversiveness of cues associated with traumatic experiences. Of these three types of avoidance, emotional avoidance (in the form of numbing or dissociation) and cognitive avoidance (in the form of dissociation) are most readily measured. Measuring behavioral avoidance is more problematic because trauma patients may be unaware that they are avoiding reminders of the trauma, and consequently, they may be unable to report behavioral avoidance. In contrast, trauma patients are typically aware when they experience dampened affect, even when they don't understand why. Similarly, cognitive avoidance in the form of dissociation is experienced and can be reported without any need for awareness on the part of the trauma survivor. Dissociative experiences typically associated with traumatic experiences include amnesia (keeping experiences that are psychologically overwhelming out of awareness), depersonalization (distortions in perceptions of oneself), and derealization (distortions in perceptions of the environment). A causal connection between trauma and dissociation recently has been demonstrated by Bremner (in press), who found elevated levels of dissociative symptoms following trauma cues in combat veterans. We believe that a similar causal connection exists between trauma and dissociation in individuals who have been abused.

High levels of dissociation have been observed in subjects who have histories of childhood abuse (American Psychiatric Association 1987; Chu and Dill 1990; Coons et al. 1989; DiTomasso and Routh 1993; Goodwin et al. 1990; Putnam 1985; Swett and Halpert 1993; van der Kolk 1987; van der Kolk and Kadish 1987). Some studies have found higher levels of dissociation in samples of abused individuals than in nonabused control subjects (Briere 1988; Briere and Runtz 1988; Chu and Dill 1990; Strick and Wilcoxon 1991). One subtype of dissociation, derealization, was associated with childhood sexual abuse in two studies of patients with borderline personality disorder (BPD) (Ogata et al. 1990; Westen et al. 1990). Another subtype of dissociation, dissociative amnesia, also has been associated with childhood abuse experiences. Briere and Conte (1993) found that a high proportion (59%) of adults who had been sexually abused as children had amnesia for their abuse for some time following the experience. Williams (1994) found amnesia for a sexual assault experience in 38% of a sample of adults who had been sexually assaulted as children.

Several aspects of traumatic experiences, or trauma factors, influence the severity of symptoms seen in those who have experienced trauma. These trauma factors include severity of the trauma, developmental level at the time of trauma, social context in which the trauma occurred and in which the person is recovering, biological factors (such as biological resilience and vulnerability), and subsequent life events (particularly additional traumatic experiences). Of these, the severity of the trauma appears to be both a strong predictor of the trauma response and readily quantifiable. In this chapter, we limit our discussion of trauma factors in order to address severity of the trauma.

The idea that the amount and intensity of traumatic experiences are closely associated with the severity of the patient's response is intuitively appealing but has been firmly established empirically only in studies of combat veterans (see Bremner et al. 1994 for a review). Study of this issue in other populations has been hampered by a relative lack of attention to quantification of traumatic experiences. In most studies, subjects are categorized as exposed to a particular traumatic experience or not exposed to that traumatic experience, and differences in the experiences of those who are exposed are not closely examined. For example, in abuse research, those who experienced one event of sexual assault (e.g., one incident of fondling) are typically grouped with those who experienced severe, long-term sexual abuse (such as several years of incestuous sexual abuse). This grouping effectively obscures important differences in the experiences and responses of individuals whose abuse was very different.

For this reason, we believe that it is important to quantify abuse experiences in a way that reflects the severity of the stressor. As it applies to abuse, the severity of the stressor variable can be conceptualized as including the extent of the abuse, nature of the abuse, duration of the abuse, and number of different abusers. In this study, we defined and measured extent of abuse by calculating an index that included both the frequency and the intensity of abuse experiences.

A few studies to date have quantified traumatic experiences so that the strength of the association between severity of trauma and PTSD symptoms can be assessed. In one study, Resnick et al. (1989) found that level of combat exposure was significantly related to PTSD symptomatology in a sample of Vietnam veterans. Sales et al. (1984) found that the degree of violence experienced during rape affected PTSD symptoms in a group of rape victims. In addition, Wilson et al. (1985) found that loss of a loved one and degree of life threat were associated with more severe PTSD symptoms in various groups of trauma survivors.

In several studies, abuse trauma was quantified and correlated with PTSD symptoms. In a study of children who had been sexually abused, D. Wolfe et al. (1994) found a relationship between the severity of sexual abuse and PTSD symptoms. Roesler and McKenzie (1994) found the same relationship in a group of adults who had been sexually abused as children. In studies of adult veterans, Rowan et al. (1994) found a relationship between the severity of sexual abuse and PTSD symptoms, and Zaidi and Foy (1994) found a relationship between the severity of physical abuse and PTSD symptoms.

Studies of several different populations have quantified abuse and related severity of abuse to level of dissociation. Several studies have found a relationship between severity of sexual abuse and later levels of dissociation in adults (Irwin 1994; Maynes and Feinauer 1994; Shearer 1994; Zatzick et al. 1994). One study also found a relationship between severity of physical abuse and later levels of dissociation in a sample of adult women with BPD (Shearer

1994). Sandberg and Lynn (1992) found that female college students with higher levels of dissociation reported greater amounts of physical and sexual abuse than did those with lower levels of dissociation. In addition, dissociation was found to be moderately correlated with severity of abuse in an inpatient adolescent psychiatric sample (Sanders and Giolas 1991).

Also of interest is the relationship between PTSD symptoms and dissociation. Finding out how these two prominent responses to trauma relate to one another may shed light on the psychological mechanisms involved in responses to trauma. Two studies to date have correlated dissociation and PTSD levels to investigate the strength of the relationship between these two symptoms. Carlson and Rosser-Hogan (1991) found that dissociation and PTSD symptoms were highly correlated in a group of Cambodian refugees. Bremner et al. (1992) found a moderately high correlation between dissociative and PTSD symptoms in a sample of Vietnam combat veterans.

In an ongoing study of a wide range of experiences and symptoms in adult psychiatric patients, we measured the extent of childhood sexual and physical abuse and current levels of post-traumatic stress and dissociative symptoms. Also, as an additional measure of dissociation, we asked subjects specifically about their past amnesia for abuse experiences.

Method

Subjects

In a large, private, nonprofit psychiatric hospital primarily serving urban and suburban areas, we sought to interview all newly admitted patients who were coherent and stable enough to be interviewed. Some patients were not approached because the admitting psychiatrist or psychologist did not respond to our request for permission to approach the patient in time for us to interview the patient before discharge. For other patients, we received permission to approach them but were unable to interview them before they were discharged.

Of 187 subjects interviewed to date, 58% were female and 42% were male. The average age of subjects was 37.8 (SD = 4.8). We sampled only subjects who were between ages 30 and 45 years to control the length of the recall period for those reporting abuse experiences. In terms of race, 82% were white, 17% black, and 1% some other race. The sample was socioeconomically diverse and diverse in terms of marital status.

Materials

Physical abuse. The Physical Force Experiences as a Child form was used to collect information about various types of violence experienced before the age of 18 years. Subjects are asked, "When you were a child, did anyone ever use physical force on you?" If they answer "yes," they are asked for information about the person who used force and then asked a series of questions about specific types of force such as "Did this person ever throw something at you?" Subjects are asked about 10 different types of physical force, including experiences such as being slapped, hit, kicked, or burned. These same questions were used by Jacobson and Richardson (1987) in their study of physical and sexual assault experiences in psychiatric inpatients and by Jacobson (1989) in a similar study of psychiatric outpatients. Jacobson and Richardson's (1987) form for physical violence was a slightly modified version of one of the Conflict Tactics Scales (CTS; Straus 1979). The CTS is widely used in studies of family violence (see Straus and Gelles 1986). In its original form, it has been shown to have good reliability (Straus et al. 1980) and validity (Straus and Gelles 1986). In modifying Straus's scale, Jacobson (1989) used only items from the Physical Violence Scale and altered the format so that data could be collected about more than one abuser. In our study, we collected information on up to four abusers. Additions were made so that the form also collects information about the age at which the abuse by each abuser began and how long it lasted (duration of abuse) and the frequency of each different type of physical force experience.

We made an additional alteration to the scale by asking for the frequency of a behavior instead of asking for a category indicating

frequency (e.g., 6–10 times, 11–20 times). Because frequency estimates would be expected to be at least as accurate (if not more) as
ordinal category estimates, the continuous data provided by the
former were preferred to the ordinal data provided by the latter.

Sexual abuse. The Sexual Experiences as a Child form was used to
collect information about a wide variety of forced sexual experiences (e.g., being touched on sexual organs, forced intercourse)
that occurred before the age of 18 years. These same questions were
used by Jacobson and Richardson (1987) in their study of physical
and sexual assault experiences in psychiatric inpatients and by Jacobson (1989) in a similar study of psychiatric outpatients. Adapta-
tions were made to this form (similar to those previously described)
to collect information for up to four abusers and to collect information about the age at which the abuse by each abuser began, the
frequency of each different type of sexual experience, and the duration of abuse by each abuser.

Improving accuracy of reports of sexual and physical force. To
maximize accuracy of reports, wording of questions about sexual
and physical force experiences was factual and neutral, and the experiences were not labeled "abuse." Similarly, the person using
physical or sexual force on the child was not labeled an "abuser."
This wording is important because many victims of abuse do not
conceptualize their experiences as "abuse" and use of that label
seems likely to make reporting less accurate.

   To further improve the accuracy of reports, several methods
were used. First, a time line for life events was constructed with
each subject at the beginning of the interview. A specific list of key
life events was used to create a life history anchored in time. This
time line was later used to locate abuse events in time relative to
anchored life events. This method is expected to increase the accuracy of the retrospective reports by decreasing distortion and tele-
scoping of time in memory and by providing memory cues to
which subjects relate events (Bradburn et al. 1987; B. Cohen et al.
1984). Consequently, we expect to obtain more accurate reports of
abuse experiences.

Another method used to improve the accuracy of reporting was the use of specific verbal cues. In measuring abuse experiences, subjects were asked about the occurrence of specific experiences rather than being asked to recall freely their abuse experiences. Specific verbal cues tend to increase reporting of events that patients may be reluctant to report, such as physical and sexual abuse experiences. These verbal cues relieve subjects of the need for free responses and allows them to respond "yes" or "no" to questions of a sensitive nature. This method was recommended by B. Cohen et al. (1984) to increase the accuracy of reports in retrospective studies.

Retesting of a subset of subjects is also being employed to establish the reliability of the abuse reports and the measures used. Unfortunately, obtaining retest data has been difficult because the majority of inpatients are discharged before it is possible to test them a second time. As a result, too few subjects have been retested at this time to conduct meaningful statistical analyses. However, preliminary retest data look promising, with subjects reporting similar experiences on both occasions.

Although we have made considerable efforts to maximize the accuracy of the reports we are collecting, we do not conceptualize these reports as factual accounts of events experienced by subjects. It is likely that some subjects overreport or distort their abuse experiences and that some subjects underreport their experiences. The important questions are what proportion of subjects will report inaccurately and how extreme will their errors be. Based on our review of the literature on retrospective reports of traumatic experiences and others' reviews (e.g., Christianson and Loftus 1987), we believe that the impact of misreporting on a large set of data will be relatively minimal. Although we expect most subjects to have inaccuracies in their reports, we expect those inaccuracies to be relatively small for most subjects. Because we transformed the data for these variables before analysis (as described in the "Results" section), these minor inaccuracies in reporting will have a negligible effect on results. In the entire data set, we expect there to be only a handful of subjects who overreport or underreport to an extreme degree. Data from these subjects will contribute error to the data, but we expect it to have a minimal impact on the overall results. Furthermore, for all analyses, we examined the raw data to ensure that outliers were not exerting undue influence on the outcomes of any statistical tests.

Extent of abuse index.   To measure the extent of each type of abuse, we used an index that combined the frequency of force experiences with the intensity of the experiences. Separate scores for extent of sexual abuse and extent of physical abuse were calculated for each subject. To calculate each extent index, items constituting major physical or major sexual assault were assigned weights of 2 and other experiences were assigned weights of 1 (using the designations of major physical abuse described by Straus et al. [1980] and comparable designations for major sexual abuse). Specifically, experiences of physical assault such as being kicked, bitten, or hit with a fist (or more severe experiences) were "doubled-counted" so that the extent index would reflect intensity as well as frequency of experiences. Experiences of sexual force, such as having one's sexual organs touched (and similar or more severe sexual experiences involving physical contact) were doubled-counted to measure extent of sexual abuse. Applying unit weights is considered a better method than deriving weights by having judges rate experiences for severity. We use this method in accordance with the "simple is better" principle espoused by J. Cohen (1990). For example, a subject might have a sexual abuse extent score of 100 when she reported 20 major sexual force experiences (weighted by 2) and 60 nonmajor sexual force experiences.

It is important to note that the frequencies used in the indexes of extent represent frequencies of each specific experience item and not occasions on which abuse occurred. Counted in this way, a higher frequency count is assigned when multiple sexual or physical force experiences occurred on the same occasion. In the example above, wherein the subject has a sexual abuse extent score of 100 (for 20 major and 60 nonmajor sexual force experiences), these experiences might have occurred during only 20 occasions (with one major and three nonmajor sexual force experiences on each occasion).

Level of PTSD.   The Structured Interview for Posttraumatic Stress Disorder (SI-PTSD; Davidson et al. 1989) was used to quantify post-traumatic stress symptoms. The SI-PTSD includes questions about experiences that compose the diagnostic criteria for PTSD from DSM-III-R and DSM-IV (Davidson et al. 1989; Davidson et al. 1990). Interviewers assign subjects a score on a 4-point scale (from 0 = absent to 4 = extremely severe) for 17 PTSD items so that the SI-PTSD score can range from 0 to 68. The SI-PTSD has been found to have good interrater reliability, good test-retest reliability, and good concurrent validity (Davidson et al. 1989; Davidson et al. 1990). SI-PTSD scores were available only for subjects who reported one or more traumatic experiences. Some subjects who had abuse histories did not report having had a traumatic experience and were not administered the SI-PTSD.

Level of dissociation.   The Dissociative Experiences Scale (DES; Bernstein and Putnam 1986) was used to quantify the dissociative symptoms of subjects. This 28-item, self-report measure includes questions about experiences of amnesia, depersonalization, derealization, absorption, and imaginative involvement. Subjects are asked to circle a number to show what percentage of the time each experience happens to them. Total scores on the scale are the average of the 28 items' scores and can range from 0 to 100. The DES is a reliable and valid measure of the frequency of dissociative experiences that has been used in more than 250 published empirical studies (Bernstein and Putnam 1986; Carlson and Putnam 1993; Waller, in press).

Abuse categorization.   To distinguish between single or isolated incidents of sexual or physical assault and more chronic abuse experiences, we developed definitions to categorize subjects in terms of their abuse experiences. We did so because we expect subjects to have different responses to isolated incidents of assault than they have to chronic abuse experiences. For some analyses, we categorized subjects as having experienced no abuse, physical abuse only, sexual abuse only, or both sexual and physical abuse.

We categorized subjects as having been physically abused if the duration of their experiences was greater than 1 month *and* if they had experienced a total of 260 or more experiences of being hit or spanked hard, a total of 25 or more (over a period of 1 year) moderately severe physical force experiences (e.g., being pushed, hit with a fist, kicked), or a total of 10 very severe physical force experiences (e.g., being burned, beaten up, or threatened with a gun or knife). These criteria were set to identify what experiences we believe clearly constitute chronic physical abuse (as opposed to harsh physical discipline) but not to imply that experiences of less severity and/or shorter duration are not abuse. In fact, few subjects fell near cutoff points for criteria: almost all subjects experienced much less physical force or much more physical force than specified by the criteria.

We categorized subjects as having been sexually abused if they were forced to have sexual experiences on 4 or more occasions over a period of 1 month or more. We set no criteria for the intensity of the experiences because we view any forced sexual experiences that meet the above duration criteria to be potentially traumatizing. These criteria were set to identify what experiences we believe clearly constitute chronic sexual abuse (as opposed to isolated sexual assault experiences) but not to imply that experiences of less frequency and/or shorter duration are not abuse.

Amnesia for abuse.   To measure amnesia for abuse experiences, we asked subjects who reported abuse whether there was any time following the abuse when they had no memory of the experiences. We also asked whether there was any time when they remembered part but not all of the experiences. In this way, we were able to categorize subjects as having no amnesia, partial amnesia, or total amnesia for their abuse at some time in the past. We asked this question separately in regard to sexual and physical abuse.

Results

In general, the range of experience of physical and/or sexual abuse by subjects was extremely varied. By using the categorization method described, 21% (39) of the subjects were categorized as having experienced no abuse, 32.6% (61) of the subjects were categorized as having experienced physical abuse only, 6.4% (12) of the subjects were categorized as having experienced sexual abuse only, and 40% (75) of the subjects were categorized as having experienced both physical and sexual abuse. Thirteen percent (25) of the subjects reported experiencing sexual abuse that was extreme enough to yield extent of sexual abuse scores over 10,000. (To put that score in perspective, a person who reported being sexually assaulted by her father 4 times per week for 6 years, with 2 major and 4 nonmajor experiences of sexual force on each occasion, would have a score of 9,984.) Twenty-six percent (49) of the subjects reported experiencing physical abuse that was extreme enough to yield extent of physical abuse scores over 10,000.

Because the distributions of the extent of physical abuse and the extent of sexual abuse variables were extremely skewed, common logarithm transformations were performed on those variables. Pearson correlations were calculated between the extent of sexual abuse and SI-PTSD and DES scores and between the extent of physical abuse and SI-PTSD and DES scores. A Pearson correlation also was calculated between SI-PTSD and DES scores. Results of these analyses are shown in Table 7–1.

When the 113 subjects who reported sexual abuse experiences were asked if they had had partial or total amnesia for their sexual abuse experiences at any time in the past, 39% (44) of the subjects reported no amnesia, 19% (22) reported partial amnesia, and 42% (47) reported total amnesia. When the 168 subjects who reported physical abuse experiences were asked if they had had partial or total amnesia for their physical abuse experiences at any time in the past, 58% (97) of the subjects reported no amnesia, 21% (36) reported partial amnesia, and 21% (35) reported total amnesia.

Analyses of variance (ANOVAs) were calculated for extent of sexual abuse, SI-PTSD scores, and DES scores across levels of amnesia for sexual abuse. Group means and results of the ANOVAs are shown in Table 7–2. ANOVAs also were calculated for extent of physical abuse, SI-PTSD scores, and DES scores across levels of amnesia for physical abuse. Group means and results of the ANO-

Table 7–1.   Correlations among abuse extents and symptoms

	SI-PTSD	n	Dissociative Experiences Scale (DES)	n
Extent of sexual abuse	.59[b]	127	.48[b]	162
Extent of physical abuse	.41[b]	144	.26[a]	182
SI-PTSD			.63[b]	148

Note. SI-PTSD = Structured Interview for Posttraumatic Stress Disorder;
DES = Dissociative Experiences Scale.
[a]$P < .005.$ [b]$P < .00001.$

VAs are shown in Table 7–3. The maximum number of subjects available for each analysis is limited to the number of subjects who reported abuse experiences (110 for sexual abuse and 165 for physical abuse). These numbers differ from the abuse categorization numbers given above because some who reported abuse experiences did not meet the abuse criteria (usually because they experienced isolated assaults, not chronic abuse). The number of subjects differs across ANOVAs in Tables 7–2 and 7–3 because some subjects were unable to quantify abuse and some subjects were not administered the SI-PTSD because they reported no traumatic experiences.

Discussion

The results indicate that there are strong relationships between the extent of abuse experienced and later symptoms of PTSD and dissociation. Most noteworthy was an extremely large correlation between PTSD and extent of sexual abuse. This correlation seems to indicate that these PTSD symptoms are a primary response to childhood sexual abuse and that symptoms persist well into adulthood. The correlation between the extent of physical abuse and PTSD symptoms was also fairly high, indicating that PTSD symptoms are strongly associated with physical abuse trauma and that this response persists into adulthood. These findings are consistent with those of previous studies linking severity of abuse trauma to

Table 7–2.   Group means and analysis of variance results across levels of amnesia for sexual abuse experiences

	None	*n*	Partial	*n*	Total	*n*	*F*	df	*P*
Extent of sexual abuse	1.6	(40)	2.8	(21)	3.9	(31)	28.2	2, 89	.00001
SI-PTSD	27	(30)	30	(22)	40	(44)	7.9	2, 93	.0007
DES	29	(44)	32	(22)	45	(47)	6.4	2, 110	.002

Note.   SI-PTSD = Structured Interview for Posttraumatic Stress Disorder; DES = Dissociative Experiences Scale.

level of PTSD symptoms (Roesler and McKenzie 1994; Rowan et al. 1994; D. Wolfe et al. 1994; Zaidi and Foy 1994).

The correlation between the extent of sexual abuse experienced and dissociation was very high, whereas the correlation between the extent of physical abuse experienced and dissociation was moderate. These correlations seem to indicate that dissociation (in addition to PTSD symptoms) is a primary response to sexual abuse trauma but that it is less strongly associated with physical abuse experiences. The results also indicate that for many subjects the dissociative response to abuse trauma persists into adulthood. These findings, too, are consistent with those of previous studies linking severity of abuse trauma to level of dissociative symptoms (Irwin 1994; Maynes and Feinauer 1994; Sandberg and Lynn 1992; Sanders and Giolas 1991; Shearer 1994; Zatzick et al. 1994).

The high correlation between scores on the SI-PTSD and the DES seems to indicate that these two responses to trauma tend to co-occur. We interpret the relationship in this way because the two measures overlap little in the content of their questions. But further analyses need to be done to understand the extent to which the instruments (and the constructs they are meant to measure) overlap conceptually. The criteria on which the SI-PTSD is based, namely the DSM-III-R and DSM-IV criteria for PTSD, are ambiguous conceptually because they combine a variety of symptoms that may represent different psychopathological constructs. For example, the PTSD criteria include symptoms of autonomic

Table 7–3. Group means and analysis of variance results across levels of amnesia for physical abuse experiences

	None	n	Partial	n	Total	n	F	df	P
Extent of physical abuse	3.0	(97)	3.3	(35)	4.0	(31)	10.8	2,160	.00001
SI-PTSD	22	(73)	33	(29)	41	(32)	18.9	2,131	.00001
DES	22	(97)	36	(36)	51	(35)	29.1	2,165	.00001

SI-PTSD = Structured Interview for Posttraumatic Stress Disorder; DES = Dissociative Experiences Scale.

hyperarousal, cognitive hyperarousal, emotional numbing, cognitive avoidance, behavioral avoidance, cognitive intrusion, diminished cognitive functioning, anhedonia, and aggression. Three of these symptoms, emotional numbing, cognitive avoidance, and cognitive intrusion, could be conceptualized as aspects of dissociation. Although the measures do not overlap in actual content, their conceptual overlap may drive the strong relationship between scores. On the other hand, the measures' conceptual overlap may not be sufficient to account for the strong relationship between the scores. In either case, the set of symptoms we now call PTSD and the symptoms we now consider dissociative seem to co-occur in response to abuse trauma. Furthermore, both responses frequently persist long after the traumatic experience.

Results shown in Tables 7–2 and 7–3 indicate that higher levels of amnesia for abuse experiences are associated with higher extents of sexual and physical abuse and with higher levels of PTSD symptoms and dissociation. It is not surprising that those who experienced very severe abuse were more likely to have amnesia for the abuse. Similarly, it is not surprising that those who had more amnesia (and more severe abuse) also had higher levels of PTSD symptoms and dissociative symptoms. These findings are consistent with our findings of relationships between extent of sexual abuse and dissociation, between extent of physical abuse and dissociation, and between PTSD symptoms and dissociation. They also are consistent with Briere and Conte's (1993) findings of a rate of total amnesia of 59% among adults who were sexually abused as children.

It is also interesting to note the diversity in experience of amnesia across subjects, particularly the proportion of subjects who report that they have had no amnesia or only partial amnesia for their abuse at any time in the past. Most of the subjects reported remembering all or part of the abuse they had experienced. In the ongoing controversy about the prevalence of total amnesia for abuse, these findings may be helpful in establishing the actual rates of such reports. It is significant that these amnesia reports are from an inpatient population because it is one of the most disordered, and probably the most amnestic, populations of subjects.

Furthermore, because these reports were not elicited in the context of therapy or legal action, motivations for misreporting or fabrication seem minimal.

Clearly, there is difficulty in accurately assessing amnesia for abuse because it is possible that some subjects who report no amnesia may have reported inaccurately if they were currently experiencing partial amnesia (amnesia for some abuse experiences) at the time of the interview, and some who report no abuse may actually have had abuse experiences for which they are totally amnestic. Although it is difficult to determine how many subjects might fall into the first category (currently experiencing partial amnesia for some abuse), we believe that few fall into the latter category (totally amnestic). This belief follows from the finding that an extremely high proportion (79%) of the inpatient subjects reported some form of abuse. It seems unlikely that any sizable proportion of those who reported no abuse could be abused persons with amnesia because, if that were the case, the proportion of inpatients who experienced abuse would rise well above what we would reasonably expect from similar studies of inpatient populations (Chu and Dill 1990; Jacobson and Richardson 1987).

Conclusion

Results to date show strong relationships between severity of abuse trauma and symptoms of PTSD and dissociation. The results suggest that childhood abuse, especially sexual abuse, plays an important role in the development of severe psychiatric problems and that the extent of childhood abuse may explain a significant proportion of the variance in the severity of PTSD and dissociative symptoms experienced by adults. Because severity of abuse is highly related to some symptoms, treatment of the symptoms may be more effective if therapists are attentive to issues such as extent of abuse experienced. It also seems likely that routine screening for PTSD and dissociative symptoms among psychiatric inpatients would lead to identification of many with undetected early trauma histories.

Further analyses in this study are focusing on several aspects of abuse and other relevant experiences to account for variance in adult symptomatology. In addition to extent of abuse, these variables include age at onset of abuse, duration of abuse, number of different abusers, nature of the relationship to abusers, social support in childhood, aspects of the childhood home environment (such as neglect and chaotic home life), and number of additional traumatic experiences. Other responses that we also are studying include anxiety, depression, somatization, aggression, and self-destructiveness. We expect multivariate analyses of the influences of these trauma-relevant variables on adult symptomatology to further expand our understanding of human responses to traumatic experiences.

References

Albach F, Everaerd W: Posttraumatic stress symptoms in victims of childhood incest. Journal of Psychotherapy and Psychosomatics 57: 143–151, 1992

American Psychiatric Association: Diagnostic and Statistical Manual of Mental Disorders, 3rd Edition, Revised. Washington, DC, American Psychiatric Association, 1987

American Psychiatric Association: Diagnostic and Statistical Manual of Mental Disorders, 4th Edition. Washington, DC, American Psychiatric Association, 1994

Bernstein EM, Putnam FW: Development, reliability, and validity of a dissociation scale. J Nerv Ment Dis 174:727–735, 1986

Bradburn NM , Rips LJ, Shevell SK: Answering autobiographical questions: the impact of memory and inference on surveys. Science 236: 157–161, 1987

Bremner JD, Southwick S, Brett E, et al: Dissociation and posttraumatic stress disorder in Vietnam combat veterans. Am J Psychiatry 149: 328–332, 1992

Bremner JD, Southwick SM, Charney DS: Etiologic factors in the development of posttraumatic stress disorder, in Stress and Psychiatric Disorders. Edited by Mazure C. Washington, DC, American Psychiatric Press, 1994, pp 149–186

Bremner JD: Measurement of dissociative states with the Clinician Administered Dissociative States Scale (CADSS). Journal of Traumatic Stress, in press

Briere J: The long-term clinical correlates of childhood sexual victimization. Ann N Y Acad Sci 528:327–334, 1988

Briere J, Conte J: Self-reported amnesia for abuse in adults molested as children. J Trauma Stress 6:21–31, 1993

Briere J, Runtz M: Multivariate correlates of childhood psychological and physical maltreatment among university women. Child Abuse Negl 12:331–341, 1988

Carlson EB, Putnam FW: An update on the Dissociative Experiences Scale. Dissociation 6:16–27, 1993

Carlson EB, Rosser-Hogan R: Trauma experiences, posttraumatic stress, dissociation, and depression in Cambodian refugees. Am J Psychiatry 148:1548–1552, 1991

Christianson S-Å, Loftus EF: Memory for traumatic events. Applied Cognitive Psychology 1:225–239, 1987

Chu JA, Dill DL: Dissociative symptoms in relation to childhood physical and sexual abuse. Am J Psychiatry 147:887–892, 1990

Cohen B, Erikson P, Powell A: How does the length of recall period affect the number of physician visits reported? in Proceedings of the Social Statistics Section of the American Statistical Association. Washington, DC, American Statistical Association, 1984, pp 593–598

Cohen J: Things I have learned (so far). Am Psychol 45:1304–1312, 1990

Coons PM, Bowman E, Pellow TA, et al: Post-traumatic aspects of the treatment of victims of sexual abuse and incest. Psychiatr Clin North Am 12:325–335, 1989

Coons PM, Cole C, Pellow TA, et al: Symptoms of posttraumatic stress and dissociation in women victims of abuse, in Incest-Related Syndromes of Adult Psychopathology. Edited by Kluft RP. Washington, DC, American Psychiatric Press, 1990, pp 205–225

Davidson JRT, Smith RD, Kudler HS: Validity and reliability of the DSM-III criteria for posttraumatic stress disorder: experience with a structured interview. J Nerv Ment Dis 177:336–341, 1989

Davidson JRT, Kudler HS, Smith RD: Assessment and pharmacotherapy of posttraumatic stress disorder, in Biological Assessment and Treatment of Posttraumatic Stress Disorder. Edited by Giller EL. Washington, DC, American Psychiatric Press, 1990, pp 205–221

DiTomasso MJ, Routh DK: Recall of abuse in childhood and three measures of dissociation. Child Abuse Negl 17:477–485, 1993

Goodwin JM, Cheeves K, Connell V: Borderline and other severe symptoms in adult survivors of incestuous abuse. Psychiatric Annals 20: 22–32, 1990

Irwin HJ: Proneness to dissociation and traumatic childhood events. J Nerv Ment Dis 182:456–460, 1994

Jacobson AJ: Physical and sexual assault histories among psychiatric outpatients. Am J Psychiatry 146:755–758, 1989

Jacobson AJ, Richardson B: Assault experiences of 100 psychiatric inpatients: evidence of the need for routine inquiry. Am J Psychiatry 144:908–913, 1987

Kiser LJ, Heston J, Millsap PA, et al: Physical and sexual abuse in childhood: relationship with post-traumatic stress disorder. J Am Acad Child Adolesc Psychiatry 30:776–783, 1991

Maynes LC, Feinauer LL: Acute and chronic dissociation and somatized anxiety as related to childhood sexual abuse. American Journal of Family Therapy 22:165–175, 1994

Ogata SN, Silk KR, Goodrich S, et al: Childhood sexual and physical abuse in adult patients with borderline personality disorder. Am J Psychiatry 147:1008–1013, 1990

Orr SP, Pitman RK, Lasko NB, et al: Psychophysiological assessment of posttraumatic stress disorder imagery in World War II and Korean combat veterans. J Abnorm Psychol 102:152–159, 1993

Pitman RK, Orr SP, Forgue DF, et al: Psychophysiologic responses to combat imagery of Vietnam veterans with posttraumatic stress disorder versus other anxiety disorders. J Abnorm Psychol 99:49–54, 1990

Putnam FW: Dissociation as a response to extreme trauma, in Childhood Antecedents of Multiple Personality. Edited by Kluft RP. Washington, DC, American Psychiatric Press, 1985, pp 65–97

Putnam FW, Helmers K, Trickett PK: Development, reliability, and validity of a child dissociation scale. Child Abuse Negl 17:731–741, 1993

Resnick HS, Foy DW, Donahoe CP, et al: Antisocial behavior and post-traumatic stress disorder in Vietnam veterans. J Clin Psychol 45: 860–866, 1989

Roesler TA, McKenzie N: Effects of childhood trauma on psychological functioning in adults sexually abused as children. J Nerv Ment Dis 182:145–150, 1994

Rowan AB, Foy DW, Rodriguez N, et al: Posttraumatic stress disorder in a clinical sample of adults sexually abused as children. Child Abuse Negl 18:51–61, 1994

Sales E, Baum M, Shore B: Victim readjustment following assault. Journal of Social Issues 40:117–136, 1984

Sandberg DA, Lynn SJ: Dissociative experiences, psychopathology and adjustment, and child and adolescent maltreatment in female college students. J Abnorm Psychol 101:717–723, 1992

Sanders B, Giolas MH: Dissociation and childhood trauma in psychologically disturbed adolescents. Am J Psychiatry 148:50–54, 1991

Shearer SL: Dissociative phenomena in women with borderline personality disorder. Am J Psychiatry 151:1324–1328, 1994

Straus MA: Measuring intrafamily conflict and violence: the Conflict Tactics Scales. Journal of Marriage and the Family 41:75–88, 1979

Straus MA, Gelles R: Societal change and change in family violence from 1975 to 1985 as revealed by two national surveys. Journal of Marriage and the Family 48:465–479, 1986

Straus MA, Gelles RJ, Steinmetz SK: Behind Closed Doors: Violence in the American Family. New York, Anchor Books, 1980

Strick FL, Wilcoxon SA: A comparison of dissociative experiences in adult female outpatients with and without histories of early incestuous abuse. Dissociation 4:193–199, 1991

Swett C, Halpert M: Reported history of physical and sexual abuse in relation to dissociation and other symptomatology in women psychiatric inpatients. Journal of Interpersonal Violence 8:545–555, 1993

van der Kolk BA: The psychological consequences of overwhelming life experiences, in Psychological Trauma. Edited by van der Kolk BA. Washington, DC, American Psychiatric Press, 1987, pp 1–30

van der Kolk BA, Kadish W: Amnesia, dissociation, and the return of the repressed, in Psychological Trauma. Edited by van der Kolk BA. Washington, DC, American Psychiatric Press, 1987, pp 173–190

Waller NG: The Dissociative Experiences Scale, in Twelfth Mental Measurements Yearbook. Edited by Conoley JC, Impara JC. Lincoln, NE, University of Nebraska Press, 1995

Warshaw MG, Fierman E, Pratt L, et al: Quality of life and dissociation in anxiety disorder

Westen D, Ludolph P, Misle B, et al: Physical and sexual abuse in adolescent girls with borderline personality disorder. Am J Orthopsychiatry 60:55–66, 1990

Williams LM: Recall of childhood trauma: a prospective study of women's memories of child sexual abuse. J Consult Clin Psychol 62:1167–1176, 1994

Wilson JP, Smith WK, Johnson SK: A comparative analysis of PTSD among various survivor groups, in Trauma and Its Wake. Edited by Figley C. New York, Brunner/Mazel, 1985, pp 142–172

Wolfe D, Sas L, Wekerle C: Factors associated with the development of posttraumatic stress disorder among child victims of sexual abuse. Child Abuse Negl 18:37–50, 1994

Wolfe VV, Gentile C, Wolfe DA: The impact of sexual abuse on children: a PTSD formulation. Behavior Therapy 20:215–228, 1989

Zaidi LY, Foy DW: Childhood abuse experiences and combat-related PTSD. J Trauma Stress 7:33–42, 1994

Zatzick DF, Marmar CR, Weiss DS, et al: Does trauma-linked dissociation vary across ethnic groups? J Nerv Ment Dis 182:576–582, 1994

Chapter 8

Peritraumatic Dissociation and Posttraumatic Stress Disorder

Charles R. Marmar, M.D., Daniel S. Weiss, Ph.D., and
Thomas Metzler, M.A.

A Brief Overview of Empirical Studies of Trauma and Dissociation

The past decade has witnessed an intense resurgence of interest in the study of trauma and dissociation. In particular, the contributions of Janet, which had been largely eclipsed by developments within modern ego psychology, have been closely reexamined. Putnam (1989b) and van der Kolk and van der Hart (1989a, 1989b) have provided a contemporary reinterpretation of the contributions of Janet to the understanding of traumatic stress and dissociation.

Paralleling the resurgence of interest in theoretical studies of trauma and dissociation has been a proliferation of research studies addressing the relationship between trauma and general dissociative tendencies. Hilgard (1970) observed that students rated as highly hypnotizable reported more frequent histories of childhood punishment than their low-hypnotizability peers. She speculated that a heightened hypnotic capacity might confer protection against reexperiencing painful childhood memories. Chu and Dill (1990) reported that psychiatric patients with a history of childhood abuse reported higher levels of dissociative symptoms than those without histories of childhood trauma. Carlson and Rosser-Hogan (1991) reported a strong relationship between the amount of trauma in Cambodian refugees and the severity of both traumatic stress response and dissociative reactions. D. Spiegel and Cardena (1991) reviewed studies linking traumatic stress response and general dissociative tendencies and reported the following: 1) retrospective studies support a strong relationship between early physical or sexual abuse and later dissociative phenomenology, 2) repeated and severe childhood abuse is more strongly associated with adult dissociative phenomena than are isolated instances of abuse, 3) dissociation at the time of childhood trauma may be a mechanism to cope with overwhelming traumatic events, and 4) adults with posttraumatic stress disorder (PTSD) have higher levels of hypnotizability than adult patients without PTSD.

Following on Hilgard's (1970) original observations concerning trauma and hypnotizability, Stutman and Bliss (1985) reported that a nonpatient population of veterans who had high levels of PTSD symptoms were more hypnotizable than their counterpart veterans who had low levels of PTSD symptoms. D. Spiegel et al. (1988) compared the hypnotizability of Vietnam veterans who had PTSD with patients who had affective disorders, generalized anxiety disorder, and schizophrenia and with a healthy control group. The group with PTSD were found to have hypnotizability scores that were higher than both the psychopathology and healthy control subjects. Hypnotizability scores in childhood have been shown to have stable traitlike characteristics, raising the possibility that traumatized individuals with higher levels of pretrauma exposure hypnotizability may be more vulnerable to developing PTSD. It is also possible that chronic PTSD results in changes in level of hypnotizability. Prospective studies are required to assess these possibilities.

Recent empirical studies have supported a strong relationship among trauma, dissociation, and personality disturbances. Herman et al. (1989) found a high prevalence of traumatic histories in patients with borderline personality disorder (BPD) who reported dissociative symptoms. Level of adult dissociative symptoms was better predicted by childhood traumatic history than even the borderline diagnostic status. Ogata et al. (1990), in a study of trauma and dissociation in BPD, found a higher frequency of childhood abuse in subjects with BPD than in depressed control subjects.

A profound association has been reported for childhood trauma and multiple personality disorder (MPD). Kluft (1993) proposes a four-factor theory to explain the causes of MPD: 1) inherent capacity to dissociate, 2) traumatic life experiences that overwhelm the adaptational capacities of the child to use nondissociative defenses, 3) role of the environment in shaping the development of fragmented aspects of personality, and 4) inadequate availability of restorative experiences by protective others. Kluft (1993) proposes that the dissociative processes underlying MPD continue to serve a defensive function for individuals who have neither the external nor internal resources to cope with traumatic experiences. Coons and Milstein (1986) reported that 85% of 20 MPD patients had documented allegations of childhood abuse. Frischholz (1985) and Putnam et al. (1986) reported rates of severe childhood abuse as high as 90% in patients with MPD. The nature of the childhood trauma in many of these cases is notable for its severity, multiple aspects of physical and sexual abuse, threats to life, bizarre elements, and profound rupture of the sense of trust and safety when the perpetrator is a primary caregiver or has another type of close relationship with the child.

Acute Dissociative Responses to Trauma: Peritraumatic Dissociation

The aforementioned studies clearly demonstrate the association between traumatic life experience and general dissociative response. One fundamental aspect of the dissociative response to trauma concerns immediate dissociation at the time the traumatic event occurs. Traumatized patients frequently report alterations in the experience of time, place, and person, which leads to a sense of unreality as the event is occurring. Dissociation during trauma may take the form of altered sense of time, with time being experienced as slowed down or rapidly accelerated; experiences of depersonalization; profound feelings of unreality that the event is occurring or that the individual is the victim of the event; out-of-body experiences; confusion and disorientation; altered body image or feelings of disconnection from one's body; tunnel vision; altered pain perception; and other experiences reflecting immediate dissociative responses to trauma. We have designated these acute dissociative responses to trauma as peritraumatic dissociation (Marmar et al. 1994; Marmar et al., 1996b; Weiss et al. 1995).

Although actual clinical reports of peritraumatic dissociation date back nearly a century, systematic investigation has occurred more recently. D. Spiegel (1993) reviews studies of detachment experiences at the time of trauma—one feature of peritraumatic dissociation. Noyes and Kletti (1977) surveyed 101 survivors of automobile accidents and physical assault. They reported that 72% experienced feelings of unreality and altered passage of time during the event, 57% experienced automatic movement, 52% experienced a sense of detachment from the event, 56% reported depersonalization, 34% reported a sense of detachment from the body, and 30% experienced derealization. Hillman (1981) reported on the experiences of 14 correctional officers held hostage during a violent prison riot. The hostage victims described employing dissociative perceptual alterations, including time distortion, to cope with the terror of their experience and psychogenic anesthesia to protect against overwhelming pain. Wilkinson (1983) investigated the psychological responses of survivors of the Hyatt Regency Hotel skywalk collapse in which 114 people died and 200 were injured. Survivors commonly reported depersonalization and derealization experiences at the time of the structural collapse. Siegel (1984) studied 31 kidnapping and terrorist hostages and found that during the hostage experience, 25.8% reported alterations in body imagery and sensations, depersonalization, and disorientation, and 12.9% reported out-of-body experiences.

Holen (1993), in a long-term prospective study of survivors of a North Sea oil-rig disaster, found that the level of reported dissociation during the trauma was a predictor of PTSD 6 months after the accident. Cardena and Spiegel (1993) reported on the responses of 100 graduate students from two different institutions in the Bay Area following the 1989 Loma Prieta earthquake. At the time the earthquake occurred, the participants reported experiencing derealization and depersonalization, time distortion, and alterations in cognition, memory, and somatic sensations. These results suggest that among nonclinical populations, exposure to catastrophic stress may trigger transient dissociative phenomena. Koopman et al. (1994), in a study of 187 survivors of the 1991 Oakland Hills firestorm, found that dissociative symptoms at the time the firestorm was occurring more strongly predicted subsequent posttraumatic symptoms than did anxiety at the time of exposure and the subjective experience of loss of personal autonomy.

These independently replicated clinical and research findings point toward an important vulnerability role for peritraumatic dissociation as a risk factor for subsequent PTSD. These findings were at first surprising, given the prevailing clinical view that dissociative responses to trauma at the time catastrophic events occur conferred a sense of distance and safety to the victim. For example, an adult survivor of childhood incest reported that during the experience of being sexually abused she would leave her body and view the assault from above, with a feeling of detachment and compassion for the helpless little child who was being assaulted sexually. Although out-of-body and other peritraumatic dissociative responses at the time of traumatic stress exposure may defend against even more catastrophic states of helplessness and terror, dissociation at the time of trauma is one of the most important risk factors for the subsequent development of chronic PTSD. Causal relationships that may mediate between peritraumatic dissociation and the heightened risk for PTSD are discussed in the section on "Proposed Mechanisms for Peritraumatic Dissociation."

Peritraumatic Dissociative Experiences Questionnaire: A Proposed Measure of Acute Dissociative Responses to Trauma

Based on the important clinical and preliminary research observations on peritraumatic dissociation as a risk factor for chronic PTSD, we initiated a series of studies to develop a reliable and valid measure of peritraumatic dissociation. We designate this measure the Peritraumatic Dissociative Experiences Questionnaire (PDEQ; Marmar et al., 1996a) (see Appendix A, this chapter, following the references). The first version of the PDEQ was a rater version consisting of nine items addressing dissociative experiences at the time the traumatic event was occurring: sense of time changing during the event; the event seeming unreal, as in a dream or play; feeling as if floating above the scene; moments of losing track or blanking out; finding the self acting on "automatic pilot," feeling disconnected from body or body distortion; not being aware of things that happened during the event that normally would have been noticed; confusion as to what was happening to the self and others; and not feeling pain associated with physical injury.

In a first study with the PDEQ, the relationship between peritraumatic dissociation and posttraumatic stress was studied in male Vietnam theater veterans (Marmar et al. 1994). Two hundred fifty-one male Vietnam theater veterans from the Clinical Examination Component of the National Vietnam Veterans Readjustment Study were investigated to determine the relationship of level of war zone stress exposure, retrospective reports of level of dissociation during the most disturbing combat trauma events, and level of general dissociative tendencies with PTSD case determination. Peritraumatic dissociation was assessed with a rater version of the PDEQ (see Appendix B, this chapter, following the references). Total score on the PDEQ was strongly associated with level of current posttraumatic stress symptoms, level of stress exposure, and level of general dissociative tendencies. Total PDEQ score was weakly associated with general psychopathology as assessed by the 10 clinical scales of the Minnesota Multiphasic Personality Inventory–2 (MMPI-2; Hathaway and McKinley 1989). Logistic regression analyses supported the incremental value of dissociation during trauma, over and above the contributions of level of war zone stress exposure and general dissociative tendencies, in accounting for PTSD case determination. These results provided preliminary support for the reliability and validity of the rater version of the PDEQ, and for a trauma-dissociation linkage hypothesis; the greater the dissociation during traumatic stress exposure, the greater the likelihood of meeting criteria for current PTSD.

In a first replication of this finding, the relationship between peritraumatic dissociation and symptomatic distress was determined in emergency services personnel exposed to traumatic critical incidents (Marmar et al., 1996b; Weiss et al., 1995). Three hundred sixty-seven emergency services personnel who had responded to either a large-scale mass disaster operation or smaller critical incident were interviewed, including emergency medical technicians (EMTs)/paramedics, fire fighters, police, and California Department of Transportation workers. One hundred fifty-four of the emergency medical service workers had been involved in the 1989 Interstate-880 Nimitz Freeway collapse that occurred during the Bay Area Loma Prieta earthquake. A variety of predictors of current symptomatic distress were measured, including level of critical incident exposure, psychological traits, locus of control, social support, general dissociative tendencies, and peritraumatic dissociation. Findings demonstrated that levels of current symptomatic distress were negatively associated with level of adjustment and positively associated with degree of exposure to the critical incident. After controlling for both exposure and adjustment, symptomatic distress could, for the most part, be predicted by social support, experience on the job, locus of control, general dissociative tendencies, and dissociative experiences at the time of the critical incident. The two dissociative variables, total score on the Dissociative Experiences Scale (DES; Bernstein and Putnam 1986) and total score on the PDEQ, were strongly predictive of symptomatic response, even after controlling for adjustment, exposure, and the three other predictors. This study added further support to the growing body of literature linking dissociative tendencies and experiences to distress as a result of exposure to traumatic stressors.

In a second replication, the relationship between peritraumatic dissociation and posttraumatic stress was investigated in female Vietnam theater veterans (Tichenor et al. 1994). Part of the rationale for this study was to assess the relationship of peritraumatic dissociation and posttraumatic stress in a female sample because the two earlier studies focused primarily on male participants. Seventy-seven female Vietnam theater veterans were interviewed by using the rater version of the PDEQ. Total score on the PDEQ was found to be associated strongly with posttraumatic stress symptomatology, as measured by the Impact of Events Scale (Horowitz et al. 1979) and also positively associated with level of stress exposure and general dissociative tendencies, as measured by the DES (Bernstein and Putnam 1986). Scores on the PDEQ were not associated with general psychiatric symptomatology, as assessed by the 10 clinical scales of the MMPI-2 (Hathaway and McKinley 1989). As in the two earlier studies, PDEQ scores were predictive of posttraumatic stress symptoms above and beyond level of exposure and general dissociative tendencies. The findings replicate the earlier results for male Vietnam veterans and emergency services personnel, providing further support for the reliability and validity of the PDEQ and additional support for a linkage between trauma and dissociation.

Recently, we have investigated the relationship between peritraumatic dissociation and posttraumatic stress response in individuals exposed to the 1994 Los Angeles area Northridge earthquake (C. R. Marmar, et al., unpublished manuscript, June 1996). Sixty adult men and women who were working for a large private insurance company and lived close to the epicenter of the earthquake were evaluated. A self-report version of the PDEQ was used to assess dissociation at the time of earthquake exposure. Reports of dissociation at the time of the traumatic event were predictive of current posttraumatic stress response symptoms, after controlling for the level of exposure, replicating the findings for male and female veterans and emergency services personnel.

Across the four studies, the PDEQ has been demonstrated to be internally consistent, strongly associated with level of stress exposure, strongly associated with measures of traumatic stress response, strongly associated with a measure of general dissociative tendencies, and unassociated with measures of general psychopathology. These studies support the reliability and convergent, discriminant, and predictive validity of the PDEQ. Strengthening these findings are two independent studies by investigators in other PTSD research programs utilizing the PDEQ. Bremner et al. (1992), using selective items from the PDEQ as part of a measure of peritraumatic dissociation, reported a strong relationship between peritraumatic dissociation and posttraumatic stress in an independent sample of Vietnam veterans. In the first longitudinal study with the PDEQ, Shalev et al. (1993) investigated the relationship between PDEQ ratings gathered in the first week following trauma exposure and posttraumatic stress symptomatology at 5 months. In this study of acute accident and terrorist attack victims admitted to an Israeli teaching hospital emergency room, PDEQ ratings at 1 week predicted stress symptomatology at 5 months, after controlling for exposure levels, Impact of Events Scale (Horowitz et al. 1979) scores, and social supports in the first week. This study is noteworthy because it is the first with the PDEQ in which ratings were gathered longitudinally. Retrospective ratings of peritraumatic dissociation months, years, or decades after traumatic events are subject to the bias that greater current distress may result in attributing greater dissociation at the time of exposure. The findings by Shalev et al. (1993) are therefore important in supporting the validity of retrospective ratings of peritraumatic dissociation.

Proposed Mechanisms for Peritraumatic Dissociation

The strong replicated findings relating peritraumatic dissociation with subsequent PTSD raises theoretically important questions concerning the mechanisms that underlie peritraumatic dissociation. Speculation concerning psychological factors underlying trauma-related dissociation date back to the early contributions of Breuer and Freud (1893–1895/1955). In their formulation, traumatic events are actively warded off from conscious experience but return in the disguised form of symptoms. The dissociated complexes have an underground life causing hysterical persons to "suffer mainly from reminiscences." Janet (1889) proposed that trauma-related dissociation occurred in individuals with a fundamental constitutional defect in psychological functioning, which he termed "la misère psychologique." Janet proposed that healthy individuals have sufficient psychological energy to bind together their mental experiences, including cognitions, sensations, feelings, memories, and volition, into an integrated synthetic whole under the control of a single personal self with access to conscious experience (see Nemiah, Chapter 1, in this volume). From Janet's perspective, peritraumatic dissociation resulted in the coexistence within a single individual of two or more discrete dissociative streams of consciousness, each with rich mental contents, including feelings, memories, and bodily sensations, and each with access to conscious experience at different times.

Contemporary psychological studies of peritraumatic dissociation have focused on individual differences in the threshold for dissociation. Adult trauma patients who dissociate during their trauma may have experienced childhood or adolescent traumatic events that lower their threshold for dissociation. It is also possible that the threshold for peritraumatic dissociation or generalized dissociative vulnerability is a heritable trait, aggravated by early trauma exposure and correlated with hypnotizability, as suggested by D. Spiegel et al. (1988). Hypnosis has been conceptualized as a controlled and structured form of dissociation (Nemiah 1985; H. Spiegel and Spiegel 1978). Three critical elements to the hypnotic experience, compartmentalization of experience, suggestibility, and absorption, share much in common with the clinical phenomena of trauma-related dissociation. Further supporting the linkage between trauma-related dissociation and hypnotizability are the findings of Stutman and Bliss (1985), who found greater hypnotizability in nonpatient veterans who had high levels of PTSD symptoms when compared with nonpatient veterans who had low levels of PTSD symptoms. D. Spiegel et al. (1988) compared patients with affective disorders, generalized anxiety disorder, schizophrenia, and PTSD and found that the PTSD group had higher hypnotizability scores than those of the other groups and control subjects. In a recent investigation of clinical dissociation, hypnotizability, and trauma in sexually abused girls and control subjects, Putnam et al. (1995) reported a positive association between hypnotizability and clinical dissociation in the trauma subjects but not in the control subjects. This study suggests that in the absence of trauma, high hypnotizability alone is not a sufficient condition for high levels of dissociation. Taken together, the studies on hypnotizability, trauma, and dissociation suggest that individuals who are constitutionally predisposed to being highly hypnotizable and who experienced trauma early in life are those with greatest vulnerability to subsequent dissociation at the time of exposure to traumatic events during adulthood. Further research is required to determine whether Janet's formulation of a genetically determined weakness in the capacity to bind and integrate psychological information may be related to a genetically determined increase in hypnotizability.

A second line of investigation concerning the underlying mechanisms for peritraumatic dissociation focuses on the neurobiology and neuropharmacology of anxiety. A study by Southwick et al. with yohimbine challenges (1993) suggests that in individuals with PTSD, flashbacks occur in the context of high-threat arousal states. It is also significant that patients with panic disorder frequently report dissociative reactions during anxiety attacks (Krystal et al. 1991). The effects of yohimbine in triggering flashbacks in PTSD patients and panic attacks in patients with panic disorder are mediated by a central catecholamine mechanism, as yohimbine serves as an α_2-adrenergic receptor antagonist, resulting in increased firing of locus ceruleus neurons. These observations suggest that the relationship between peritraumatic dissociation and PTSD may be mediated by high levels of anxiety during the trauma. The possibility that panic-level states of anxious arousal may trigger dissociation in some individuals is consistent with Moleman et al.'s report (1992) on the general relationship between high arousal and dissociation.

Marmar et al. (1996a) reported on individual differences in the level of peritraumatic dissociation during critical incident exposure in emergency services personnel. They found the following factors to be associated with greater levels of peritraumatic dissociation: higher levels of exposure during critical incident, greater subjective perceived threat at the time of critical incident, younger age, poorer general psychological adjustment, poorer identity formation, lower levels of ambition and prudence as defined by the Hogan Personality Inventory, greater external locus of control, and greater use of escape-avoidance and emotional self-control coping. Taken together, these findings suggest that emergency services personnel with more vulnerable personality structures, less work experience, higher subjective levels of perceived threat and anxiety at the time of the incident, greater reliance on the external world for an internal sense of safety and security, and greater use of maladaptive coping strategies are more vulnerable to peritraumatic dissociation.

To disentangle cause-and-effect relations in trauma-dissociation linkage, future studies are required that prospectively examine dissociative tendencies in populations subsequently exposed to trauma. In addition, twin, cross-fostering, family history, and biological marker studies will be required to determine if peritraumatic and general dissociative tendencies are characteristics that are inherited or learned early in life. It remains to be demonstrated whether trauma determines greater vulnerability to dissociative responses, both generally and specifically, with respect to peritraumatic responses. It also will be of interest to determine what factors protect against peritraumatic dissociation and determine prospectively if resilience factors reduce the risk of developing subsequent PTSD.

Treatment of Trauma-Related Dissociation

To date, no controlled clinical trials have been reported of psychosocial or pharmacological intervention specifically targeting trauma-related dissociation. Kluft (1993), in an overview of clinical reports on treatment approaches for trauma-related dissociation, recommends individual supportive-expressive psychodynamic psychotherapy, augmented as needed with hypnosis or drug-facilitated interviews.

D. Spiegel (1993) proposes eight C principles for the psychotherapy of individuals experiencing acute traumatic dissociative reactions: 1) *confrontation* of the trauma to counter depersonalization and derealization; 2) *condensation* of the traumatic experience in the form of reconstructing the memory of the traumatic event, including the technical use of hypnosis to relive the experiences and address psychogenic amnesia; 3) *confession* to address shame and guilt; 4) *consolation,* an appropriate expression of sympathy for the tragic circumstances that the patient has experienced; 5) *consciousness,* the bringing of traumatic memories and associated feelings into conscious awareness, without dissociation; 6) *concentration,* the use of hypnosis and self-hypnosis to help the patient gain conscious control over disturbing memories; 7) *control,* the further management of memories and associated affects through flexible experiencing and suppression of traumatic memories rather than dissociation; and 8) *congruence,* the integration of traumatic memories into preexisting self-concepts.

For the treatment of the most severe form of trauma-related dissociation, multiple personality disorder, Kluft (1993), drawing on the work of Braun (1986) and Putnam (1989a), outlines nine stages of a supportive-expressive psychodynamically informed treatment: 1) establishing a therapeutic alliance involving the creation of a safe atmosphere and a secure treatment frame to establish trust and realistic optimism; 2) preliminary interventions designed to gain access to the more readily reached dissociative aspects of personality, including establishing agreements with the alters against terminating treatment abruptly, self-harm, or other self-defeating behaviors; 3) history gathering and mapping of the nature of and relationships among alters to define the constellation of personalities; 4) metabolism of the trauma, which includes accessing and processing traumatic events related to the development of multiple personality disorder; 5) movements toward integration and resolution across the alters by facilitating cooperation, communication, and mutual awareness; 6) integration-resolution, involving a smooth collaboration among the alters; 7) learning new coping skills to manage stress without resorting to dissociation; 8) solidification of gains in working through the transference, including the management of anxiety related to conflicted sexual, aggressive, and dependency issues as they arise in the relationship with the therapist; and 9) follow-up to assess the stability of the outcome and to address new layers of personality that have not emerged in the prior treatment.

A number of investigators have advocated the use of hypnosis as an adjunct to the treatment of trauma-related dissociation. Van der Hart and Spiegel (1993) advocated the use of hypnosis as a way of creating a safe, calm mental state, in which the patient has control over traumatic memories, as an approach to the treatment of trauma-induced dissociative states presenting as hysterical psychosis.

Contemporary psychodynamic approaches to the treatment of trauma-related dissociation emphasize establishing the therapeutic alliance, reconstructing traumatic memories, working through of problematic weak and strong self-concepts activated by the trauma, and interpreting transference aimed at helping the patient process perceived threats in the relationship with the therapist without resorting to dissociation (Horowitz 1986; Marmar 1991; and Steinman 1994). Contemporary psychoanalytic theory emphasizes the complementarity of traumatic and structural models (Nemiah, Chapter 1, in this volume). The traumatic model addresses the fractionation of the ego into multiple dissociative elements, the pathological use of dissociation as a defense, and the abreaction and integration of dissociated traumatic memories. As the previously dissociative elements are brought into a more coherent self, Gabbard (1994) advocates the further use of traditional psychodynamic psychotherapy to solidify gains, mourn losses, and resolve conflicts through interpretation.

Future Research Directions for and Practical Clinical Applications of the Peritraumatic Dissociative Experiences Questionnaire

Future research will clarify the relationship among subjective threat appraisal, emotional distress at the time of trauma, peritraumatic dissociation, activation of central nervous system structures that regulate threat arousal, and psychophysiological arousal in the peripheral nervous system. Trauma patients can be challenged by reminders of their traumatic events and assessed for level of peritraumatic dissociation by their nonverbal behavior, including facial expressions, and changes in central nervous system activity determined with brain imaging procedures, event-related potential studies, and peripheral psychophysiological assessment.

Specific treatment interventions for peritraumatic dissociation, and dissociative responses that occur in the course of uncovering traumatic memories, will depend on rapid identification of those experiencing peritraumatic dissociation and advances in understanding the psychological and neurobiological factors underlying trauma-related dissociation. The PDEQ can be used to screen for acute dissociative responses at the time of exposure to traumatic stress. From a neuropharmacological point of view, R. Pitman (personal communication, November 1995), has advocated using medications to lower threat-arousal levels at the time of trauma. α_2-Adrenergic agonists, β-blockers, or other nonsedating antiarousal agents could be provided to emergency services personnel to aid in the modulation of arousal responses to life-threatening or gruesome exposure. Advances in critical incident stress debriefing procedures may lead to psychological interventions that lower immediate threat arousal and consequently reduce the likelihood of sustained peritraumatic dissociation. The PDEQ can be used to determine the effectiveness of novel pharmacological or psychotherapeutic interventions in reducing acute dissociative response to trauma.

The PDEQ additionally can be used as part of a standard assessment battery for individuals presenting for treatment with acute or chronic PTSD symptoms. Higher PDEQ scores in acute trauma patients support the need for active intervention. Higher PDEQ scores in those individuals presenting for treatment years to decades following traumatic exposure support the validity of subjective complaints of PTSD and also alert clinicians to the risks for patients' reentry into dissociative states during the uncovering phase of psychotherapy.

References

Bernstein EM, Putnam FW: Development, reliability, and validity of a dissociation scale. J Nerv Ment Dis 174:727–734, 1986

Braun BG: Issues in the psychotherapy of multiple personality, in Treatment of Multiple Personality Disorder. Edited by Braun BG. Washington, DC, American Psychiatric Press, 1986, pp 1–28

Bremner JD, Southwick S, Brett E, et al: Dissociation and posttraumatic stress disorder in Vietnam combat veterans. Am J Psychiatry 149: 328–332, 1992

Breuer J, Freud S: Studies on hysteria (1893–1895), in The Standard Edition of the Complete Psychological Works of Sigmund Freud, Vol 2. Translated and edited by Strachey J. London, Hogarth Press, 1955, pp 1–319

Cardena E, Spiegel D: Dissociative reactions to the San Francisco Bay area earthquake of 1989. Am J Psychiatry 150:474–478, 1993

Carlson EB, Rosser-Hogan R: Trauma experiences, posttraumatic stress, dissociation, and depression in Cambodian refugees. Am J Psychiatry 148:1548–1552, 1991

Chu JA, Dill DL: Dissociative symptoms in relation to childhood physical and sexual abuse. Am J Psychiatry 147:887–892, 1990

Coons PM, Milstein V: Psychosexual disturbances in multiple personality. J Nerv Ment Dis 47:106–110, 1986

Frischholz EJ: The relationship among dissociation, hypnosis, and child abuse in the development of multiple personality disorder, in Childhood Antecedents of Multiple Personality. Edited by Kluft RP. Washington, DC, American Psychiatric Press, 1985, pp 99–126

Gabbard GO: Psychodynamic Psychiatry in Clinical Practice: The DSM-IV Edition. Washington, DC, American Psychiatric Press, 1994

Hathaway SR, McKinley JC: Minnesota Multiphasic Personality Inventory–2. Minneapolis, MN, University of Minnesota, 1989

Herman JL, Perry JC, van der Kolk BA: Childhood trauma in borderline personality disorder. Am J Psychiatry 146:490–495, 1989

Hilgard ER: Personality and Hypnosis: A Study of Imaginative Involvement. Chicago, University of Chicago Press, 1970

Hillman RG: The psychopathology of being held hostage. Am J Psychiatry 138:1193–1197, 1981

Holen A: The north sea oil rig disaster, in International Handbook of Traumatic Stress Syndromes. Edited by Wilson JP, Raphael B. New York, Plenum, 1993

Horowitz MJ: Stress Response Syndromes, 2nd Edition. Northvale, NJ, Jason Aronson, 1986

Horowitz MJ, Wilner NR, Alvarez W: Impact of Events Scale: a measure of subjective distress. Psychosomatic Medicine 41:208–218, 1979

Janet P: l'Automatisme Psychologique. Paris, Balliere, 1889

Kluft RP: Multiple personality disorder, in Dissociative Disorders: A Clinical Review. Edited by Spiegel D. Lutherville, MD, Sidran Press, 1993

Koopman C, Classen C, Spiegel D: Predictors of posttraumatic stress symptoms among survivors of the Oakland/Berkeley, California, firestorm. Am J Psychiatry 151:888–894, 1994

Krystal J, Woods S, Hill C, et al: Characteristics of panic attack subtypes: assessment of spontaneous panic, situational panic, sleep panic, and limited symptom attacks. Compr Psychiatry 32:474–480, 1991

Marmar CR: Brief dynamic psychotherapy of post-traumatic stress disorder. Psychiatric Annals 2:404–414, 1991

Marmar CR, Weiss DS, Schlenger WE, et al: Peritraumatic dissociation and posttraumatic stress in male Vietnam theater veterans. Am J Psychiatry 151:902–907, 1994

Marmar CR, Weiss DS, Metzler TJ, et al: Characteristics of emergency services personnel related to peritraumatic dissociation during critical incident exposure. Am J Psychiatry 153:94–102, 1996a

Marmar CR, Weiss DS, Metzler TJ, et al: Stress responses of emergency services personnel to the Loma Prieta earthquake Interstate-880 freeway collapse and control traumatic incidents. Journal of Traumatic Stress 9:63–85, 1996b

Moleman N, van der Hart O, van der Kolk BA: Dissociation and hypnotizability in posttraumatic stress disorder. J Nerv Ment Dis 180: 271–272, 1992

Nemiah JC: Dissociative disorders, in Comprehensive Textbook of Psychiatry/IV, 4th Edition, Vol 1. Edited by Kaplan HI, Sadock BJ. Baltimore, MD, Williams & Wilkins, 1985, pp 942–957

Noyes R, Kletti R: Depersonalization in response to life-threatening danger. Comparative Psychiatry 18:375–384, 1977

Ogata SN, Silk KR, Goodrich S, et al: Childhood sexual and physical abuse in adult patients with borderline personality disorder. Am J Psychiatry 147:1008–1013, 1990

Putnam FW: The Diagnosis and Treatment of Multiple Personality Disorder. New York, Guilford, 1989a

Putnam FW: Pierre Janet and modern views of dissociation. J Trauma Stress 2:413–429, 1989b

Putnam FW, Guroff JJ, Silberman EK, et al: The clinical phenomenology of multiple personality disorder: review of 100 recent cases. J Clin Psychiatry 47:285–293, 1986

Putnam FW, Batson R, van der Kolk B, et al: Treatment of PTSD: implications of working with dissociative phenomena in the treatment of PTSD (abstract). Plenary symposium conducted at the meeting of the International Society for Traumatic Stress Studies, Chicago, IL, November 1994

Putnam FW, Helmers K, Horowitz LA, et al: Hypnotizability and dissociativity in sexually abused girls. Child Abuse Negl 19:1–11, 1995

Shalev AP, Peri T, Schreiber S, et al: Early predictors of PTSD among recent trauma victims (abstract). Abstracts of the Tenth Annual Meeting of the International Society for Traumatic Stress Studies, Chicago, November 1994

Siegel RK: Hostage hallucinations. J Nerv Ment Dis 172:264–272, 1984

Southwick SM, Krystal JH, Morgan CA, et al: Abnormal noradrenergic function in posttraumatic stress disorder. Arch Gen Psychiatry 50: 266–274, 1993

Spiegel D: Dissociation and trauma, in Dissociative Disorders: A Clinical Review. Edited by Spiegel D. Lutherville MD, Sidran Press, 1993

Spiegel D, Cardena E: Disintegrated experience: the dissociative disorders revisited. J Abnorm Psychol 100:366–378, 1991

Spiegel H, Spiegel D: Trance and Treatment: Clinical Uses of Hypnosis. New York, Basic Books, 1978

Spiegel D, Hunt T, Dondershine HE: Dissociation and hypnotizability in posttraumatic stress disorder. Am J Psychiatry 145:301–305, 1988

Steinman I: Psychodynamic treatment of multiple personality disorder. Paper presented at the tenth annual meeting of the International Society for Traumatic Stress Studies, Chicago, IL, November 1994

Stutman RK, Bliss EL: Posttraumatic stress disorder, hypnotizability, and imagery. Am J Psychiatry 142:741–743, 1985

Tichenor V, Marmar CR, Weiss DS, et al: The relationship of peritraumatic dissociation and posttraumatic stress: findings in female Vietnam theatre veterans. J Consult Clin Psychol 64:1054–1059, 1996

van der Hart O, Spiegel D: Hypnotic assessment and treatment of trauma-induced psychoses: the early psychotherapy of H. Breukink and modern views. Int J Clin Exp Hypn 41:191–209, 1993 van der Kolk BA, van der Hart O: Pierre Janet and the breakdown of adaptation in psychological trauma. Am J Psychiatry 146:1530–1540, 1989a

van der Kolk BA, van der Hart O: Pierre Janet on posttraumatic stress. J Trauma Stress 2:265–378, 1989b

Weiss DS, Marmar CR, Metzler TJ, et al: Predicting symptomatic distress in emergency services personnel. J Consult Clin Psychol 63:361–368, 1995

Wilkinson CB: Aftermath of a disaster: the collapse of the Hyatt Regency Hotel skywalks. Am J Psychiatry 140:1134–1139, 1983

Appendix A

Peritraumatic Dissociative Experiences Questionnaire— Self-Report Version

Instructions: Please complete the items below by circling the choice that best describes your experiences and reactions **during the _____ and immediately afterward.** If an item does not apply to your experience, please circle "Not at all true."

1. I had moments of losing track of what was going on—I "blanked out" or "spaced out" or in some way felt that I was not part of what was going on.

1	2	3	4	5
Not at all true	Slightly true	Somewhat true	Very true	Extremely true

2. I found that I was on "automatic pilot"—I ended up doing things that I later realized I hadn't actively decided to do.

1	2	3	4	5
Not at all true	Slightly true	Somewhat true	Very true	Extremely true

3. My sense of time changed—things seemed to be happening in slow motion.

1	2	3	4	5
Not at all true	Slightly true	Somewhat true	Very true	Extremely true

4. What was happening seemed unreal to me, like I was in a dream or watching a movie or play.

1	2	3	4	5
Not at all true	Slightly true	Somewhat true	Very true	Extremely true

5. I felt as though I were a spectator watching what was happening to me, as if I were floating above the scene or observing it as an outsider.

1	2	3	4	5
Not at all true	Slightly true	Somewhat true	Very true	Extremely true

6. There were moments when my sense of my own body seemed distorted or changed. I felt disconnected from my own body or that it was unusually large or small.

1	2	3	4	5
Not at all true	Slightly true	Somewhat true	Very true	Extremely true

7. I felt as though things that were actually happening to others were happening to me—like I was being trapped when I really wasn't.

1	2	3	4	5
Not at all true	Slightly true	Somewhat true	Very true	Extremely true

8. I was surprised to find out afterward that a lot of things had happened at the time that I was not aware of, especially things I ordinarily would have noticed.

1	2	3	4	5
Not at all true	Slightly true	Somewhat true	Very true	Extremely true

9. I felt confused—that is, there were moments when I had difficulty making sense of what was happening.

1	2	3	4	5
Not at all true	Slightly true	Somewhat true	Very true	Extremely true

10. I felt disoriented—that is, there were moments when I felt uncertain about where I was or what time it was.

1	2	3	4	5
Not at all true	Slightly true	Somewhat true	Very true	Extremely true

Appendix B

Peritraumatic Dissociative Experiences Questionnaire— Rater Version

Instructions: I'd like you to try to recall as best you can how you felt and what you experienced at the time (most upsetting event) happened, including how you felt the few minutes just before. Now, I'm going to ask you some specific questions about how you felt at that time. *Note:* DK = don't know; 01 = absent or false; 02 = subthreshold; 03 = threshold.

1. (At that time) Did you have moments of losing track of what was going on—that is, did you "blank out," "space out," or in some other way not feel that you were part of the experience?   **DK 01 02 03**

2. (At that time) Did you find yourself going on "automatic pilot"—that is, doing something that you later realized you had done but hadn't actively decided to do?   **DK 01 02 03**

3. (At that time) Did your sense of time change during the event—that is, did things seem unusually speeded up or slowed down?   **DK 01 02 03**

4. (At that time) Did what was happening seem unreal to you, as though you were in a dream or watching a movie or a play?   **DK 01 02 03**

5. (At that time) Were there moments when you felt as though you were a spectator watching what was happening to you—for example, did you feel as if you were floating above the scene or observing it as an outsider?   **DK 01 02 03**

6. (At that time) Were there moments when   **DK   01   02   03**
    your sense of your own body seemed
    distorted or changed—that is, did you feel
    yourself to be unusually large or small, or did
    you feel disconnected from your body?

7. (At that time) Did you get the feeling that   **DK   01   02   03**
    something that was happening to someone
    else was happening to you? For example, if
    you saw someone being injured, did you feel
    as though you were the one being injured,
    even though that was not the case?

8. Were you surprised to find out after the event   **DK   01   02   03**
    that a lot of things had happened at the time
    that you were not aware of, especially things
    that you felt you ordinarily would have
    noticed?

9. (At that time) Were there moments when you   **DK   01   02   03**
    had difficulty making sense of what was
    happening?

10. (At that time) Did you feel disoriented—that   **DK   01   02   03**
    is, were there moments when you felt
    uncertain about where you were or what time
    it was?

Chapter 9

Treatment of Dissociative Disorders

Onno van der Hart, Ph.D., Bessel A. van der Kolk, M.D., and Suzette Boon, Ph.D.

F or more than a century, people's reactions to overwhelming experiences have been understood in terms of an alternate consciousness paradigm; the study of traumatized patients, such as "shell-shocked" soldiers and "hysterics," has consistently provided us with information that traumatized individuals may have one or more alternate states of consciousness that contain the memories of the trauma (Crabtree 1993; Ellenberger 1970). For example, the British psychiatrist Charles Samuel Myers (1940), reflecting on his clinical observations of shell-shocked soldiers during World War I, stated:

> The recent emotional experiences of the individual have the upper hand and determine his conduct: the normal has been replaced by what we may call the "emotional" personality. Gradually or suddenly an "apparently normal" personality returns—normal save for the lack of all memory of events directly connected with the shock [i.e., trauma], normal save for the manifestation of other ("somatic") hysteric disorders indicative of mental dissociation. (p. 67)

Myers (1940) ascribed the shifting appearances of the emotional (traumatic) personality state and the apparently normal personality state to the phenomenon of dissociation. Dissociation refers to a compartmentalization of experience: elements of an experience are not integrated into a unitary whole but are stored in memory as isolated fragments. In recent years, it has become increasingly clear that dissociative processes play a critical role in the development of trauma-related psychological problems; clinical investigators have empirically documented the link between psychological trauma and dissociative symptoms (Briere and Conte 1993; Marmar et al. 1994; Spiegel and Cardena 1991). Dissociation occurs both peritraumatically, that is, at the time of the traumatic event (Bremner et al. 1992; Marmar et al. 1994), and posttraumatically, as a long-term consequence of traumatic exposure (Bremner et al. 1992, 1993; Chu and Dill 1990).

DSM-IV (American Psychiatric Association 1994) also recognizes the dissociative nature of people's reactions to a traumatic event, which is now codified as acute stress disorder (ASD). Paradoxically, the DSM-IV Task Force decided to subsume posttraumatic stress disorder (PTSD) under the anxiety disorders, despite strong scientific support for categorizing it as a dissociative disorder. Dissociation is a way of organizing information. Depending on the severity, chronicity, developmental level at which the trauma occurs, temperament, and posttrauma environment, people may adapt to their dissociative responses to a traumatic experience by developing a variety of Axis I and II disorders. In some individuals, the dissociated fragments of a traumatic experience may be buried without markedly interfering with overall personality development, whereas others organize their character development around dealing with the aftermath of the trauma. Patients with borderline personality disorder (BPD) or dissociative identity disorder (DID or multiple personality disorder) in most cases are people whose character is organized around traumatic reexperiences.

Although high levels of dissociation have been noted in patients with somatization disorder, BPD, and PTSD, DSM-IV created a separate category for dissociative disorders to capture the notion of alternate consciousness (characterized by "a disruption in the usually integrated functions of consciousness, memory, identity, or perception of the environment" [American Psychiatric Association 1994, p. 477]). DSM-IV thereby created a category that describes a way of processing information, without capturing the various personality organizations that are part and parcel of the adaptation to trauma. Therefore, it is critical for clinicians who treat patients with the primary diagnosis of somatization disorder, BPD, or PTSD to be thoroughly familiar with the diagnosis and treatment of dissociation and that clinicians who focus on dissociation are conversant with the complexities of treating patients with severe personality disorders.

Levels of Dissociation

Patients who have dissociative disorders almost invariably have histories of severe trauma. Moreover, the younger they were when they were traumatized, and the longer the trauma lasted, the more severe their dissociative disorder is likely to be. The word *dissociation* currently is used to refer to four distinct, but related, mental phenomena (van der Kolk and Fisler 1995).

Primary Dissociation

Many children and adults confronted with overwhelming threat are unable to integrate the totality of the experience into consciousness. Sensory and affective fragments of the experience may not be integrated into personal memory and identity and therefore remain isolated from ordinary consciousness. The experience is split into its isolated somatosensory elements, without integration into a personal narrative (as measured by the Traumatic Memory Inventory [TMI; van der Kolk and Fisler 1995]). This fragmentation is accompanied by states of mind that are distinct from the normal state of consciousness. This condition is characteristic of PTSD, the most obvious symptoms of which consist of expressions of the dissociated traumatic memory, such as reexperiencing the event in the form of intrusive recollections, nightmares, and flashbacks and concomitant emotional constriction (numbing, detachment, and feelings of isolation).

Secondary Dissociation

Once an individual is in a traumatic (dissociated) state of mind, further disintegration of elements of the personal experience can occur. A "dissociation between observing ego and experiencing ego" (Fromm 1965) has been described in incest survivors, traffic accident victims, and combat soldiers: they report mentally leaving their bodies at the moment of the trauma and observing what happens from a distance (Gelinas 1983; Noyes et al. 1977). The distancing maneuvers of secondary dissociation allow individuals to observe the traumatic experience as a spectator and to limit their pain or distress; secondary dissociation protects them from being aware of the full impact of the event. Whereas primary dissociation limits people's cognitions regarding the reality of their traumatic experience and allows them temporarily to go on as if nothing happened (e.g., Spiegel 1988), secondary dissociation puts people out of touch with the feelings and emotions related to the trauma— they are anesthetized. In recent publications, secondary dissociation has been labeled *peritraumatic dissociation* (Marmar et al. 1994), which can be measured with the Peritraumatic Dissociative Experiences Questionnaire (PDEQ; Marmar et al. 1994) or the Stanford Acute Stress Reaction Questionnaire (Koopman et al. 1994).

Tertiary Dissociation

When people develop distinct ego-states that contain the traumatic experience and consist of complex identities with distinct cognitive, affective, and behavioral patterns, it is called tertiary dissociation. Different ego-states may contain the pain, fear, or anger related to particular traumatic experiences, and ego states that are unaware of the trauma and its concomitant affects are able to carry out routine functions of daily life. Examples are the multiple dissociated identity (alter) fragments in DID, some of which experience different aspects of one or more traumatic incidents, whereas others remain unaware of these unbearable experiences. To the degree that dissociative amnesia allows them to, these patients typically report chronic and intense sexual, physical, and psychological abuse that started at a very early age (Boon and Draijer 1993; Loewenstein and Putnam 1990; Putnam et al. 1986). The use of dissociative responses on a day-to-day basis is best measured by the Dissociative Experiences Scale (DES; Bernstein and Putnam 1986, and the encapsulation of traumatic experiences in separate states of consciousness is best measured by the Dissociative Disorders Interview Scale (DDIS; Ross et al. 1989) or the Structured Clinical Interview for DSM-IV Dissociative Disorders (SCID-D; Steinberg 1993).

Treatment Goals

The essence of the treatment of all trauma-induced dissociation was well summarized by Myers (1940):

> . . . [to] deprive the "emotional" personality of its pathological, distracted, uncontrolled character, and . . . [to] effect . . . its union with the "apparently normal" personality hitherto ignorant of the emotional experiences in question. When this re-integration has taken place, it becomes immediately obvious that the "apparently normal" personality differed widely in physical appearance and behaviour, as well as mentally, from the completely normal personality thus at last obtained. (p. 69)

In other words, in order to recover from an "illness of synthesis," as Janet (1907) called dissociative disorders, the traumatic memories need to be integrated and "owned" by one unified personality state (Kluft 1987, 1993b; Putnam 1989; Ross 1989).

Patients with dissociative disorders have a multitude of clinical presentations, ranging from patients showing high levels of personal and professional functioning, with isolated dissociative memories or ego states, to patients whose identity and perceptions are so fragmented that they are unable to live outside of institutional settings. Therefore, the diagnosis of a dissociative disorder always needs to be accompanied by an assessment of 1) patients' current personal and professional functioning, including the capacity to form a therapeutic alliance, to abide by contractual arrangements, to understand and tolerate other people's points of view, to form supportive relationships with significant others, and to check their impulses, as well as their general capacity for self-care; 2) presence of other Axis I and Axis-II disorders, including affective disorders, panic, PTSD, and self-injurious behavior; 3) substance abuse; and 4) ongoing trauma, such as abusive relationships.

Ever since clinicians have treated patients with dissociative disorders, they have emphasized the need to first stabilize them and only then gradually approach the dissociated parts of the personality, including the traumatic memories (D. Brown and Fromm 1986; W. Brown 1918; Kardiner and Spiegel 1947; Kluft 1984; Myers 1940; Putnam 1989; Ross 1989). Generally, the less time that has elapsed since the emergence of the dissociative symptoms, the sooner the symptoms will be resolved.

Principles of Treatment

The treatment of both acute and chronic trauma has three principal components: 1) controlling and mastering physiological and biological stress reactions; 2) processing and coming to terms with the horrifying, overwhelming experience; and 3) reestablishing secure social connections and personal, as well as interpersonal, efficacy. As long as traumatized people dissociate, and are plagued by involuntary intrusions of fragments of the trauma, the emphasis in treatment needs to be on self-regulation and rebuilding. Early exploration and abreaction of traumatic experiences, without having established the capacity for restabilization, are likely to lead to negative therapeutic outcomes. Therefore, therapy needs to focus on reestablishing a sense of security and predictability and active engagement in adaptive action.

The standard of care for treating patients with dissociative psychopathology includes some form of phase-oriented treatment. Such an approach was first described by Pierre Janet (van der Hart et al. 1989) and has subsequently been reinvented by many contemporary clinicians (e.g., D. Brown and Fromm 1986; Herman 1992; McCann and Pearlman 1990; van der Hart and Friedman 1995). The basic phase-oriented model consists of three stages of treatment, each with its own treatment foci and procedures: 1) stabilization and symptom reduction, 2) treatment of traumatic memories, and 3) reintegration and rehabilitation. In complex dissociative disorders, these various stages often need to be revisited several times during the course of the treatment (Horevitz and Loewenstein 1994; Kluft 1993c; Ross 1989). Following Janet (1904), we propose the following major treatment foci for the respective treatment phases: 1) overcoming the phobia of dissociative states:

stabilization and symptom reduction, 2) overcoming the phobia of traumatic memories: treatment of traumatic memories, and 3) overcoming the phobia of ordinary life: reintegration and rehabilitation (Nijenhuis and van der Hart 1994). In simple dissociative disorders, these various phobias have not yet coalesced into distinct problems.

This phase-oriented treatment takes place against the backdrop of careful attention to affective and characterological issues as they shift and are activated during treatment. No uncovering should occur before adequate stabilization has been accomplished because patients may become overwhelmed by the emerging traumatic memory, which may reinforce their fear of the memory and even precipitate suicide attempts (Abeles and Schilder 1935; Gudjonsson and Haward 1982; Stengel 1941; Takahashi 1988).

Stage 1: Stabilization and Symptom Reduction

Like treatment for all patients with PTSD, the first condition for effective treatment of patients with dissociative disorders consists of establishing personal safety and self-care. When they first come to the attention of mental health professionals, patients with dissociative amnesias often are disorganized, neglectful of their personal hygiene, have irregular sleeping and eating habits, and engage in self-destructive behaviors. They habitually may "space out" or become unresponsive under stress and may engage in substance abuse and various dangerous reenactment behaviors. These problems often necessitate an initial hospitalization, whereby patients and therapists can begin to take an inventory of what is going on in their lives and work on the principles of stabilization.

Stabilization needs to include attention to the patient's safety, establishment of regular day and night rhythms, appropriate self-care (including adequate food and rest), structuring of daily activities, establishment of an "emotional 911" (people or institutions that the patient can reliably turn to in times of extreme distress), and prescription of appropriate medications.

Although many patients who suffer from dissociative disorders may be competent in some areas of functioning, they often exhibit poor judgment, particularly in unstructured situations that are reminiscent of their original traumas, in which trust, aggression, or sexuality plays a significant role. Confronted with such situations, they often rely on dissociation as an ongoing way of coping with stress. Therefore, it is important to establish the triggers of a particular patient's irrational behaviors, which, over time, the patient and therapist may come to understand as representing fragmented traumatic reexperiences. This reliving of experiences may or may not have visual flashback components, without which it is difficult to make a direct connection between the flashbacks and the particular traumatic events in the patient's life. It is critical for the therapist to help focus the patient on the *facts* of what is happening and to bolster the capacity to attend to the details of living while developing adequate problem-solving strategies.

Many therapists of patients with dissociative disorders have found that hypnotic techniques using the metaphoric imagery of placing a memory inside some imaginary safe, vault, or box are helpful in fostering containment of traumatic memories (see the discussion on "Teaching Techniques for Coping With Reactivated Traumatic Memories"). Additional hypnotic suggestions may be given for creating an imaginary "safe place," serving as a base from which the dissociated memories eventually may be approached (D. Brown and Fromm 1986; Hammond 1990; Spiegel 1988; van der Hart et al. 1990).

The therapeutic relationship.   Central to a good therapeutic outcome is the therapeutic alliance—the element of trust between patients and therapists. Patients who have dissociative disorders often are unsure about the validity of their perceptions, are not firmly rooted in a continuous sense of self (i.e., who they are from moment to moment), and their lives have been marked by sudden, terrifying breaches of predictability and safety. Therefore, their relationship with their therapists is the anchor of the work of therapy. As Kluft (1993a) points out, this does not necessarily mean that patients need to feel safe with their therapists. After betrayal and victimization by others, it is unrealistic and naive to expect that patients will trust their therapists. The best that can be hoped for is that therapists will provide clear rules, will be predictable, and will be respectful of their patients' need to protect themselves against further victimization. Within the therapeutic relationship, old attachment patterns certainly will be activated. In the treatment of patients with dissociative disorders, therapists are bound to encounter trauma-related interpersonal crises such as 1) fear of abandonment, 2) an apparently insatiable need for contact with the therapist, 3) fear of rejection and lack of understanding, and 4) issues of trust, which often are expressed in hostile crises or self-destructive behaviors. The boundaries of the relationship need to be unambiguously defined, including frequency of contact, payment, crises calls, coverage, vacations, and extratherapy telephone contact (Kluft 1993a).

Psychoeducation. Psychoeducation is an important element of treatment. Emotions need to be labeled, reality clarified, and daily structure reintroduced. Psychoeducation may need to include an explanation of dissociative amnesia as a failure of the mind to tolerate the unbearable. The nature of the therapeutic relationship needs to be defined: treatment is a collaborative effort between patient and therapist to establish a safe base from which they can start understanding the personal meaning of the apparently alien phenomena that intrude in the patient's life. The therapist needs to explain that any concern that the patient has about approaching hidden memories should be taken seriously and should be examined before attempts at uncovering these memories are undertaken.

Usually, dissociative problems are accompanied by PTSD symptoms, and patients also will experience intrusive recollections of nondissociated aspects of the traumatic experience, as well as hyperarousal, sleep disturbances, and episodes of anxiety and uncontrolled or inhibited anger. Therefore, patients need to be educated about the whole spectrum of PTSD and dissociative symptoms and how the symptoms are interrelated. Creating a cognitive framework for understanding the patients' problems as expectable reactions forms one of the pillars of rational psychotherapy for dissociative disorders.

Stage 2: Treatment of Traumatic Memories

In patients who have simpler forms of dissociation, adequate stabilization often can effect a spontaneous remission (Loewenstein, in
press). In those cases, the amnestic barrier will loosen and the dissociated memories will spontaneously emerge. Hypnosis has been
used successfully for two centuries as an effective treatment for dissociated memories. Because of a recent popular confusion between
the therapeutic benefits of hypnosis and its adequacy for use in forensic settings, there has been an unfortunate prejudice against its
use. Clearly, patients should be informed that although hypnosis
may be beneficial for the mental integration of traumatic memories,
memories retrieved under hypnosis are not necessarily accurate
and that hypnosis is likely to make these memories inadmissible as
evidence in a court of law (Scheflin and Shapiro 1989; Spiegel and
Scheflin 1994).

One hypnotic technique for well-paced memory recovery includes using an imaginary television screen (D. Brown and Fromm
1986; Spiegel 1981; van der Hart et al. 1990). D. Brown and Fromm
(1986) instruct patients to watch a safe scene on an imaginary television screen. When they feel ready, they may switch to the channel where the traumatic event, including the episode for which
amnesia exists, can be watched. When the patients become too af-
fectively overwhelmed, they are encouraged to switch back to the
safe program. A variant was developed by Spiegel (1981) who suggests using a two-part television screen: patients may watch safe
images on one half while watching the traumatic event on the
other. At the end of such a hypnotic procedure, it may be suggested that patients take with them into their ordinary waking
state only what is safe for them to remember. Eventually, they
should be able to process the formerly dissociated memories in
their waking state.

The purpose of these approaches is to help patients regulate
their emotional arousal, gaining access to the cognitive elements
of the traumatic experience (Hammond 1990; van der Hart 1985).
Regulating emotional arousal involves 1) reconnecting the affective, cognitive, and somatic aspects of the traumatic experience

(which we call "synthesis," or fusion with the traumatized person-ality state); and 2) "realizing" the event and thereby making it part of the autobiographical memory of patients (Janet 1919/1925).

Stage 3: Reintegration and Rehabilitation

Making the unconscious memory conscious includes integrating it into the totality of the personality. Often, formerly dissociated trau-matic memories are relevant to current circumstances; there may be many situations or relationships that patients learn to avoid in order not to trigger intense emotional states and traumatic flash-backs. Similar to exposure therapy for well-medicated patients with panic disorder, individuals with a dissociative disorder also need to actively expose themselves to situations that formerly were imbued with a sense of dread. Because of this, it is important to provide adequate follow-up after integrating the traumatic memories. Dur-ing this period, patients need to work on developing new coping skills and not dissociating when faced with threatening situations. Group psychotherapy may be particularly helpful at this stage.

Loewenstein (1991) has noted that most reports on patients with acute amnesia lack long-term follow-up data. He postulates that in many patients the dissociative amnesia was actually part of a more complex dissociative disorder such as DID.

Treatment of Tertiary Dissociation: Dissociative Identity Disorder

People with severe childhood trauma may organize their traumatic experiences in different ego-states that contain the memories of those experiences, which are ordinarily inaccessible to other parts of the self. Recent studies have shown that full-blown DID (for-merly called multiple personality disorder) occurs in about 5% of psychiatric inpatients (Saxe et al. 1993) and is accompanied by markedly increased somatization and problems with affect regula-tion (van der Kolk et al. 1996). Essentially, the three-stage treatment model outlined earlier in this chapter can bring relief in a relatively short time for patients with uncomplicated dissociative disorders;

can take years to bring relief in the more complicated forms of the disorder, such as DID and dissociative disorder not otherwise specified (DDNOS); and the cycle of going through the three different stages usually is completed numerous times.

During the initial contacts with patients who have severe dissociative disorders, it often is not clear if patients eventually will be capable of integrating the traumatic past and of establishing an identity that is capable of responding primarily to the demands of the present. Even after an extensive treatment period focused on stabilization and symptom reduction, many DID patients remain vulnerable to extreme states of physiological arousal and may not develop the capacity for self-regulation necessary to integrate the traumatic past. Research data on these issues show that DID is a heterogeneous condition in which patients have very different prognoses. Three groups can be delineated:

1. *High-functioning DID patients.* High-functioning DID patients have little Axis II comorbidity, possess a significant capacity to tolerate both positive and negative affects without acting on them, and are capable of using the therapeutic alliance for self-regulation.

2. *Patients who have complicated dissociative disorders with comorbid Axis II conditions.* Patients who have more complicated dissociative disorders tend to have poor affect tolerance, engage in pathological self-soothing behaviors, and have poor judgment in their interpersonal relationships, in which they tend to reenact their traumas. Treatment of these patients necessarily is much slower, and full integration may not be achieved.

3. *Patients who are unable to use the therapeutic relationship to achieve some self-soothing and to appraise their contributions to their problems.* Patients who cannot use the therapeutic relationship for self-soothing and self-appraisal remain embedded in their trauma. They tend to engage in abusive relationships, have a "dissociative" lifestyle, and actively participate in self-destructive and/or antisocial behaviors and habits. These patients have a poor therapeutic prognosis and can be treated most effectively when therapy is geared toward symptom sta-

bilization and crisis management rather than the uncovering and integration of identities (Horevitz and Loewenstein 1994; Kluft 1994b; Groenendijk and van der Hart 1995).

The factors that are thought to play a role in determining long-term prognosis include 1) duration and severity of a patient's trauma, 2) capacity to use attachment figures for self-soothing, 3) propensity to reenact the trauma in adult life, 4) nature and severity of comorbid psychiatric conditions, 5) capacity to attend to stimuli without cognitive or affective distortion, 6) intellectual endowment, and 7) degree of primary identity as patient or victim.

Basic Principles in Treating Patients With Dissociative Identity Disorder

Basic principles in treating DID patients are not different from the principles that form the backbone of therapy for all patients: 1) honesty, 2) clear communication, 3) clear boundaries and limits, 4) negotiation of treatment goals and process, and 5) flexibility. Adhering to these principles with DID patients promotes predictability, which is especially important because these patients often have family backgrounds that were extremely authoritarian and/or unpredictable and chaotic.

Psychoeducation about dissociative identity disorder.   DID patients look for help for a wide range of symptoms or complaints, but they seldom seek help for the core symptoms that characterize DID: amnestic episodes, a sense that their personality is not functioning as a whole, and confusion about their identity. Making the right diagnosis is not the only necessary precondition for adequate treatment. It also is important that patients learn to understand the symptoms of DID (just as it would be extraordinarily difficult to treat manic-depressive patients who do not understand the basic nature of their disorder). DID is a disorder of secrecy. During their initial intake interview, few patients will mention spontaneously that they have different internal identities; often, it takes a long time before patients feel sufficiently secure in the therapeutic relationship to disclose this shameful fact. When they feel more or less safe, some patients will report that they know that there are different identities; sometimes these different identities have their own name. These patients generally feel relieved by the therapist's explanation of the nature of DID: their problem has a name, and treatment is possible. However, DID patients present a wide spectrum in regards to the degree to which their dissociative identities are conscious of each other's existence. Patients who have little or no coconsciousness have a great deal of trouble accepting their diagnosis and are particularly concerned about being "found out" for doing things that the presenting personality is not aware of.

Confronting the fact that there are parts of one's personality that one is not familiar with and that lead lives of their own is a threatening realization. It evokes fear, not only to be labeled as crazy by others, including helping professionals, but also for losing control and doing terrible things, without possibly knowing about it. Even when patients are aware of dissociative phenomena, such as amnesia and identity alterations, they often tend to downplay it. "I seem to have a thing with clothes," said one DID patient, who reported being aware of closets full of clothes that she could not remember buying, but she refused to delve any deeper in trying to find an explanation. In short, there exists a phobia for dissociative states (Nijenhuis and van der Hart 1994) accompanied by cognitive avoidance strategies. Psychoeducation, particularly when it is regularly refreshed, is an important antidote. It may include clear descriptions and explanations of dissociative symptoms, the nature and functions of different types of identities (if indicated), the relationship between trauma and dissociation as survival strategy, and the difference between DID and schizophrenia. These repeated explanations may reduce feelings of fear and shame and be a first step in learning how to take control.

Also relevant is an explanation of DID as an "attachment disorder" (Barach 1991), which may explain the difficulty that many of these patients have in establishing a therapeutic alliance. Issues regarding attachment that frequently come up in the therapy of these patients are 1) fear of abandonment; 2) an apparently insatiable longing for merger and closeness, usually carried out by child identities, and a simultaneous terror of closeness and dependency; 3) fear of rejection and lack of understanding; and 4) extremely ambivalent feelings toward the therapist, often divided among different identities and manifested in a pattern of attraction and rejection.

Boundary issues require special attention; it is likely that key persons in a patient's past have made extreme boundary transgressions. These transgressions have interfered with the development of a clear sense of what is private and what is public, what can be shared and what needs to be guarded, and when it is appropriate to ask for help and when others need to be left alone. In patients with DID, there may be identities that surrender themselves much too easily, whereas other identities may be on guard against all social entanglements. Similarly, having not learned the rules of engagement, some identities may transgress the boundaries of other people, including those of the therapist. Therapy will be more effective if these issues are kept in focus, even before crises actually occur, because during times of crises, problems with shame and rage may interfere with the capacity to deal effectively with these issues. As Kluft (1993a) has noted, these patients suffer from a multiple reality disorder, meaning that the therapist frequently has to articulate the basic issues involved in the patients' creating a road map of their lives.

Fostering cooperation between identities participating in daily life. When a patient has achieved a reasonable degree of stabilization and when there is a general agreement between patient and therapist about the nature of the problems, the therapist may begin to establish contact with the patient's different states of mind. Some therapists of patients with DID tend to contact as many identities as possible to map the inner system of identities and to gain a sense of what to expect later in treatment. However, we think that this approach may cause too much upheaval, and we tend to focus more on the states of mind that play an active role in a patient's daily life. Apart from this, we try to establish a good working relationship with so-called inner "helpers" and "leaders."

The inner system of identities in adult DID patients seems to have a surprising degree of consistency from one patient to another: certain types of identities seem to be present in most patients with DID. Following a trauma, or more commonly a series of traumas, these different identities evolve to fulfill different functions within the system. There are usually a number of adult identities, who may know little about a patient's past traumatic experiences; they usually are in charge of the patient's occupational life and, if they have children, the care of their offspring. Conventionally, the personality state that is most apparent and in charge of daily "business transactions" is called the "host." Among the different identities, some tend to be interested in the therapeutic process, whereas others usually are resistant. In addition to these more "adult" states, which are generally quite capable of articulating their points of view, there usually are younger identities that "hold" the traumatic memories. They tend to be fearful and often suffer from traumatic reexperiences. Among them may be suicidal, self-destructive, and self-mutilating identities. To prevent reactivation of traumatic memories in these child identities, helpers within the system may try to shield them from triggers that activate traumatic memories. These helpers are able to take the position of observers. When willing and able to cooperate with the therapist, they may provide information to the therapist about various aspects of the inner world of the patient. Some patients have inner helpers who serve as a "good mother," who takes care of the child identities. Such helpers also may cooperate with the therapist to prevent dysregulation of the patient by preventing reactivation of traumatic memories. Other ego-states are those that have developed from introjects of the perpetrators who abused the patient. They often try to sabotage treatment and give destructive orders to other identities (e.g., to mutilate or starve themselves or to make suicide attempts), particularly after child identities have disclosed "forbidden" information to the therapist.

Within the system of identities, there may be one-way or two-way amnesias (compare Ellenberger 1970; Janet 1907). Identities tend to be grouped around certain themes or traumas. In very complex cases, there may be multiple systems of identities, with considerable amnesias between systems. Sometimes, inner "historians" may have knowledge about one entire system, but they are ignorant of others. When therapists interact only with identities that participate in daily life, they more or less explicitly invite the inner helpers and leaders to listen.

Building a working alliance with persecutory states of mind. Treatment goes much better if the therapist is able to engage persecutory identities as allies or at least can persuade them to listen and postpone their destructive actions. Regardless of the level of therapeutic intervention, it is important to discuss with the patient how difficult it is to deal with anger when he or she feels hurt, frightened, and humiliated and that the tasks of these identities seem to deal precisely with these complex emotions. The therapist may address hostile states of mind indirectly by respectfully talking about them with the identity that is "out." The therapist often already has heard from these hostile identities by having been told about the presence of threatening or punishing auditory hallucinations; these voices are generally found to belong to identities that came into being to protect the patient against abuse. Although these ego-states may sound like the original perpetrators themselves, they seem to have come into being in an attempt to help the patient survive. One of their functions seems to be to keep the patient's rage about the abuse under control. The therapist needs to show understanding that the persecutory identities sometimes lose control in response to reactivated traumatic fears because they have not yet found other ways of dealing with that fear and humiliation. Intermittently, persecutory identities tend to direct their rage against themselves, even though they may "experience" it as if it were directed against others (i.e., other identities).

The therapist and patient may gradually discover alternative ways of coping with anger. The therapist needs to repeatedly point out to the patient that the motivation of hostile identities is not to live out their sadism against other identities, but that they have not yet developed other ways of dealing with their rage. By approaching these ego-states respectfully, they tend to become allies in the therapeutic process. They slowly will begin to understand that certain steps that are therapeutic for the rest of the system of identities also are beneficial for them. Creating imaginary safe places for fearful identities, for instance, helps to prevent them from acting on their fears when traumatic memories are reactivated. Providing clear explanations about the function of their behaviors and their problems tolerating issues that remind them of their traumas can help the patient not to sabotage the therapeutic process.

Contacting identities. Identities may spontaneously appear during sessions. When that occurs, the therapist may inquire about the reasons why they seem to be appearing at a particular time, their names, and what their function might be in the system of identities. Contacting an identity that is not out during a particular session is usually quite easy. The patient is simply asked to let the identity come forward that, for instance, has written in a diary about a particular issue, that is in charge of running daily activities, or that is instructing the patient to commit suicide. Direct contact and negotiations between therapist and identities may form the basis for helping these ego-states to communicate, negotiate, and collaborate. One way of motivating them to do so is to explain that they are already cooperating *implicitly* (e.g., by having identities automatically do their particular jobs in particular situations). Because this implicit cooperation is still fraught with failure (e.g., having an unprepared identity take an examination), *explicit* cooperation involving negotiating and agreeing on specific goals would be a major improvement.

Teaching techniques for coping with reactivated traumatic memories. When the patient has some understanding of the nature of dissociative symptoms and the existence of different identities, the next step is teaching him or to obtain more control over traumatic reexperiences and related symptoms. The first step is learning to identify reactivating stimuli (triggers). A patient may be triggered by a large range of stimuli, such as 1) sensory experiences, 2) stimuli related to anniversaries, 3) daily life events, 4) events during the therapeutic sessions, 5) emotions, 6) physiological states, 7) stimuli that evoke memories of being intimidated by a perpetrator, and 8) current trauma (van der Hart and Friedman 1992). Often, internal helpers, who know about the traumas without suffering from them themselves, can help inform the therapist about existing triggers, what they try to do to keep other identities at a distance from them, and what has worked and what has not. This information may help the therapist negotiate with the patient alternative ways of coping with triggers, techniques for preventing traumatic reexperiences, and techniques for faster reorientation in the here and now once a reexperience takes place.

The following procedures, discussed elsewhere in more detail (see van der Hart and Friedman 1992), may be helpful: 1) removing or neutralizing the reactivating stimulus; 2) emphasizing the safe present and cue conditioning to return to the present; 3) suggesting temporary amnesia for, or creating more mental distance from, the traumatic memory (e.g., by placing it in an imaginary safe); 4) creating imaginary safe places in which traumatized identities can seek shelter (e.g., D. Brown and Fromm 1986); and 5) protecting traumatized identities from reactivating stimuli by creating dissociative barriers. Hypnotic techniques may be helpful with these procedures.

Cognitive therapy.   Dissociated identities have, by definition, a limited and often distorted perspective of themselves, other identities, and the outside world, and these distorted perspectives may be responsible for actions that are based on faulty understanding. For instance, some identities are convinced that they live in a different body from the other identities and therefore feel free to assail that body, as if it did not belong to them. These perspectives may be quite rigid, and the different identities are often quite impervious to new information. Many of their ideas have developed in the context of traumatic experiences (e.g., "it is my fault that my uncle had sex with me"), and they remain fixed along with the traumatic memories. These cognitive distortions also tend to incorporate any number of rigid notions and overgeneralizations (e.g., that no man, or woman, can ever be trusted). After the therapist gains a thorough understanding of the cognitive and perceptual organization of the patient, cognitive interventions constitute an important part of stabilization and symptom reduction (Fine 1988, 1991; McCann and Pearlman 1990; Ross 1989). Naturally, such faulty cognitions have the best chance to be changed if the patient is in an environment in which he or she has experiences that contradict those cognitions (Epstein 1991).

Family and couples therapy.   If the patient is a victim of chronic intrafamilial abuse, family therapy with the family of origin usually cannot be recommended. If the DID patient is a child, the first task is to stop the abuse, which often includes out-of-home placement. Family therapy in the foster families in which these children are placed can be helpful (Fagan and McMahon 1984). Adult DID patients and their partners and children may benefit from supportive couples or family therapy. Individual treatment of DID patients may be so demanding of the therapist that attention to and care for the couple (if there is any) or current family may be too much to handle. However, education of the partner and family members about the nature of DID is important; they need support during times of crisis as well. It is important to explain to the partner (and sometimes to the children) to regard the patient as one person and to realize that he or she has a relationship with that complete person, not just with some of the patient's identities. Furthermore, it is important not to see DID as the problem of the relationship or family but as a complicating factor (Panos et al. 1990).

Medications.   Many DID patients benefit from some form of psychopharmacological intervention. Prescribing medication to these patients can be a complicated affair. The effect of medication differs from patient to patient and from identity to identity within one patient. Pharmacotherapy with patients is a matter of trial and error because many have highly idiosyncratic responses and no double-blind studies are available. Putnam and Loewenstein (1993) report some success with antidepressants and anxiolytics. Van der Kolk has found serotonin reuptake inhibitors useful in many patients with DID, as well as anticonvulsants such as valproate and Neurontin. Currently, we are investigating the validity of the observation by Dr. Thomas Jobe (personal communication, November 1995) that H_2

blockers, such as mesoridazine besylate (Serentil) and doxepin, may have unique therapeutic actions in these patients.

The therapist should always be aware of the possibility that there are identities that hoard medications for an eventual suicide attempt and that DID patients often stop taking the medication on their own initiative and without consultation. Naturally, the chance of success is higher when the identities collaborate with each other.

Developing a protocol for crisis intervention, including short-term psychiatric admissions. Despite all interventions geared toward stabilization and symptom reduction, a crisis cannot always be prevented; therefore, it is most important to have a protocol for crisis intervention ready. Such a protocol may include instructions for a short-term stay in a crisis center or psychiatric hospital. It is advisable to develop the protocol together with the patient and to reach an agreement about its contents. One way to reduce the chance of crises during a therapist's leaves of absence is the enlistment of a deputy therapist, who also should be fully informed about the protocol.

Overcoming the phobia of traumatic memories. Traumatic memories are usually kept by traumatized child and adolescent identities. When the DID patient is becoming aware of the traumatic memories, it is usually in the form of traumatic imagery and reexperiences in the form of nightmares and flashbacks. Often, these experiences are preceded by confusing and terrifying feelings of panic and fear and intense somatic sensations (van der Kolk and Fisler 1995). Some authors discuss these various forms of traumatic reexperiences in terms of abreactions, which is criticized by van der Hart and Brown (1992) as being conceptually inadequate. When memories of trauma primarily intrude into consciousness in the form of sensory impressions and intense affect states, with little personal narrative, the patient is considered not to have "realized" the traumatic event (Janet 1935; van der Hart et al. 1993). Realization requires putting the event into words, relating it as a narrative, and reconciling the experience within the personality, thereby restoring continuity to the individual's personal history (van der Hart et al. 1993).

To effect realization, the dissociated aspects of the traumatic memories need to be reactivated in a safe therapeutic setting, lived through, and "brought together." This technique is based on the older literature (e.g., Myers 1920), emphasizing alleviation of traumatic dissociation as the essential stepping stone "toward realization and integration of the trauma memory." Therapeutic synthesis of traumatic memories is a purposeful mental action based on a conscious decision either by the whole personality or by the identities involved in the traumatic experience. For this endeavor to succeed, the patient, or the identities involved, need the full support of the therapist not only through his or her sharing in the experience, but also through encouragement and guidance.

The treatment of traumatic memories can be divided into three phases: preparation, synthesis, and realization/integration.

1. *Preparation.* Preparation addresses 1) safety factors; 2) controlling or containing reactivated traumatic memories, which are also part of stabilization and symptom reduction; 3) exploring traumatic memories; 4) correcting cognitive errors and distortions, which also took place during the previous phase; 5) careful explaining and planning of synthesis sessions; and 6) dealing with resistances.

Explanation is essential in building the necessary cognitive context for synthesis. The therapist explains the prninciples of trauma treatment and the forms it can take. This explanation sometimes takes two rounds (i.e., the first round with adult identities and the second with traumatized [child] identities involved in specific traumatic memories). When the explanation of treatment of a particular traumatic memory meets "resistance," it is most important to respect this resistance and consider the one or more important reasons identities may have to advise against trauma work or to be wary of it. These issues deserve careful and systematic exploration before moving on to the exploration of the traumatic memory and subsequent synthesis.

Exploration of the traumatic memories consists of 1) charting the context of the trauma, 2) completing the story of the trauma, and 3) identifying the identities involved and their role in the trauma. Because the host identity, with whom the therapist often is in contact, usually knows little about the trauma and the identities involved, it may be a good practice to request the relevant information from an observer identity, who has watched what happened "from a distance." To prevent unnecessary flashback experiences, the therapist suggests that other identities withdraw to (imaginary) safe places. The purpose of the ensuing inquiry is to become aware of all the dissociated elements, or "pathogenic kernels" (van der Hart and Op den Velde 1991), which must be synthesized to neutralize the traumatic memory. Often, the personal meaning in these pathogenic kernels is more important than the objective factual details.

Related to these pathogenic kernels are the cognitive distortions that developed during the actual trauma; they often contain the essence of the patient's personal experience. The trauma is encoded within a specific cognitive schema and continues to be interpreted within this context by the patient until the therapist assists in the construction of new assumptions, beliefs, and expectations about self and others. Resistances, which should be carefully explored as previously advised, often emanate from deeply embedded beliefs about the trauma (e.g., about the experience: "It lasted forever"; about the perpetrator: "He'll know if I ever tell," and about the self: "It was my fault" or "It didn't happen to me") (van der Hart et al. 1993).

2. *Synthesis.* Synthesis of a traumatic memory involves its controlled reactivation in a collaborative effort by the therapist and the patient. The involved identities reexperience and share their respective parts of the trauma with each other and with other identities not involved in the trauma. In this way, existing dissociations are relieved. The therapist helps the patient to stay in touch with the safe present and with the therapist, while the patient, and the identities involved, returns to the traumatic experience. At the end of synthesis, the therapist helps the patient to make a smooth transition to being completely in

the present. It has been determined in advance in what way the patient returns home and what kind of support and aftercare are available. This transformation requires both acceptance of the memory as real and a conciliation between this narrative memory and the patient's personality. Janet (1935) called this conciliation "realization" of the event and its consequences.

3. *Realization/integration.* The goal of successful synthesis is for the traumatic memory to stop operating at a sensorimotor level. The traumatic memory has now been transformed from an intrusive reexperiencing to a trauma-related narrative. Realization is the formulation of a belief about what happened (the trauma), when it happened (in the past), and to whom it happened (to self). The trauma becomes personalized, relegated to the past, and takes on symbolic rather than sensorimotor properties. Realization also involves an experiencing of one's history as one's own. With grief and mourning as the intermediate stages, realization involves the gradual assimilation or integration into the patient's personality.

The therapist's first task during this phase is to listen empathically to the narration of the story, repeatedly, if need be. Telling the story is an important component of realization and integration. The narrative makes the story more real and personal, and it shifts the trauma from an autistic reexperiencing to a relational sharing and linking in the therapeutic alliance. Cognitive work also should continue during this phase (Ross 1989). The patient develops more insights into the origins of cognitive distortions, and the affective and behavioral realms follow suit.

Overcoming the phobia of ordinary life.   Traumatic memories obstruct fusions between identities concerned, and a successful treatment of traumatic memories frees the way for it. With each fusion, another milestone toward integration of the personality is reached. Often, the fusion that patient and therapist regard as the last one (i.e., when unification has taken place) is not. Only when the dissociative symptoms have not reappeared after more than 2 years, Kluft (1987) states, may this fusion indeed be regarded as the final one. Integration is fostered first by stimulating identities to collaborate and negotiate with each other (the preparation phase).

When identities have learned to know each other, have shared their respective life histories and experiences, and have resolved their mutual conflicts and problems, then they are more clearly on the way to personal unity. The most frank way in which this happens is the fusion of two or more identities who are ready for it. There are DID patients who, even when all traumatic experiences seem to be integrated, continue living with a certain number of identities instead of aiming for unification. In our limited clinical practice, however, it appears that this decision always implies the existence of some other traumatic memories with which the patient tried to avoid dealing.

The third treatment phase, realization/integration, involves guiding the patient to build a new "culture," a new lifestyle (i.e., as belonging to a unified personality). We call this "ordinary life," and one of the resistances against this goal may be the patient's phobia of an ordinary life (Nijenhuis and van der Hart 1994). There is an all-pervasive fear that the patient is unable to cope with life without other identities to fall back on or to withdraw behind. This fear may be linked to the existence of unresolved traumatic cognitions (e.g., "I am always the victim"), which, however negative they may be, may give the patient something to live by. The certainty of a negative but familiar cognitive schema and related survival strategies is preferred above the uncertainty of an unknown ordinary life. However, Kluft (1993b) shows that fully integrated patients suffer less relapse and are more stress resistant than those who are not.

The implication that the patient has a phobia of ordinary life is not to push the patient toward final integration but to help the patient first to increase the capacity for self-care, self-confidence, and self-esteem; to acknowledge personal needs; and to change trauma-induced cognitions into more flexible ones. The patient is stimulated to take an active role in creating an environment in which trust, healthy independence, autonomy, power, esteem, and intimacy can flourish (McCann and Pearlman 1990). Ordinary life is a life with a sense of continuity, continuity of the present with the past as well as with the future. Many patients express feelings that they deserve to exist or even to live for the first time. A core sense of shame dissolves as the therapist provides a positive identification for patients in the context of the therapeutic alliance. Patients are urged to conclude that they have a right to selfhood and can begin building on that foundation (van der Hart et al. 1993).

Transference and Countertransference

A good working alliance, as the basis for effective psychotherapy, can be severely compromised by transference and countertransference reactions. As described by Kluft (1984, 1994a), Loewenstein (1993), Putnam (1989), and Spiegel (1986), among others, a traumatic (or posttraumatic) transference is usually the predominant mode in patients with DID and other trauma-induced disorders such as PTSD. This means that the patients consciously or subconsciously perceive the therapist as someone belonging to the traumatic experience and act toward him or her in a fitting manner. Thus, they may attribute to the therapist characteristics belonging to the perpetrator of the abuse or other violent crime they suffered, or those belonging to a neglectful caregiver. Patients with DID usually have a concomitant history of childhood abuse and neglect. Loewenstein (1993) discusses the following important transference themes: lack of trust in the therapist, fear that the therapist will use or abuse the patient for his or her own purposes, and desire to be healed through the therapist's love, attention, and care (associated with idealizing the therapist). Wilbur (1988) remarks that patients' transference can become extremely complicated because it contains admixtures of many forms of transference (which belong to different personality states all responding to the therapist). Barach (1991) describes the transference reactions of DID patients as attachment disorders and regards these various forms of transference as reactivations of their traumatic attachments in the past. The therapeutic relationship inevitably acts as a trigger for patients with DID (Loewenstein 1993); they experience flashbacks, which seriously cloud their realistic appraisal of the therapist.

The treatment of DID also can evoke strong countertransference responses in the therapist. (1994a) mentions as inevitable countertransferential phenomena an initial fascination and over-involvement with the patient, followed by a sense of discouragement, exhaustion, and burnout. Various authors emphasize the risk of secondary PTSD in therapists of traumatized patients (compare Wilson and Lindy 1994). This risk is rather high in the treatment of patients with DID. The inevitability of strong countertransference, which may impede therapy, is one of the reasons that therapists working in the DID field should not do their work alone but join groups of colleges for supervision or case consultation. When personal weaknesses are touched too often, or too intensely, seeking personal psychotherapy may be necessary.

References

Abeles M, Schilder P: Psychogenic loss of personal identity. Archives of Neurology and Psychiatry 34:587–604, 1935

American Psychiatric Association: Diagnostic and Statistical Manual of Mental Disorders, 4th Edition. Washington, DC, American Psychiatric Association, 1994

Barach P: Multiple personality disorder as an attachment disorder. Dissociation 4:117–123, 1991

Boon S, Draijer N: Multiple Personality Disorder in the Netherlands. Lisse, The Netherlands, Swets & Zeitlinger, 1993

Bremner JD, Southwick SM, Brett E, et al: Dissociation and posttraumatic stress disorder in Vietnam combat veterans. Am J Psychiatry 149: 328–333, 1992

Bremner JD, Steinberg M, Southwick SM, et al: Use of the Structured Clinical Interview for DSM-IV Dissociative Disorders for systematic assessment of dissociative symptoms in posttraumatic stress disorder. Am J Psychiatry 150:1011–1014, 1993

Briere J, Conte J: Self-reported amnesia for abuse in adults molested as children. J Trauma Stress 6:21-31, 1993

Brown D, Fromm E: Hypnotherapy and Hypnoanalysis. Hillsdale, NJ, Lawrence Erlbaum, 1986

Brown W: The treatment of cases of shell shock in an advanced neurological centre. Lancet 17:197–200, 1918

Chu JA, Dill DL: Dissociative symptoms in relation to childhood physical and sexual abuse. Am J Psychiatry 147:887–892, 1990

Crabtree A: From Mesmer to Freud: Magnetic Sleep and the Roots of Psychological Healing. Princeton, NJ, Princeton University Press, 1993

Ellenberger HF: The Discovery of the Unconscious. New York, Basic Books, 1970

Epstein S: The self-concept, the traumatic neurosis, and the structure of personality, in Perspectives on Personality, Vol 3. Edited by Ozer D, Healy JM, Stewart AJ. London, Jessica Kingsly, 1991

Fagan J, McMahon PP: Incipient multiple personality disorder in children: four cases. J Nerv Ment Dis 172:26–36, 1984

Fine CG: Thoughts on the cognitive-perceptual substrates of multiple personality disorder. Dissociation 1:5–10, 1988

Fine CG: Treatment stabilization and crisis intervention: pacing the therapy of the multiple personality disorder patient. Psychiatr Clin North Am 14:661–675, 1991

Fromm E: Hypnoanalysis: theory and two case excerpts. Psychotherapy: Theory, Research and Practice 2:127–133, 1965

Gelinas DJ: The persisting negative effects of incest. Psychiatry 46: 312–332, 1983

Groenendijk I, van der Hart O: Treatment of DID and DDNOS patients in a regional institute for ambulatory mental health care in the Netherlands: a survey. Dissociation 8:73–83, 1995

Gudjonsson GH: The psychology of Interrogations, Confessions and Testimony. New York, Wiley, 1992

Gudjonsson GH, Haward LRC: Hysterical amnesia as an alternative to suicide. Med Sci Law 22:68–72, 1982

Hammond DC (ed): Handbook of Hypnotic Suggestions and Metaphors. New York, WW Norton, 1990

Herman JL: Trauma and Recovery. New York, Basic Books, 1992

Horevitz RP, Loewenstein RJ: The rational treatment of multiple personality disorder, in Dissociation: Clinical and Theoretical Perspectives. Edited by Lynn SJ, Rhue JW. New York, Guilford, 1994, pp 289–316

Janet P: L'amnésie et la dissociation des souvenirs par l'émotion. Journal de Psychologie 1:417–453, 1904

Janet P: The Major Symptoms of Hysteria. London, Macmillan, 1907

Janet P: Les médications psychologiques (1919). Translation in Psychological Healing. New York, Macmillan, 1925

Janet P: Réalisation et interprétation. Ann Med Psychol (Paris) 93: 329–366, 1935

Kardiner A, Spiegel H: War Stress and Neurotic Illness. New York, Hoeber, 1947

Kluft RP: Aspects of the treatment of multiple personality disorder. Psychiatric Annals 14:51–55, 1984

Kluft RP: An update of multiple personality disorder. Hospital and Community Psychiatry 38:363–373, 1987

Kluft RP: Basic principles in conducting the psychotherapy of multiple personality disorder, in Clinical Perspectives on Multiple Personality Disorder. Edited by Kluft RP, Fine CG. Washington, DC, American Psychiatric Press, 1993a, pp 19–50

Kluft RP: Clinical approaches to the integration of personalities, in Clinical Perspectives on Multiple Personality Disorder. Edited by Kluft RP, Fine CG. Washington, DC, American Psychiatric Press, 1993b, pp 101–133

Kluft RP: The initial stages of psychotherapy in the treatment of multiple personality disorder patients. Dissociation 6:145–161, 1993c

Kluft RP: Countertransference in the treatment of multiple personality disorder, in Countertransference in the Treatment of Posttraumatic Stress Disorder. Edited by Wilson JP, Lindy JD. New York, 1994a, pp 122–150

Kluft RP: Treatment trajectories in multiple personality disorder. Dissociation 7:63–76, 1994b

Koopman C, Classen C, Spiegel D: Predictors of posttraumatic stress symptoms among survivors of the Oakland/Berkeley, California, firestorm. Am J Psychiatry 151:888–894, 1994

Loewenstein RJ: Psychogenic amnesia and psychogenic fugue: a comprehensive review, in American Psychiatric Press Review of Psychiatry, Vol. 10. Edited by Tasman A, Goldfinger SM. Washington, DC, American Psychiatric Press, 1991, pp 189–222

Loewenstein RJ: Posttraumatic and dissociative aspects of transference and countertransference in the treatment of multiple personality disorder, in Clinical Perspectives on Multiple Personality Disorder. Edited by Kluft RP, Fine CG. Washington, DC, American Psychiatric Press, 1993, pp 51–85

Loewenstein RJ: Dissociative amnesia and dissociative fugue, in Treatments of Psychiatric Disorders, 2nd Edition. Edited by Gabbard GO. Washington, DC, American Psychiatric Press,1995, pp 1569–1597

Loewenstein RJ, Putnam FW: The clinical phenomenology of males with multiple personality disorder. Dissociation 3:135–143, 1990

McCann IL, Pearlman LA: Psychological Trauma and the Adult Survivor. New York, Brunner/Mazel, 1990

Marmar CR, Weiss DS, Schlenger WE, et al: Peritraumatic dissociation and posttraumatic stress in male Vietnam theatre veterans. Am J Psychiatry 151:902–907, 1994

Myers CS: The revival of emotional memories and its therapeutic value, III. Br J Med Psychol 1:20–22, 1920

Myers CS: Shell Shock in France 1914–1918. Cambridge, England, Cambridge University Press, 1940

Noyes R, Hoenck PR, Kupperman BA: Depersonalization in accident victims and psychiatric patients. J Nerv Ment Dis 164:401–407, 1977

Nijenhuis ERS, van der Hart O: Dissociatieve stoornissen, in Handboek Klinische Psychologie. Houten, The Netherlands, Bohn Stafleu Van Loghum, 1994

Panos PT, Panos A, Allred GH: The need for marriage therapy in the treatment of multiple personality disorder. Dissociation 3:10–14, 1990

Putnam FW: Diagnosis and Treatment of Multiple Personality Disorder. New York, Guilford, 1989

Putnam FW, Guroff JJ, Silberman EK, et al: The clinical phenomenology of multiple personality disorder. J Clin Psychiatry 47:285–293, 1986

Ross CA: Multiple Personality Disorder. New York, Wiley, 1989

Ross CA, Heber S, Norton GR, et al: The Dissociative Disorders Interview Schedule: a structured interview. Dissociation 2:169–189, 1989

Saxe GN, van der Kolk BA, Berkowitz R, et al: Dissociative disorders in psychiatric inpatients. Am J Psychiatry 150:1037–1042, 1993

Scheflin AW, Shapiro L: Trance on Trial. New York, Guilford, 1989

Spiegel D: Vietnam grief work using hypnosis. Am J Clin Hypn 24:33–40, 1981

Spiegel D: Dissociation, double binds, and posttraumatic stress in multiple personality disorder, in Treatment of Multiple Personality Disorder. Edited by Braun BG. Washington, DC, American Psychiatric Press, 1986

Spiegel D: Dissociation and hypnosis in the treatment of victims of sexual abuse. Psychiatr Clin North Am 12:295–306, 1988

Spiegel D, Cardena E: Disintegrated experience: the dissociative disorders revisited. J Abnorm Psychol 100:366–378, 1991

Spiegel D, Scheflin AW: Dissociated or fabricated? psychiatric aspects of repressed memory in criminal and civil cases. Int J Clin Exp Hypn 42:411–432, 1994

Steinberg M: Structured Clinical Interview for DSM-IV Dissociative Disorders (SCID-D). Washington, DC, American Psychiatric Press, 1993

Takahashi Y: Aokigahara-jukai: suicide and amnesia in Mt. Fuji's black forest. Suicide Life Threat Behav 18:164–175, 1988

van der Hart O: Metaphoric and symbolic imagery in the hypnotic treatment of an urge to wander: a case report. Australian Journal of Clinical and Experimental Hypnosis 13:83–95, 1985

van der Hart O (ed): Trauma, Dissociatie en Hypnose. Lisse, The Netherlands, Swets & Zeitlinger, 1995

van der Hart O, Brown P: Abreaction re-evaluated. Dissociation 5: 127–140, 1992

van der Hart O, Friedman B: A reader's guide to Pierre Janet on dissociation: a neglected intellectual heritage. Dissociation 2:8–16, 1989

van der Hart O, Friedman B: Trauma, dissociation and triggers: their role in treatment and emergency psychiatry, in Emergency Psychiatry Today. Edited by van Luyn JB t al. New York, Elsevier, 1992

van der Hart O, Op den Velde W: Traumatische herinneringen [traumatic memories], in Trauma, Dissociatie en Hypnose. Edited by van der Hart O. Lisse, The Netherlands, Swets & Zeitlinger, 1995, pp 79–102

van der Hart O, Boon S, van Everdingen GB: Writing assignments and hypnosis in the treatment of traumatic memories, in Creative Mastery in Hypnosis and Hypnoanalysis: A Festschrift for Erika Fromm. Edited by Fass ML, Brown D. Hillsdale, NJ, Lawrence Erlbaum, 1990, pp 231–253

van der Hart O, Steele K, Boon S, et al: The treatment of traumatic memories: synthesis, realization and integration. Dissociation 6:162–180, 1993

van der Kolk B, Fisler R: Dissociation and the fragmentary nature of traumatic memories. Journal of Traumatic Stress 8:505–525, 1995

van der Kolk BA, Pelcovitz I, Roth S, et al: Dissociation, somatization and affect: the complexity of adaptation of trauma. Am J Psychiatry 153:83–93, 1996

Wilbur CA: Multiple personality disorder. Dissociation 1:73–76, 1988

Wilson JP, Lindy JD (eds): Countertransference in the Treatment of Posttraumatic Stress Disorder. New York, Guilford, 1994

Chapter 10

Effects of Flooding on Memories of Patients With Posttraumatic Stress Disorder

Philip A. Saigh, Ph.D.

To date, a host of flooding trials involving patients with post-traumatic stress disorder (PTSD) have appeared in the clinical literature. Most of these reports have used outcome measures involving self-report indexes of anxiety or cardiovascular indicators of reactivity to traumatic stimuli. More recently, a great deal of interest has been focused on the memory alterations of PTSD patients. This interest raises the question of whether treatments such as flooding may influence the memories of individuals who have been exposed to extreme stress. In view of these points, I review in this chapter the single-case, quasi-experimental, and experimental studies that examine the effects of flooding on memory.

History

Although flooding has gained considerable currency as an effective treatment for anxiety disorders since the late 1960s, variants of this modality have been used for centuries. Goethe, for example, provided the following description of his self-initiated remedy for acrophobia:

> I ascended quite alone the highest pinnacle of the cathedral spire, and sat in the so-called neck under the knob or crown, as it is called, for a quarter of an hour, before I ventured to step out again into the open air, where, on standing on a platform, scarcely an ell square, without anything particular to hold on to, one sees before one the

boundless land, while the nearest objects and ornaments conceal the church and everything on which and above which one stands. It is exactly as if one saw oneself carried up into the air in a balloon. Such anxiety and pain I repeated so often until the impression became quite different to me, and I have therefore derived great advantage from these practices in mountain travels and on geological studies, and on great buildings, where I have viewed with the carpenters in running over the freeflying beams and the cornices of the building, and even in Rome, where one must run similar risks in order to obtain a nearer view of important works of art. (Goethe 1770, quoted in Boudewyns and Shipley 1983, p. 3)

Examined from a more contemporary perspective, Herzberg (1941) treated a 31-year-old agoraphobic female by advising her to complete a series of progressively longer walks in a park that was adjacent to her residence. Although the patient experienced considerable distress, she completed 18 exposure sessions. Following treatment, Herzberg reported that the patient could "go everywhere without fear or weakness" (p. 26).

Similarly, Malleson (1959) described a course of in vitro or imaginal flooding that was used in the treatment of a test-phobic Indian student who was studying in Great Britain for an important qualifying exam. The student was characterized as " . . . classically panic stricken . . . sobbing and fearful, bewailing his fate, and terrified of the impending examination . . . " (p. 225). Malleson's treatment consisted of advising the student to "tell of the awful consequences that he felt would follow his failure—derision from his colleagues in India, disappointment from his family and financial loss" (p. 225). Moreover, the student was advised that "whenever he felt a little wave of spontaneous alarm, he was not to push it aside, but was to augment it, to try to experience it more profoundly and more vividly" (p. 225).

Although the procedure was associated with considerable distress, the student practiced assiduously and reported that he was almost unable to feel frightened as the date of the exam approached. He passed the exam without difficulty.

In 1961, Stampfl, in an unpublished manuscript titled "Implosive Therapy: A Learning Theory Derived Psychodynamic Technique," coined the term *implosive therapy* to characterize a regimen that "may be regarded as a synthesis between Freudian-oriented and Mowrerian[1] approaches to psychotherapy" (p. 1). Stampfl and Levis (1967) devised an elaborate description of the procedure and theoretical rationale to account for its efficacy. They noted that the initial objective of implosive therapy involves the identification of the exteroceptive and interoceptive conditioned stimuli or cues that are being avoided. It was hypothesized that fear-inducing cues are apparent in a variety of forms (e.g., auditory, tactile, and cognitive). They also theorized that these stimuli are interdependent and ordered in a serial hierarchy as a function of the degree of avoidance. Cues are said to be selected from subjective experiences wherein "objects or situations are known to have high-anxiety eliciting value, as in specific traumatic situations, material produced by dreams or symbolism of a psychoanalytic nature" (Stamfl and Levis 1967, p. 502). Once recognized, cues are presented in a sequential order by instructing patients to imagine and verbalize significant symptom-contingent cues until extinction takes place.

Rachman (1966) introduced the term *flooding* to the clinical literature. It is of interest to note that Rachman attributed the term to Pollin (1959) who used it to describe the aversive component of an infrahuman laboratory trial involving extinction. Although Rachman's (1966) article concluded that systematic desensitization was more effective than flooding in the treatment of phobic individuals, he acknowledged that the patients who were treated had not received more than 2 minutes of anxiety-inducing stimulation at a time and that it was "possible therefore that the crucial element omitted in the present technique is prolonged exposure" (p. 6). Shortly thereafter, a number of studies involving prolonged expo-

---

[1]Oval Herbert Mowrer (1907–1987) was an American psychologist who applied learning theory to complex behavioral problems. He is recognized for rephrasing psychoanalysis precepts in operational terms and for experimentally testing Freudian notions. His two-factor formulation of learned anxiety has been highly influential in behavioral psychology (Rachman 1990).

sure (i.e., 40–60 minutes of stimulation) were conducted (compare I. A. Marks 1972). In contrast to Rachman's (1966) report, these studies demonstrated efficacy across a wide range of patients with simple and social phobias. For example, Barrett (1969) compared the effects of systematic desensitization and implosive therapy relative to the avoidance behaviors and fear ratings of a sample of undergraduates with a snake phobia. Although no significant variations were observed between the experimental groups immediately after treatment and at a 6-month follow-up, both groups evinced significantly less avoidance and lower self-reported fear estimates than a nontreated control group. Barrett (1969) also observed that implosive therapy was appreciably faster than systematic desensitization (i.e., implosive therapy was completed in 45% of the time that was required to complete systematic desensitization).

By 1972, a considerable number of flooding trials had been performed across a host of heterogeneous cases. Based on an extensive review of these reports, I. A. Marks (1972) formulated an important definition for the flooding process:

> Flooding is not a fixed technique but comprises a range of procedures that merge into one another. Flooding is at one end of a continuum of approach to distressing situations, at the opposite end of which is desensitization. The difference between the two is largely one of degree. The more sudden the confrontation, the more it is prolonged, and the greater the emotion that accompanies it, the more apt is the label *flooding* for that procedure. (p. 154, italics in original)

Continuing from the 1970s to date, a number of studies have been done on flooding as a treatment for a wide range of phobic individuals (Boudewyns 1975; Boudewyns and Shipley 1983; Hogan and Kirchner 1967; Horne and Matson 1977; Jacobson 1991; I. Marks et al. 1975; Sellick and Peck 1981; Smith and Sharpe 1970; Yule et al. 1974). Although it is beyond the scope of this chapter to present a detailed review of this literature, it may be said that flooding in one form or another has been used effectively to treat a wide variety of phobias.

Imaginal Flooding and Posttraumatic Stress Disorder

Drawing from the exposure-based anxiety disorder therapeutic literature, Fairbank et al. (1981) used a multifaceted flooding package in the treatment of an accident victim. As this investigation was actually conducted before PTSD was recognized as a psychiatric disorder in 1980, the patient was described as having "a persistent posttraumatic startle response" (Fairbank et al. 1981, p. 321). The report involved a 32-year-old female survivor of a motor vehicle collision. The patient and two of her daughters experienced multiple physical injuries (i.e., one child was rendered unconscious after striking her head against the windshield, and the patient received a number of lacerations). Although the patient recovered from her injuries and was able to drive again, she experienced acute anxiety attacks whenever she attempted to drive a motor vehicle. She also reported a shortness of breath and a proclivity to tug the steering wheel to the right whenever she saw an oncoming vehicle. Using a treatment package involving directed relaxation, self-monitoring, and imaginal exposure to traumatic scenes, Fairbank et al. (1981) eliminated the startle reaction and appreciably reduced the woman's self-rated anxiety estimates following five treatment sessions. These impressive improvements continued to be seen at 1-, 4-, and 6-month follow-up assessments.

Keane and Kaloupek (1982) subsequently published a frequently cited paper involving imaginal flooding in the treatment of posttraumatic stress disorder. Their article described the treatment of a 36-year-old veteran of the Vietnam conflict who developed PTSD following a series of war-related incidents. Keane and Kaloupek (1982) identified a number of traumatic experiences that reoccurred in the form of intrusive and highly arousing thoughts, nightmares, and dissociative flashbacks. Nineteen flooding sessions were used wherein the patient was instructed to imagine the traumatic events for approximately 40 minutes. Keane and Kaloupek (1982) reported significant reductions in self-reported anxiety and reductions in heart rate reactivity as measured during traumatic simulations. The patient also reported that his sleep and work-related efficacy had significantly improved. In keeping with the scientist-practitioner tradition, follow-up assessments were performed and continued efficacy was demonstrated 3 and 12 months after the last therapeutic session.

In a host of single-case research, inferences are generally made about the efficacy of an intervention by comparing data points that are collected as different conditions are presented to one or more subjects. According to Kazdin (1992), single-case experimental designs require continuous assessment (before, during, and after therapy), as well as the presence of a stable rate of performance at baseline (i.e., the absence of a trend or slope and little variability in performance). Flooding trials involving PTSD patients subsequently appeared in the clinical literature (e.g., Black and Keane 1982; Fairbank and Keane 1982; Fairbank et al. 1983; McCaffrey and Fairbank 1985; Saigh 1987a, 1987b, 1987c, 1989a, 1989b). Three quasi-experimental studies (Richards et al. 1994; R. K. Pitman, S. P. Orr, B. Altmann, R. E. Longprel, R. E. Poir, M. L. Macklin, and G. S. Steketee: "Emotional Processing During Flooding Therapy of Vietnam Veterans With PTSD," unpublished study, November 1995; P. A. Saigh: "The Effects of Imaginal Flooding on the Short Term Memory, Concentration, and Self-Reported Distress of Child-Adolescent Posttraumatic Stress Disorder Patients," unpublished study, 1995) and three experimental studies (Cooper and Clum 1989; Keane et al. 1989; Boudewyns and Hyer 1990) involving the use of flooding with PTSD patients have been published. Inasmuch as this book deals with PTSD and memory, this chapter reviews the single-case, quasi-experimental, and experimental studies that examine the effects of flooding on memory. Particular attention is afforded to studies that consider the effects of flooding on trauma-related thoughts or nightmares. Attention also is afforded to investigations that employ standardized indicators of memory and concentration. Although primary consideration is given to the effects of flooding on the parameters of memory as specified within this chapter, attention also is given to indicators of psychological and psychophysiological adjustment. Inasmuch as the external validity of similar treatments may vary as a function of the design characteristic (Barlow and Hersen 1984; Kazdin 1992), the single-case, quasi-experimental, and experimental flooding reports are reviewed separately.

The Effects of Therapeutic Flooding on Memory Functions

Single-Case Studies

Within the context of single-case studies that employed traumatic recollections as a treatment outcome variable, Fairbank et al. (1983) initially presented a course of flooding to a Vietnam combat veteran with PTSD (age and duration of time since stress exposure were not reported). Therapy consisted of nine flooding sessions (15 minutes of relaxation exercises followed by 60–70 minutes of imaginal exposure). Fairbank et al. (1983) reported that the patient had been experiencing 2–5 nightmares per week as denoted by self-monitored frequencies that were recorded for 6 consecutive days before the treatment. Posttreatment anecdotal comments indicated that "the subject continued to think about the traumatic event on a daily basis, but he noted that the recollections were no longer as distressing as prior to the treatment" (p. 565). Although the posttreatment frequency of war-related nightmares was not reported, a 6-month follow-up assessment determined that he had only 1 combat-related nightmare during the previous months. In addition, Fairbank et al. (1983) observed significant reductions in motor reactions (e.g., rapid respiration, arm and leg movements, crying, and facial expression) to traumatic stimuli over the course of the therapeutic regimen. Clinically significant reductions also were noted on the Hamilton Depression Rating Scale (Hamilton 1960) and a locally developed DSM-III (American Psychiatric Association 1980) 15-category PTSD checklist at posttreatment and 6-month follow-up.

Rychtarik et al. (1984) subsequently described using imaginal flooding with a 22-year-old female incest victim. The patient reported that between the ages of 12 and 15 years, her father had repeatedly forced her to experience a number of incestuous activities. Her presenting symptoms included anxiety-evoking incest-related thoughts, isolation, sleep disturbance, and alcohol abuse. Treatment consisted of 9 sessions that involved 10 minutes of therapist-directed relaxation exercises and 80–90 minutes of imaginary exposure to incestuous scenes. Rychtarik et al. (1984) observed that the incidence of self-monitored incest-related thoughts and nightmares that were fairly prominent before treatment were virtually nonexistent after therapy. Similar results were observed at a 6-month follow-up. Clinically significant reductions in self-reported anxiety as measured by the State Trait Anxiety Inventory (STAI; Spielberger et al. 1968) were observed at 6- and 8-week follow-ups. Six- and 8-week follow-up assessments also evidenced clinically significant reductions on skin conductance levels that were recorded during the imaginal exposures to incest-reminiscent material.

McCaffrey and Fairbank (1985) went on to describe the treatment of a 31-year-old male witness to a fatal helicopter crash and a 28-year-old female motor vehicle accident victim. Eighteen to 20 months after their respective experiences, the subjects met DSM-III criteria for PTSD. The first subject received four 120-minute treatment sessions that consisted of relaxation training, as well as imaginal exposure and an unspecified number of in vivo exposure sessions to trauma-reminiscent stimulus cues. The second subject received a comparable regimen involving eight imaginal and in vivo exposure sessions.

To gauge the efficacy of the therapeutic package, the subjects self-monitored the number of nightmares, as well as the amount of sleep, that they experienced before and after therapy. The total number of self-monitored trauma-related dreams decreased from two to zero for the first subject and from six to two for the second. It is of considerable interest to observe that the second subject "reported for the first time that she neither awakened in a cold sweat nor avoided returning to sleep following a nightmare" (McCaffrey and Fairbank 1985, p. 412). Clinically significant posttreatment gains denoting increased self-reported anxiety and increased sleep were reported. Pre- and posttreatment heart rate and skin resistance levels were monitored as the subjects watched videotaped simulations of trauma-reminiscent scenarios. Although the first subject's pre- and posttreatment heart rate and skin resistance levels were essentially similar, the second subject's basal level of cardiovascular reactivity markedly decreased.

Given the absence of information involving the effects of flooding on traumatized youth and a pressing need to provide services for traumatized youth during the Lebanese crisis, Saigh effected a number of single-case flooding trials at the American University of Beirut Medical Center. Initially, Saigh (1987a) described the treatment of a 14-year-old Lebanese boy who had been abducted and tortured. Six months after the incident, the boy met diagnostic criteria for PTSD as denoted by the Children's Posttraumatic Stress Disorder Inventory (Saigh 1989a). Before the treatment, the Wechsler Intelligence Scale for Children—Revised(WISC-R) Coding and Digit Span subtests were administered because these measures provide norm-referenced estimates of short-term memory and concentration. The boy also marked the STAI (Spielberger et al. 1968), the Rathus Assertiveness Schedule (RAS; Rathus 1973), and the Beck Depression Inventory (BDI; Beck et al. 1961). A 12-item Behavioral Avoidance Test (BAT; Saigh 1987a) was developed in order to measure the quantitative aspects of his trauma-related avoidance behaviors. In effect, the BAT involved a 10-minute behavioral walk wherein the boy left his home and proceeded along the route that he had taken to the place where the abduction occurred.

Four anxiety-evoking scenes were initially identified through a series of clinical interviews. These scenes were indicative of the chronological sequence of traumatic events that the youth had experienced (e.g., being stopped, forced into a car at gunpoint, blindfolded, and driven away). The imaginal flooding process consisted of 10 minutes of therapist-directed deep-muscle relaxation exercises that were followed by 60 minutes of therapeutic stimulation wherein the youth was instructed to imagine the particular details of the anxiety-evoking scenes according to a multiple baseline across traumatic scenes design (Fairbank and Keane 1982). Emotional distress relative to the traumatic scenes that were presented during the imaginal stimulations was evaluated through subjective units of disturbance (SUDs) ratings. In so doing, subjective levels of anxiety relative to each scene were rated according to a 0- to 10-point scale, with 0 denoting "no discomfort" and 10 denoting "maximum discomfort." SUDs ratings were elicited at 2-minute intervals during each of the aversive scene presentations. The youth's SUDs levels appreciably decreased after seven flooding sessions. As may be noted from Figure 10–1, his multiple baseline SUDs ratings appreciably decreased over time. A 4-month follow-up revealed that the youth experienced almost no distress as measured by trauma-specific SUDs ratings.

Clinically significant pre- and posttreatment gains were observed on the WISC-R Coding and Digit Span subtests. Posttreatment and 4-month follow-up assessments also reflected clinically significant treatment gains with respect to self-reported anxiety, depression, and misconduct. Although the youth only completed one-third of the BAT (Saigh 1987a) items before the treatment, 100% of the BAT activities were completed following the final treatment session. These improvements also were apparent during a 4-month follow-up evaluation.

Saigh (1987b, 1987c, 1987d, 1989b) went on to conduct four single-case replications wherein flooding was used in the treatment of traumatized youth. In each instance, traumatic scenes were identified and verbally presented according to a multiple baseline across traumatic scenes design. Examined in this context, Table 10–1 presents the transcript of a flooding session involving a 10-year-old Lebanese female who developed PTSD after being exposed to an artillery barrage (Saigh 1987b). As may be noted from Table 10–1, stimulus and response imagery cues were employed throughout the flooding process. Stimulus cues involved the visual, auditory, olfactory, and tactile components of each scene. Response cues involved the behavioral and cognitive aspects of the scene.

In two of the Lebanese reports (Saigh 1987b, 1987c), the frequency of unwanted and intrusive trauma-related thoughts (excluding the ones that were induced in therapy) were self-monitored on pocket frequency counters (i.e., the Knit Tally, Boyle Needle Company). Figure 10–2 presents the frequency of sponta-

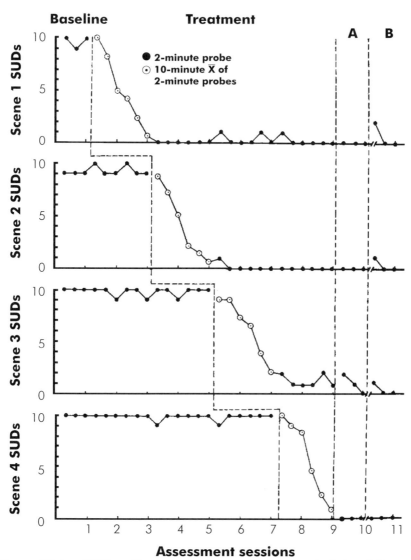

Figure 10–1. SUDs ratings across traumatic scenes. A, 3-day follow-up. B, 6-month follow-up.
Reprinted from Saigh PA: "In Vitro Flooding of a Childhood Posttraumatic Stress Disorder." *School Psychology Review* 16:203–211, 1987. Copyright 1987 by the National Association of School Psychologists. Reprinted by permission of the publisher.

Table 10–1.	Example of imaginal flooding process with a 10-year-old female
Therapist:	Imagine that you are playing in a neighborhood garden in the afternoon. Imagine the color of the grass and the plants. Imagine the people slowly walking by. Can you picture this?
Mariam:	Yes.
Therapist:	Imagine running after the ball that your mother threw. Now, imagine that you are looking at the shrubs. Imagine how you are separating the shrubs in search of the ball. Can you imagine yourself doing this?
Mariam:	Yes.
Therapist:	Now I want you to keep on imagining that you are leafing through the shrubs. Imagine the texture of them against your hands. Imagine the color of the underside of the leaves. Can you imagine this?
Mariam:	Yes.
Therapist:	According to the scale that we discussed, how much does this bother you?
Mariam:	Seven.
Therapist:	Very good. Keep on picturing this (10-second pause). Now imagine that you can hear loud noises that sound like thunder in the distance as you are looking for the ball. Can you imagine these noises?
Mariam:	Yes.
Therapist:	Good. Now I want you to imagine that you are still looking for the ball in the shrubs (10-second pause). Suddenly, you hear a very loud explosion nearby. Imagine that you are looking up. People are running away. Imagine how everyone is running. Can you do this?
Mariam:	Yes.
Therapist:	How much does it bother you?
Mariam:	Ten.

(continued)

Table 10–1.	Example of imaginal flooding process with a 10-year-old female *(continued)*
Therapist:	Keep on imagining how people are running away. Imagine that you are turning away from the shrub. You want to find your mother. Imagine looking at the place where your mother had been. She is not there. Imagine that you suddenly hear a very loud explosion. Imagine that you are starting to run to the place where your mother had been. Can you picture this?
Mariam:	Yes. It's very bad.
Therapist:	How disturbing is it?
Mariam:	Ten.

Source. Reprinted from Saigh PA: "In Vitro Flooding of a Childhood Posttraumatic Stress Disorder." *School Psychology Review* 16:203–211, 1987. Copyright 1987 by the National Association of School Psychologists. Reprinted by permission of the publisher.

neous trauma-specific thoughts, which were self-monitored by the youth who experienced the artillery barrage (Saigh 1987b). As may be noted from Figure 10–2, treatment was associated with a brief exacerbation of intrusive trauma-related thoughts. It may also be seen that the frequency of these traumatic memories appreciably decreased over time. Similar patterns of arousal and habituation were noted in a follow-up study involving three Lebanese children with war-related PTSD (Saigh 1987c).

Clinically significant pre- and posttreatment variations were observed on the WISC-R Digit Span and Coding subtests in all of the Saigh single-case studies. Likewise, significant reductions in self-reported reactivity to the traumatic scenes were evident on the SUDs ratings that were monitored before therapy, during therapy, at posttreatment, and at follow-up assessments. Moreover, clinically significant gains were observed across a number of self-report measures of anxiety and depression. Four of the Lebanese child-adolescent reports (Saigh 1987b, 1987c, 1987d, 1989b) included performance measures. In each of these instances, appreciably less avoidance was evident as measured by BAT performance at posttreatment and follow-up assessments. Finally, the

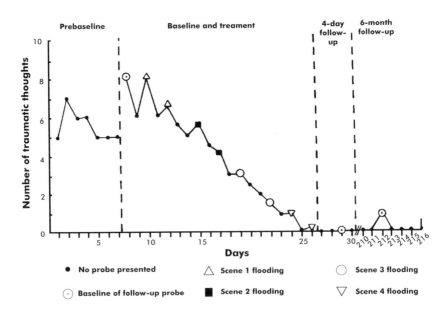

Figure 10–2.   Self-monitored frequency of traumatic thoughts.
Reprinted from Saigh PA: "In Vitro Flooding of a Childhood Posttraumatic Stress Disorder." *School Psychology Review* 16:203–211, 1987. Copyright 1987 by the National Association of School Psychologists. Reprinted
by permission of the publisher.

subjects' anecdotal comments supported the social validity
(Schwartz and Bear 1991; Wolf 1978) of the interventions because
they stated that the treatment outcome was worth the temporary
discomfort that they experienced.

Quasi-Experimental Studies

Within the context of group studies that did not involve a control
group, Richards et al. (1994) presented a regimen of imaginal and in
vivo flooding packages to 13 patients who met DSM-III-R (American Psychiatric Association 1987) criteria for PTSD. Their sample involved 9 women and 4 men with a mean age of 32 years. The
average duration of time between trauma exposure and treatment
was 2 years. Nine patients had survived the sinking of a cruise ship,

three were the victims of criminal assaults, and one was a survivor of a storm-related accident. Treatment consisted of four weekly hour-long sessions of imaginal exposure that were followed by four weekly hour-long in vivo exposures. Imaginal exposure involved asking patients to relate verbally their traumatic experiences in the first person. This process was repeated until within-session habituation occurred. In vivo exposure consisted of having the patients expose themselves (in the company of a therapist) to trauma-related situations that had been avoided. In addition, patients were assigned homework that involved listening to their audiotaped exposure sessions, as well as repeated actual exposures (in the company of a relative) to trauma-related stimuli.

Data analysis determined that posttreatment and follow-up assessments at 1, 3, 6, and 12 months were associated with significant gains on the Intrusion (an index of unwanted trauma-related memories) and Avoidance (an index of trauma-specific avoidance) scales of the Revised Impact of Event Scale (Horowitz et al. 1979). Significant pretreatment, posttreatment, and follow-up gains were also noted on a PTSD symptom checklist that denoted the frequency of trauma-related intrusive thoughts. Comparable gains were noted for self-reported avoidance and hyperarousal. Comparable significant gains were observed on the BDI (Beck et al. 1961), Fear Questionnaire (I. M. Marks and Matthews 1979), General Health Questionnaire (Goldberg and Williams 1988), and Work and Social Adjustment (I. M. Marks 1986).

Pitman et al. (" Emotional Processing During Flooding Therapy of Vietnam Veterans With PTSD," unpublished study, November 1995) went on to conduct a one-group pretest-posttest flooding study involving Vietnam veterans with war-related PTSD. Subjects were 20 men with a mean age of 42.5 years. Although the mean interval between stress exposure and therapy was not reported, the authors indicated that the subjects were symptomatic for 20 years. Treatment was preceded by a 10-minute baseline psychophysiological recording session and 10 minutes of relaxation and pleasant imagery exercises. The subjects went on to receive seven to eleven 10-minute imaginal flooding sessions. Each session concluded with a brief discussion of what had transpired during the simulations. Pitman and his colleagues observed a significant reduction in the number of self-monitored combat-related memories as measured before treatment and immediately after the treatment was concluded. In addition, significant reductions were observed on the Intrusion and Avoidance indexes of the Revised Impact of Event Scale (Horowitz et al. 1979). On the other hand, Pitman and his colleagues observed nonsignificant effects on the Mississippi Scale for Combat-Related Posttraumatic Stress Disorder (Keane et al. 1988) and the Symptom Checklist—90—Revised Global Symptom Inventory (SCL-90-R-GSI; Derogatis 1983).

Because the efficacy of flooding with traumatized youth rested on a handful of single-case reports, I conducted a quasi-experimental analysis (P. A. Saigh: "The Effects of Imaginal Flooding on the Short Term Memory, Concentration, and Self-Reported Distress of Child-Adolescent Posttraumatic Stress Disorder Patients," unpublished study, 1995) of the research involving Lebanese youth. The subject pool involved 8 patients (5 males and 3 females) with a mean age of 11 years. The mean duration between stress exposure and treatment was 2 years. Although different outcome measures were employed in a number of these trials (e.g., the Revised Children's Manifest Anxiety Inventory [RCMAI; Reynold and Richmond 1978], the STAI [Spielberger et al. 1968], the Reynolds Adolescent Depression Scale, the Children's Depression Inventory, and the BDI [Beck 1961]), all these elements used the WISC-R Digit Span and Block Design subtests, as well as SUDs ratings that were recorded during the simulations. Moreover, all the Lebanese single-case trials used treatment packages that involved relaxation (10–15 minutes), imaginal exposure to traumatic scenes (24–60 minutes), and additional relaxation (5–10 minutes). Data analysis determined that imaginal flooding was associated with statistically significant gains on standardized indexes of short-term memory and concentration at posttreatment (i.e., the Digit Span and Coding subtests). Significant posttreatment reductions also were noted on the trauma-specific indicators of emotional distress. Four- to 6-month follow-up assessments also were associated with statistically significant WISC-R Digit Span and Coding gains and significant SUDs reductions.

Experimental Studies

Although three experimental studies explored the efficacy of flooding in Vietnam veterans with combat-related PTSD (Boudewyns and Hyer 1990; Cooper and Clum 1989; Keane et al. 1989), only two of these reports (Cooper and Clum 1989; Keane et al. 1989) employed indicators of memory function as outcome variables. Viewed in this context, Cooper and Clum (1989) randomly assigned eight Vietnam veterans with PTSD to a flooding group and eight others to a "standard" Veterans Administration treatment program for PTSD. Subjects were matched relative to age, marital status, race, comorbid psychiatric diagnosis, and psychotropic medication. The actual flooding process consisted of ten to twelve 50-minute sessions of therapeutic stimulation. In addition, the experimental and control groups received 1 hour per week of individual therapy involving general discussions of war-related experiences and 2 hours per week of insight-oriented group psychotherapy.

A posttreatment assessment and a 3-month follow-up revealed that the frequency of war-related nightmares of the flooding group was significantly lower than that of the control group. Comparable effects were observed on the STAI state scores and self-reported reactivity to noise (i.e., startle response). Flooding was associated with significantly less avoidance on a war-related BAT. On the other hand, no significant differences were observed on the STAI trait scores and BDI. Heart rate estimates that were recorded when a BAT was attempted were not significantly different.

Similarly, Keane et al. (1989) randomly assigned a sample of 11 Vietnam veterans to an experimental (imaginal flooding) group and 13 others to a wait-list control group. Both groups met DSM-III criteria through a series of clinical interviews. As in the case of the Cooper and Clum (1989) study, groups were comparable with regard to race, marital status, age, education, and degree of combat exposure. The experimental subjects received 14 sessions of imaginal flooding. After two to three sessions of guided relaxation, a multifacilitated flooding package was presented (i.e., 15 minutes

of discussion, 10 minutes of relaxation, 45 minutes of traumatic imagery, 10 minutes of relaxation, and 10 minutes of debriefing). Because of ethical concerns, 10 of the 13 patients who were assigned to
the wait-list control group received a regimen of anxiolytic medication. Treatment efficacy was judged according to posttreatment and
6-month follow-up scores on a PTSD checklist as well as standardized self-report measures of anxiety and depression. In terms of
memory function, posttreatment and 6-month follow-up assessments determined that the flooding group had significantly fewer
trauma-reexperiencing symptoms than the control group. Therapist ratings also indicated that the flooding group had significantly
fewer startle reactions, less self-reported guilt, and less memory impairment as compared with the wait-list control subjects. The flooding group had significantly lower scores on the STAI State and Trait
scales, Fear Survey Schedule (Geer 1965), BDI, and Zung Depression Scale (Zung 1965). Nonsignificant differences were observed
on a therapist's ratings of sleep disturbance and psychic numbing,
as well as on a self-rated index of social adjustment. Significantly
lower scores were observed on the Minnesota Multiphasic Personality Inventory PTSD subscale (Keane et al. 1984).

Table 10–2 summarizes the single-case, quasi-experimental, and
experimental flooding studies that employed indicators of memory and related outcome variables. Examined comprehensively,
these studies on flooding regimens apparently have reduced
traumatic memories, facilitated adjustment, and enhanced
nontrauma-related memory. Despite these rather salutary observations, a number of clinical, ethical, and methodological concerns
also are apparent.

Clinical and Ethical Considerations

Although this chapter is not intended to serve as a clinical guide
(detailed flooding procedures with adults as well as children and
adolescents have been reported elsewhere (Keane et al. 1985; Saigh
1992; Saigh et al., in press-b), a number of clinical and ethical concerns warrant consideration.

Table 10–2. Single-case, quasi-experimental, and experimental flooding studies

Author/ date	Type of study	Subject characteristics	Treatment	Outcomes
Fairbank et al. 1983	1	Male Vietnam veteran; age and exposure-treatment interval not specified	Nine sessions (10 min relaxation followed by 60–70 min imaginal flooding)	Fewer traumatic recollections, nightmares, behavioral reactions during simulations; reduced scores on Hamilton Depression Rating Scale and PTSD checklist
Rychtarik et al. 1984	1	22-year-old female incest victim; presented 7 years posttrauma	Nine sessions (10 min relaxation followed by 80–90 min imaginal flooding)	Fewer and less aversive traumatic recollections and nightmares; reduced STAI scores
McCaffrey and Fairbank 1985	1	31-year-old male witness of helicopter crash; presented 20 months posttrauma	Four 2-hr imaginal flooding sessions involving relaxation followed by exposure and unspecified number of in vivo exposures	Fewer and less aversive traumatic recollections, fewer nightmares, less self-reported anxiety; heart rate and skin resistance during simulations unchanged

(continued)

Table 10–2.	Single-case, quasi-experimental, and experimental flooding studies (continued)			
Author/date	Type of study	Subject characteristics	Treatment	Outcomes
		28-year-old female motor vehicle accident survivor; presented 18 months posttrauma	Seven 2-hr. imaginal flooding sessions involving relaxation followed by exposure and unspecified number of in vivo exposures	Fewer and less aversive traumatic recollections, fewer nightmares, less self-reported anxiety; heart rate and skin resistance during simulations appreciably lower at posttreatment
Saigh 1987a	1	14-year-old Lebanese male; presented 6 months posttrauma	Six flooding sessions (10 min relaxation, 60 min imaginal flooding, and 10 min relaxation)	Posttreatment gains on the WISC-R Digit Span and Coding subtests; reduced SUDs ratings during simulations, STAI, BDI, and CTRS scores; enhanced performance on BAT
Saigh 1987b	1	10-year-old Lebanese female; presented 38 months posttrauma	Nine flooding sessions (10 min relaxation, 60 min imaginal flooding, and 5 min relaxation between scenes)	Posttreatment gains on the WISC-R Digit Span and Coding subtests; reduced SUDs ratings during simulations, RCMAS, CDI, and CTRS scores, self-monitored trauma-related ideation; enhanced performance on BAT

Saigh 1987c	1	11-year-old Lebanese female; presented 32 months posttrauma	Ten flooding sessions (10 min relaxation, 60 min imaginal flooding, and 5 min relaxation between scenes)	Posttreatment gains on the WISC-R Digit Span and Coding subtests; reduced SUDs ratings during simulations, self-monitored trauma-related ideation, RCMAS, CDI, and CTRS score; improved performance on BAT
		11-year-old Lebanese female; presented 36 months posttrauma	Nine flooding sessions (10 min relaxation, 60 min imaginal flooding, and 5 min relaxation between scenes)	Posttreatment gains on the WISC-R Digit Span and Coding subtests; reduced SUDs ratings during simulations, self-monitored trauma-related ideation, RCMAS, CDI, and CTRS score; improved performance on BAT
		12-year-old Lebanese male; presented 28 months posttrauma	Ten flooding sessions (10 min relaxation, 60 min imaginal flooding, and 5 min relaxation between scenes)	Posttreatment gains on the WISC-R Digit Span and Coding subtests; reduced SUDs ratings during simulations, self-monitored trauma-related ideation, RCMAS, CDI, and CTRS scores; improved performance on BAT
Saigh 1987d	1	6.5-year-old Lebanese male; presented 25 months posttrauma	Eleven flooding sessions (15 min relaxation, 24 min imaginal flooding, and 10 min relaxation)	Posttreatment gains on the WISC-R Digit Span and Coding subtests; reduced SUDs ratings during simulations, RCMAS, CDI, and CTRS scores

(continued)

Table 10–2. Single-case, quasi-experimental, and experimental flooding studies *(continued)*

Author/date	Type of study	Subject characteristics	Treatment	Outcomes
Saigh 1989b	1	13-year-old Lebanese female; presented 14 months posttrauma	Thirteen flooding sessions (10 min relaxation, 60 min imaginal flooding, and 10 min relaxation)	Posttreatment gains on the WISC-R Digit Span and Coding subtests; reduced SUDs ratings during simulations, self-monitored trauma-related ideation, RCMAS, CDI, and CTRS scores; improved performance on BAT
		14-year-old Lebanese male; presented 16 months posttrauma	Twelve flooding sessions (10 min relaxation, 60 min imaginal flooding, and 10 min relaxation)	Posttreatment gains on the WISC-R Digit Span and Coding subtests; reduced SUDs ratings during simulations, self-monitored trauma-related ideation, RCMAS, CDI, and CTRS scores; improved performance on BAT
Richards et al. 1994	2	Four females and 9 males, mean age 32 years; 2-year exposure-treatment interval	Four 1-hr imaginal exposures, 4 1-hr in vivo exposures, unspecified number of home-based imaginal and in vivo exposures	Significantly reduced Impact of Event Intrusion and Avoidance scores, symptoms of trauma-related thoughts, BDI, General Health Questionnaire, Fear Questionnaire, and Work and Social Adjustment scores

Study		Sample	Treatment	Results
Pitman et al.[a]	2	Twenty male Vietnam veterans, mean age 42.5 years; symptomatic for 20 years	Seven to 11 sessions (10 min relaxation and 10 min imaginal exposure)	Significantly reduced trauma-related thoughts, Impact of Event Intrusion and Avoidance scores; nonsignificant effects on the Mississippi Scale for Combat-Related PTSD and SCL-90-R-GSI
Saigh 1995	2	Three females and 5 males, mean age 11 years; 2-year mean exposure-treatment interval	Six to 13 sessions (10–15 min relaxation, 24–60 min imaginal exposure, 5–10 min relaxation)	Significant gains on the WISC-R Digit Span and Coding subtests; reduced and significant reductions on SUDs ratings during simulations
Cooper and Clum 1989	3	Eight male Vietnam veterans, mean age 39.6 years; exposure treatment interval not specified	Ten to 12 sessions involving 50 min imaginal simulation	Flooding group had significantly fewer nightmares, STAI State scores, self-reported startle response, and enhanced performance on BAT; no significant group differences were evident on STAI Trait, BDI, or heart rates during simulations
		Eight male Vietnam veterans, mean age 39.3 years; exposure treatment interval not specified	Ten to 12 sessions of "standard Veterans Administration treatment" of unreported duration	

(continued)

Table 10–2. Single-case, quasi-experimental, and experimental flooding studies *(continued)*

Author/ date	Type of study	Subject characteristics	Treatment	Outcomes
Keane et al. 1989	3	Eleven male Vietnam veterans, mean age 34.7 years; exposure treatment interval not specified Thirteen male Vietnam veterans, mean age 34.5 years; exposure treatment interval not specified	Fourteen imaginal flooding sessions (15 min discussion, 10 min relaxation, 45 min imaginal flooding, 10 min relaxation, and 10 min debriefing) Ten of 13 control subjects received anxiolytic medications	Flooding group had significantly fewer trauma reexperiencing symptoms, startle reactions, self-reported guilt, and less memory impairment; flooding group had significantly lower STAI State and Trait, BDI, and Fear Survey Schedule scores; nonsignificant group differences on therapist ratings of sleep disturbance and social adjustment and on MMPI PTSD subscale

Note. 1 = single-case design; 2 = quasi-experimental design; 3 = experimental design. PTSD = posttraumatic stress disorder; STAI = State Trait Anxiety Inventory; WISC-R = Wechsler Intelligence Scale for Children—Revised; SUDs = subjective units of disturbance; BDI = Beck Depression Inventory; BAT = Behavioral Avoidance Test; RCMAI = Revised Children's Manifest Anxiety Inventory; CDI = Children's Depression Inventory; SCL-90-R-GSI = Symptom Checklist—90—Revised Global Symptom Inventory; MMPI = Minnesota Multiphasic Personality Inventory.
[a]"Emotional Processing During Flooding Therapy of Vietnam Veterans With PTSD," November 1995.

Because flooding is a demanding process, efforts should be made to protect the rights of patients (particularly children, adolescents, and individuals with limited mental ability). Therapists should actively strive to educate traumatized patients about the actual procedures that occur throughout the flooding process and candidly answer questions that may arise. Of course, informed consent (preferably written) should be obtained before flooding is attempted. Families, mental health practitioners, and medical staff should be advised that PTSD symptoms may increase during the early stages of therapy (see Saigh et al., in press-b).

The ethical guidelines of the Association for the Advancement of Behavior Therapy (AABT 1977) are relevant because they provide operational recommendations, and these recommendations address a number of issues that are germane to the needs of flooding candidates. The AABT recommends that therapists ensure voluntary participation by reviewing possible sources of coercion and by ensuring that patients can withdraw from treatment without reprimand. Likewise, when the competence of a subordinate patient (e.g., a child or adolescent or an adult with limited mental ability) is limited, it is advised that efforts be made to ensure that the "client as well as the guardian participate in treatment discussions to the extent that the client's ability permits" (AABT 1977, p. vi). The AABT further advocates that the patients' understanding of the treatment goals should be determined by asking them to restate the goals verbally or in writing. The AABT guidelines also recommend that the choice of treatment methods should be adequately considered. Given that PTSD may spontaneously remit over time (Saigh and Fairbank, in press), therapists may initially consider using time-limited supportive counseling or anxiolytic medications.

It should be clearly understood that exposure-based paradigms for PTSD must occur within the context of a supportive therapeutic milieu (Fairbank and Nicholson 1987; Resick and Schnicke 1993). It also should be realized that flooding regimens for PTSD have been conducted within comprehensive treatment plans that targeted the multiple dimensions of PTSD (Saigh 1992). Although flooding has been associated with favorable outcomes, supportive counseling and educational interventions may offset pathological self-efficacy expectations (Saigh et al., in press-c), impaired interpersonal relations (Cooper and Clum 1989), and PTSD-related functional impairments, such as academic problems (Saigh and Mroweh 1993).

The information in Table 10–2 shows that flooding may be less effective when the interval between stress exposure and the intervention is protracted. The flooding regimen that Richards et al. (1994) presented to 13 adults, with a mean interval of 2 years between exposure and treatment, was associated with a 75%–80% improvement across PTSD-specific measures and a 65%–80% improvement across indicators of depression, fear, general health, and social adjustment. Analogously, my study (P. A. Saigh: "The Effects of Imaginal Flooding on the Short Term Memory, Concentration, and Self-Reported Distress of Child-Adolescent Posttraumatic Stress Disorder Patients," unpublished study, 1995) observed that the flooding packages presented to children and adolescents, with a mean duration of 2 years between exposure and treatment, were associated with a 46% improvement at posttreatment and a 50% improvement at 4- to 6-month follow-up assessments. On the other hand, a comparable study by Pitman and his colleagues (" Emotional Processing During Flooding Therapy of Vietnam Veterans With PTSD," November 1995) involving Vietnam veterans with a 20-year history of psychiatric morbidity was associated with a 12%–17% improvement across 7 outcome measures. In view of these findings and because epidemiological research suggests that PTSD may have a chronic course (Kulka et al. 1990; Sack et. al. 1993, 1994, 1995; Saigh 1984a, 1984b, 1985, 1988), it would seem that the early provision of therapeutic flooding is clinically warranted.

Although the flooding literature has been marked largely by favorable results, exposure may not always be the treatment of choice (Saigh 1992). Flooding may be contraindicated in cases involving comorbidity (i.e., psychosis, limited mental ability, depression, personality disorders, conduct disorder, attention-deficit/hyperactivity disorder, or substance abuse/dependence). A record of noncompliance, difficulty in establishing and/or maintaining mental images, reduced reexperiencing symptoms, and focused compensation-seeking efforts were listed by Litz et al. (1990) as reasons for not prescribing flooding. In instances where flooding is not advisable, alternative psychological procedures, such as supportive counseling, family therapy, or psychopharmacological regimens, are recommended alternatives.

Methodological Considerations

Whereas a modicum of the flooding studies employed standardized measures of short-term memory and concentration, the need to explore the effects of flooding as denoted by multiple indicators of memory is apparent. It is of interest that a number of case-control investigations reported that veterans with PTSD had significantly lower scores on standardized measures of memory as compared to veterans without PTSD. Sutker et al. (1991) compared Korean and World War II prisoners of war to matched cohorts of combat veterans who had not been interned and observed that the prisoners of war were deficient on the Wechsler Adult Intelligence Scale—Revised (WAIS-R; Wechsler 1981) Digit Span and the Wechsler Memory Scale—Revised (Wechsler 1987) Immediate Memory Index. Similarly, Bremner et al. (1993) compared matched samples of combat veterans with and without PTSD and observed that the PTSD subjects had significantly lower scores on the Wechsler Memory Scale—Revised logical memory (verbal) component measures of immediate and delayed recall. Bremner et al. (1993) also reported that the Selective Reminding Test (Hannay and Levin 1985) scores of the PTSD group were significantly lower than the scores of the control group. Clearly, adopting outcome measures such as the Wechsler Memory Scale—Revised may facilitate our understanding of the effects of flooding across multiple parameters of memory. Moreover, providing scaled and standard scores that are afforded by these measures would permit performance comparisons by age.

Given the apparent success of the single-case, quasi-experimental, and experimental trials, a randomized experimental flooding

study involving traumatized youth would be of exceptional interest because the clinical literature on children is currently limited to
a few single-case trials and one quasi-experimental study.
Whereas Saigh (1987a, 1987b) reported that systematic desensitization (i.e., an exposure-based modality that momentarily stops
aversive stimulations as soon as undue anxiety is experienced)
was not effective in the treatment of child-adolescent PTSD, Kipper (1977) successfully used a form of systematic desensitization to
reduce the war-related fears of Israeli veterans. Because the as-
signment of traumatized youth to no-treatment, waiting-list, or
nonspecific control conditions may not be feasible or ethically de-
fensible, the use of randomized active treatment designs (Kazdin
1992) is regarded as the preferred procedure. Investigators may
wish to compare the effects of flooding (i.e., the treatment of interest) to a variety of well-established behavioral procedures
such as systematic desensitization. It also would be of interest to
explore the comparative effects of in vitro participant modeling
(Bandura et al. 1974) because this approach would not call for
imaginal exposure and because young children who are unable
to imagine traumatic scenes may benefit from this form of therapeutic exposure.

Research designed to identify patient, treatment, family, and
therapist factors that are associated with successful outcome is
clearly needed. Morris and Kratochwill's (1983) review of the systematic desensitization and flooding literature concluded that investigators should attempt to identify patient variables that are
associated with treatment efficacy (i.e., age, ability to imagine,
quality of visual imagery, ability to follow verbal instruction, ability to relax, and threshold for fatigue). There also is a need to identify comorbid conditions that occur during the developmental
period (e.g., oppositional defiant disorder, conduct disorder,
attention-deficit/hyperactivity disorder, or substance abuse),
which may influence therapeutic outcomes. Likewise, the influence of moderator variables such as the quality of therapeutic relationships and qualitative aspects of family support warrant
systematic examination. Clinical investigators also should attempt
to demonstrate the integrity of these treatments because the ex-

perimental investigations that were reviewed did not control for these variables.

Conclusion

It is apparent that exposure-based paradigms have had a long and colorful history. Since Goethe's 1770 autobiography, actual or imaginal exposure has been effectively used to treat an assortment of fear reactions. Shortly before PTSD was recognized as a formal psychiatric classification, Fairbank et al. (1981) effectively employed a course of imaginal flooding to eliminate the "persistent posttraumatic startle response" of a 32-year-old motor vehicle accident victim. Since that time, the outcomes of eight single-case studies have been associated with fewer traumatic memories (Fairbank et al. 1983; McCaffrey and Fairbank 1985; Rychtarik et al. 1984) or reduced subjective disturbance estimates during trauma-reminiscent simulations (Saigh 1987a, 1987b, 1987c, 1987d, 1989b). Five single-case studies that employed the WISC-R Digit Span and Coding subtests determined that imaginal flooding was associated with meaningful gains on these indexes of memory and concentration (Saigh 1987a, 1987b, 1987c, 1987d, 1989b). The single-case results also indicate that flooding was associated with decreased self-reported anxiety (McCaffrey and Fairbank 1985; Rychtarik et al. 1984; Saigh 1987a, 1987b, 1987c, 1987d, 1989b) and depression (Fairbank et al. 1983; Rychtarik et al. 1984; Saigh 1987a, 1987b, 1987c, 1987d, 1989b). All of the single-case studies that used measures of behavioral avoidance were associated with appreciable posttreatment gains (Saigh 1987a, 1987b, 1987c, 1989b).

Three quasi-experimental studies reported significantly lower scores on the Revised Impact of Event Intrusion scale (Richards et al. 1994; Pitman et al.: "Emotional Processing During Flooding Therapy of Vietnam Veterans With PTSD," November 1995), significant gains on the WISC-R Digit Span and Coding subtests and significantly reduced subjective disturbance estimates during simulations (P. A. Saigh: "The Effects of Imaginal Flooding on the Short Term Memory, Concentration, and Self-Reported Distress of Child-Adolescent Posttraumatic Stress Disorder Patients," unpublished study, 1995) and self-reported trauma-related ideation (Richards et al. 1994; Pitman et al.: "Emotional Processing During Flooding Therapy of Vietnam Veterans With PTSD," November 1995). These studies also evidenced significant reductions on the Revised Impact of Event Avoidance scale (Pitman et al.: "Emotional Processing During Flooding Therapy of Vietnam Veterans With PTSD," November 1995; Richards al. 1994), General Health Questionnaire, and Fear Questionnaire (Richards et al. 1994). On the other hand, one study did not observe significant pre- and posttreatment differences on the Mississippi Scale for Combat-Related Posttraumatic Stress Disorder or the SCL-90-R-GSI (Pitman et al.: "Emotional Processing During Flooding Therapy of Vietnam Veterans With PTSD," November 1995).

Although the single-case and quasi-experimental reports generally denote efficacy (particularly on measures of traumatic ideation and norm-referenced indicators of memory and concentration) across different subjects, therapeutic settings, and therapists, these designs do not provide the same level of external validity that is associated with true experimental designs. Therefore, it is relevant that two randomized experimental flooding studies determined that imaginal exposure was associated with significantly fewer trauma-related thoughts (Keane et al. 1989), nightmares (Cooper and Clum 1989), startle reactions, and STAI State scores (Cooper and Clum 1989; Keane et al. 1989). Flooding was associated with lower STAI Trait, BDI, and Fear Survey Schedule scores (Keane et al. 1989). Flooding also was associated with significantly enhanced performance on a BAT (Cooper and Clum 1989) and with significantly less guilt and enhanced memory (Keane et al. 1989). On the other hand, Cooper and Clum (1989) failed to denote significant variations on the STAI Trait scale, BDI, and heart rate monitored during simulations. Keane et al. (1989) reported nonsignificant differences relative to sleep disturbance, social adjustment, and the Minnesota Multiphasic Personality Inventory PTSD subscale. Considering these studies in toto, it is apparent that flooding regimens have reduced traumatic memories, facilitated emotional adjustment, and enhanced nontrauma-related memory.

References

American Psychiatric Association: Diagnostic and Statistical Manual of Mental Disorders, 3rd Edition. Washington, DC, American Psychiatric Association, 1980

American Psychiatric Association: Diagnostic and Statistical Manual of Mental Disorders, 3rd Edition, Revised. Washington, DC, American Psychiatric Association, 1987

Association for the Advancement of Behavior Therapy: Ethical issues for human services. Behavior Therapy 8:v–vi, 1977

Bandura A, Jeffery R, Wright E: Efficacy of participant modeling as a response to instructional aids. J Abnorm Psychol 83:56–64, 1974

Barlow DH, Hersen M: Single-Case Research Design: Strategies for Studying Behavior Change, 2nd Edition. New York, Pergamon, 1984

Barrett L: Systematic desensitization versus implosive therapy. J Abnorm Psychol 74:587–592, 1969

Beck AT, Ward CH, Mandelson M, et al: An inventory for measuring depression. Arch Gen Psychiatry 4:561–-571, 1961

Black JL, Keane TM: Implosive therapy in the treatment of combat related fears in a World War II veteran. J Behav Ther Exp Psychiatry 13:163–165, 1982

Boudewyns PA: Implosive therapy and desensitization with inpatients: a five year follow-up. J Abnorm Psychol 84:159–160, 1975

Boudewyns PA, Hyer I: Physiological response to combat memories and preliminary treatment outcome in Vietnam veteran PTSD patients treated with direct therapeutic exposure. Behavior Therapy 21:63–87, 1990

Boudewyns PA, Shipley RH: Flooding and Implosive Therapy. New York, Plenum, 1983

Bremner DJ, Scott TM, Dalaney RC: Deficits in short term memory in posttraumatic stress disorder. Am J Psychiatry 150:1015–1019, 1993

Cooper NA, Clum GA: Imaginal flooding as a supplementary treatment for PTSD in combat veterans: a controlled evaluation. Behavior Therapy 20:381–391, 1989

Derogatis LR: SCL-90-R: Administration, Scoring, and Procedures Manual II. Towson, MD, Clinical Psychometric Research, 1983

Fairbank JA, Keane TM: Flooding for combat-related stress disorders: assessment of anxiety reduction across traumatic memories. Behavior Therapy 13:499–510, 1982

Fairbank JA, Nicholson RA: Theoretical and empirical issues in the treatment of posttraumatic stress disorder in Vietnam veterans. J Clin Psychol 43:44–55, 1987

Fairbank JA, DeGood DD, Jenkins CW: Behavioral treatment of a persistent post-traumatic startle response. J Behav Ther Exp Psychiatry 12:321–324, 1981

Fairbank JA, Gross RT, Keane TM: Treatment of posttraumatic stress disorder: evaluating outcome with a behavioral code. Behav Modif 7: 557–568, 1983

Geer JH: The development of a scale to measure fear. Behav Res Ther 3:45–53, 1965

Goldberg DP, Williams P: A user's guide to the General Health Questionnaire. Windsor, England, NFER-Nelson, 1988

Hamilton M: A rating scale for depression. J Neurol Neurosurg Psychiatry 23:56–62, 1960

Hannay HJ, Levin HS: Selective Reminding Test: an examination of equivalence across forms. J Clin Exp Neuropsychol 7: 251–263, 1985

Herzberg A: Short treatment of neuroses by graduated tasks. Br J Med Psychol 19:19–36, 1941

Hogan RA, Kirchner JH: Preliminary report on the extinction of learned fears via short term therapy. J Abnorm Psychol 72:106–109, 1967

Horne AM, Matson J: A comparison of modeling, desensitization, flooding, study skills, and control groups for reducing test anxiety. Behavior Therapy 8:1–15, 1977

Horowitz MJ, Wilner N, Alverez W: Impact of Event Scale: a measure of subjective stress. Psychosom Med 41:209–218, 1979

Jacobson PB: Treating a man with a needle phobia who requires daily injections of medication. Hospital and Community Psychiatry 42: 877–879, 1991

Kazdin A: Research Designs in Clinical Psychology, 2nd Edition. New York, Macmillan, 1992

Keane TM, Kaloupek DG: Imaginal flooding in the treatment of posttraumatic stress disorder. J Consult Clin Psychol 50:138–140, 1982

Keane TM, Malloy P, Fairbank JA: Empirical development of an MMPI subscale for the assessment of combat-related posttraumatic stress disorder. J Consult Clin Psychol 52:888–891, 1984

Keane TM, Fairbank JA, Caddell JM, et al: A behavioral approach to assessing and treating post-traumatic stress disorder in Vietnam veterans, in Trauma and Its Wake. Edited by Figley C. New York, Brunner/Mazel, 1985, pp 257–294

Keane T, Caddell JM, Taylor KL: The Mississippi Scale for Combat-Related Posttraumatic Stress Disorder: three studies in reliability and validity. J Consult Clin Psychol 56:85–90, 1988

Keane TM, Fairbank JA, Caddell JM, et al: Implosive (flooding) therapy reduces symptoms of PTSD in Vietnam combat veterans. Behavior Therapy 20:245–260, 1989

Kipper DA: Behavior therapy for fears brought on by war experiences. J Consult Clin Psychol 45:216–221, 1977

Kulka RC, Schlenger WE, Fairbank JA, et al: Trauma and the Vietnam Generation: Report of Findings From the National Vietnam Veterans Readjustment Study. New York, Brunner/Mazel, 1990

Litz BT, Blake DD, Gerardi RG, et al: Decision making guidelines for the use of direct therapeutic exposure in the treatment of posttraumatic stress disorder. The Behavioral Therapist 13:91–93, 1990

Malleson N: Panic and phobia: a possible method of treatment. Lancet 1:225–227, 1959

Marks I: Flooding (implosion) and allied treatments, in Behavior Modification: Principles and Applications. Edited by Argas S. Boston, Little, Brown, 1972, pp 151–211

Marks I: Behavioral Psychotherapy: Maudsley Pocket Book of Clinical Management. Bristol, England, Wright, 1986

Marks IM, Matthews A: Brief standard self-rating for phobic patients. Behav Res Ther 17:263–267, 1979

Marks IM, Viswanathan R, Lipsedge MS, et al: Enhanced relief of phobics by flooding during waning diazepam effect. Br J Psychiatry 121:493–505, 1975

McCaffrey RJ, Fairbank JA: Behavioral assessment and treatment of accident-related posttraumatic stress disorder: two case studies. Behavior Therapy 16:406–416, 1985

Morris RJ, Kratochwill TR: Treating Children's Fears: A Behavioral Approach. New York, Pergamon, 1983

Pollin AT: The effects of flooding and physical suppression as extinction techniques on an anxiety motivated avoidance locomotor response. J Psychol 7:235–245, 1959

Rachman SJ: Studies in desensitization, II: flooding. Behav Res Ther 4:1–6, 1966

Rachman SJ: Fear and Courage, 2nd Edition. New York, WH Freeman, 1990

Rathus SA: A 30-item schedule for assessing assertive behavior. Behavior Therapy 4:398–406, 1973

Resick PA, Schnicke MK: Cognitive Processing Therapy for Rape Victims: A Treatment Manual. Newbury Park, CA, Sage, 1993

Reynolds C, Richmond B: What I think and feel: a revised measure of children's manifest anxiety. J Abnorm Child Psychol 6:271–280, 1978

Richards DA, Lovell K, Marks IM: Post-traumatic stress disorder: evaluation of a behavioral treatment program. J Trauma Stress 7:669–680, 1994

Rychtarik RG, Silverman WK, Van Landingham WP: Treatment of an incest victim with implosive therapy: a case study. Behavior Therapy 15:410–420, 1984

Sack WH, Clarke G, Him C, et al: A six year follow-up of Cambodian adolescents. J Am Acad Child Adolesc Psychiatry 32:3–15, 1993

Sack WH, McSharry S, Clarke GN, et al: The Khmer adolescent project: epidemiologic findings in two generations of Cambodian refugee. J Nerv Ment Dis 182:387–395, 1994

Sack WH, Clarke GN, Kinney R, et al: The Khmer adolescent project, II: functional capacities in two generations of Cambodian adolescents. J Nerv Ment Dis 183:177–181, 1995

Saigh PA: An experimental analysis of delayed posttraumatic stress. Behav Res Therapy 22:679–682, 1984a

Saigh PA: Pre- and postinvasion anxiety in Lebanon. Behavior Therapy 15:185–190, 1984b

Saigh PA: Adolescent anxiety following varying degrees of war stress in Lebanon. Journal of Clinical Child Psychology 4:210–221, 1985

Saigh PA: In vitro flooding of an adolescent's posttraumatic stress disorder. Journal of Clinical Child Psychology 16:147–150, 1987a

Saigh PA: In vitro flooding of a childhood posttraumatic stress disorder. School Psychology Review 16:203–211, 1987b

Saigh PA: In vitro flooding of childhood posttraumatic stress disorders: a systematic replication. Professional School Psychology 2:133–145, 1987c

Saigh PA: In vitro flooding in the treatment of a 6-year-old boy's posttraumatic stress disorder. Behav Res Ther 24:685–688, 1987d

Saigh PA: Anxiety, depression, and assertion across alternating intervals of stress. J Abnorm Psychol 97:338–342, 1988

Saigh PA: The development and validation of the Children's Posttraumatic Stress Disorder Inventory. International Journal of Special Education 4:75–84, 1989a

Saigh PA: The use of in vitro flooding in the treatment of traumatized adolescents. Journal of Behavioral and Developmental Pediatrics 10: 17–21, 1989b

Saigh PA: The behavioral treatment of child and adolescent posttraumatic stress disorder. Advances in Behavioural Research and Therapy 14: 247–275, 1992

Saigh PA, Fairbank JA: War-related posttraumatic stress disorder among children and adolescents, in Stressful Life Events, 2nd Edition. Edited by Miller T. Madison, CT, International Universities Press, in press

Saigh PA, Mroweh A: Scholastic impairments among traumatized adolescents, in Current Research on Child and Adolescent Posttraumatic Stress Disorder. Chaired by Saigh PA. Symposium presented at the Lake George Research Conference on Posttraumatic Stress Disorder, Bolton Landing, New York, January 1993

Saigh PA, Green B, Kroll M: The history and epidemiology of posttraumatic stress disorder with special reference to children and adolescents. J School Psychol, in press-a

Saigh PA, Yule W, Inamder SC: Imaginal flooding of traumatized children and adolescents. Journal of School Psychology, in press-b

Saigh PA, Mroweh A, Zimmerman B, et al: Self-efficacy expectations among traumatized adolescents. Behav Res Ther, in press-c

Schwartz IS, Bear DM: Social validity assessments: is current practice the state of the art? J Appl Behav Anal 24:189–204, 1991

Sellick KJ, Peck CL: Behavioral treatment of fear in a child with cerebral palsy using flooding. Arch Phys Med Rehabil 62:398–400, 1981

Smith RE, Sharpe TM: Treatment of a school phobia with implosive therapy. J Consult Clin Psychol 35:239–243, 1970

Spielberger CD, Gorsuch RL, Lushane RE: Manual for the State Trait Anxiety Inventory. Palo Alto, CA, Consulting Psychologists Press, 1968

Stampfl TG, Levis DJ: Essentials of implosive therapy: a learning-based psychodynamic behavioral therapy. J Abnorm Psychol 72:496–503, 1967

Sutker PB, Winstead DK, Galina ZH, et al: Cognitive deficits and psychopathology among former prisoners of war and combat veterans of the
Korean conflict. Am J Psychiatry 148:67–72, 1991

Wechsler D: Wechsler Adult Intelligence Scale—Revised. San Antonio,
TX, Psychological Corporation, 1981

Wechsler D: Wechsler Memory Scale—Revised. San Antonio, TX, Psychological Corporation, 1987

Wolf MM: Social validity: the case of subjective measurement or how applied behavior analysis is finding its heart. J Appl Behav Anal 11:
315–329, 1978

Yule W, Sacks B, Hersov L: Successful flooding treatment of a noise phobia in a 11-year-old boy. J Behav Ther Exp Psychiatry 5:209–211, 1974

Zung WA: A self-rating depression scale. Arch Gen Psychiatry 12:63–70,
1965

Chapter 11

The Emerging Neurobiology of Dissociation: Implications for Treatment of Posttraumatic Stress Disorder

John H. Krystal, M.D., J. Douglas Bremner, M.D.,
Steven M. Southwick, M.D., and Dennis S. Charney, M.D.

D espite progress in identifying, characterizing, and quantita- tively assessing dissociative states, there has been surpris- ingly little study of their neurobiology. Associated with the failure to elucidate a unique neurobiology for dissociative states, there have been few placebo-controlled pharmacotherapy trials for dis- sociative disorders and no specific antidissociative drugs devel- oped. The absence of antidissociative pharmacotherapies contrasts with the development of anxiolytics, antiobsessionals, antipsychot- ics, mood-stabilizing agents, and antidepressants. In light of the paucity of research in this area, the commonly held view that core features of dissociative disorders are unresponsive to pharmaco- therapy is not surprising (Kluft 1987).

In this chapter, we review recent progress made in studying the neurobiology of dissociative states in posttraumatic stress disorder (PTSD) patients. It is possible, given the elevated prevalence of early traumatic experiences in other dissociative disorders, that

This work was supported by funds from the Department of Veterans Affairs to the National Center for Posttraumatic Stress Disorder, the Veterans Administration-Yale Alcoholism Research Center, and the Merit Review Grant Program (JHK).

studies of dissociation in PTSD patients will have broader implications for patients with other dissociative disorders (see Chapter 12 in this volume). In this chapter, we focus on studies that have produced dissociative states in healthy individuals and patients with PTSD or other neurological disorders. In doing so, we attempt to highlight bridges between the neurobiology and treatment of PTSD.

Guided Recollection: Narcosynthesis and the Amytal Interview

The medical facilitation of traumatic memory recall and flashbacks in traumatized individuals began in World War II as part of a therapeutic approach called narcosynthesis or, more recently, the "Amytal interview." This approach combined barbiturates and guided recollection of traumatic memories (Bartemeier et al. 1946; Grinker and Spiegel 1945; Sargent and Slater 1940). The use of barbiturates to facilitate traumatic memory recall was illustrated by a case reported by Grinker (1944):

> That afternoon I gave him 0.25 Gm. of pentothal sodium intravenously. He was then told that he was up in the air on a strafing mission and that the man on his wing was aflame. . . . Immediately he [shouted] to his friend . . . "pull up and bail out. Why doesn't he pull up and bail out?" . . . he went over and over the traumatic situation, crying and sobbing. As this reaction subsided he was allowed to close his eyes and sleep . . . [upon awakening] He stated "I must have been asleep. I had a dream about [my friend]". . . . (pp. 142-143)

Facilitating traumatic memory recall by barbiturates and benzodiazepines is paradoxical; drugs with prominent amnestic effects improve aspects of memory function. These drugs impair attention and memory in humans (Kirk et al. 1990; Krystal et al. 1995). However, their amnestic effects arise primarily through interfering with memory encoding rather than memory storage or retrieval (Ghoneim and Mewaldt 1990). Mechanisms through which barbiturates and benzodiazepines facilitate the recollection of traumatic memories and flashbacks are poorly understood. They enhance the actions of gamma-aminobutyric acid (GABA) at the GABA$_A$ receptor (Olsen 1981), and barbiturates additionally block the actions of glutamate at non-N-methyl-D-aspartate (non-NMDA) receptors (Collins and Anson 1987; Morgan et al. 1991). However, barbiturates are not specific in their capacity to facilitate recollection of traumatic memories in that ether, ethanol, nitrous oxide, and scopolamine-morphine combinations also appear to facilitate the recall of inaccessible memories (Erickson 1945; Rosen and Meyers 1947).

The prodissociative effects of these drugs are indirect. Benzodiazepines, for example, do not increase scores on scales measuring dissociation in healthy individuals (J. H. Krystal, L. P. Karper, D. C. D'Souza, et al: "Interactive Effects of Subanesthetic Ketamine and Lorazepam in Humans: Psychotomimetic, Dissociative, Cognitive, and Neuroendocrine Responses," unpublished manuscript, 1997). Clinical observations suggest that the sedating and anxiolytic medications employed in narcosynthesis reduce anxiety and thus may lessen the resistance to recalling anxiety-associated memories (Grinker and Spiegel 1945). This view is consistent with a patient who experienced flashbacks during relaxation training (Fitzgerald and Gonzalez 1994). Alternatively, these medications, viewed as "truth serums" by the popular press, may suppress involuntary mechanisms responsible for reducing voluntary access to traumatic memories (Kardiner and Spiegel 1947). Related to this hypothesis, recent physiological research has provided additional evidence of a neural basis for directed forgetting and other processes associated with reduced voluntary access to established memories (Geiselman et al. 1983; Paller 1990). A recent case study evaluating the neuropsychological consequences of psychogenic amnesia supported the view that guided recollection under the influence of Amytal reduced the capacity of active processes outside of voluntary control to reduce the level of awareness of learned information or memory of events (Kopelman et al. 1994).

Pharmacological Challenge Studies in Patients With Posttraumatic Stress Disorder

Flashbacks have been precipitated in Vietnam veterans with chronic PTSD following the intravenous administration of sodium lactate (Rainey et al. 1987), yohimbine (Southwick et al. 1993), and metachlorophenylpiperazine (m-CPP; Southwick et al. 1991). Administration of each of these substances produces panic attacks in a significant proportion of patients with either panic disorder (Charney et al. 1984, 1987; Pitts and McClure 1967) or PTSD (Rainey et al. 1987; Southwick et al. 1991, 1993) but not other patient groups. However, PTSD patients are the first group studied to experience flashbacks following administration of these substances.

Rainey et al. (1987) compared the response to intravenous sodium lactate, isoproterenol, and a dextrose placebo in seven Vietnam combat veterans, six of whom also met criteria for panic disorder. All seven patients experienced flashbacks following lactate, two patients also experienced flashbacks after isoproterenol infusion, and one patient experienced a flashback during placebo infusion. The authors described these flashbacks as similar to those occurring naturally as part of PTSD. Six of the seven lactate-induced flashbacks, both isoproterenol flashbacks, and the dextrose flashback were followed by paniclike states. However, the absence of reported anxiety ratings makes it impossible to determine whether subpanic increases in anxiety preceded the flashbacks. The overlap of panic disorder and PTSD in patients in this study was another limitation because it raised concerns that lactate-induced flashbacks were a property of panic disorder and not independently associated with PTSD. Little is known about the mechanisms through which lactate produces panic attacks and flashbacks in PTSD patients.

The precipitation of flashbacks and panic attacks in PTSD patients by yohimbine linked noradrenergic systems, implicated in fear and arousal regulation, to the symptoms of PTSD (Southwick et al. 1993). Yohimbine activates central noradrenergic neurons through blockade of α_2 receptors located on noradrenergic neurons. These α_2 receptors mediate, in part, feedback inhibition of noradrenergic neurons (Starke et al. 1975). Following yohimbine, 40% (8 of 20 patients) experienced flashbacks and 70% (14 of 20 patients) experienced panic attacks. No panic attacks and only one flashback emerged following placebo administration. Although 45% of the patients in this study also met DSM-III-R (American Psychiatric Association 1987) criteria for panic disorder, 43% of the yohimbine-induced panic attacks occurred in individuals without panic disorder. The risk of a yohimbine-induced panic attack was increased in patients with panic disorder relative to those without comorbid panic disorder (89% versus 43%). However, history of panic disorder did not appear to influence the likelihood of experiencing a yohimbine-induced flashback.

The following vignette illustrates features of a yohimbine-induced flashback:

10:00 A.M.: [Initiation of yohimbine infusion]

10:05 A.M.: Subject reports hot and cold flashes, goose bumps, palpitations

10:10 A.M.: Subject reports clammy hands, he asked the nurse to move away from him . . . in case he felt like running. "I feel like I'm picking up dead bodies . . . the centrifuge sounds like a helicopter . . . A chopper is shooting at us, we're trying to shoot back at it! One of the guys' head is shot off! Brains are coming at me! I smell burnt flesh . . . I feel scared, I can't hear what's going on . . . ."

The operational definition for flashback employed in Southwick et al. (1993) led to the exclusion of many dissociative states produced by yohimbine in the PTSD patients. The following criteria were employed to define a drug-induced flashback: 1) the reexperiencing of a past traumatic event during drug infusion, 2) the reexperiencing must involve one or more sensory modalities, and 3) for patients with a history of flashbacks, the drug-induced state must be similar to naturally occurring flashbacks. Despite the expedient characterization of flashbacks as being present or absent, yohimbine actually produced a continuum of dissociative phenomena. Patients experienced varying degrees of derealization and depersonalization that were often accompanied by other dissociative symptoms. Yohimbine also elicited a range of altered perceptual experiences, some of which were fragmentary or vague. For example, one patient perceived the shadow produced by a sink in the testing facility to be the shadow made by a tank turret. In addition to stimulating flashbacks, yohimbine significantly increased the recall of traumatic memories. Although yohimbine produced symptoms of autonomic arousal in many patients, these symptoms were not the sole predictor of flashbacks within a session. Yohimbine also significantly increased the recall of traumatic memories. In some cases, symptoms of autonomic arousal followed or were coincident with the reported retrieval of traumatic memories (S. M. Southwick, personal communication, May 1994). Thus, it appeared that noradrenergic systems might be involved in the elicitation of dissociative symptoms as a direct consequence of the central pharmacological actions of yohimbine on neural circuitry contributing to dissociation and memory retrieval. These data contrasted with models in which noradrenergic contributions to PTSD symptoms were entirely mediated by peripheral autonomic systems.

The yohimbine study suggested that activation of noradrenergic systems by yohimbine produced panic attacks and flashbacks in a subset of PTSD patients. One question raised by this study was whether the elicitation of flashbacks by yohimbine reflected a specific response to α_2 receptor blockade or whether all anxiogenic drugs produce flashbacks in PTSD patients. To investigate this question, yohimbine and m-CPP effects were compared in this population (Southwick et al. 1991). This study found that both m-CPP and yohimbine produced flashbacks and other dissociative states in veterans with combat-related PTSD. Preliminary analyses indicated that patients tended to experience panic attacks following yohimbine or m-CPP, but not both medications. As with the initial study, drug-induced traumatic memories, autonomic activation, and anxiety states could be associated with the induction of flashbacks, although no single response preceded flashbacks in all cases. These observations raised the possibility that yohimbine and m-CPP caused flashbacks by modulating a final common pathway that has yet to be identified or that multiple mechanisms might lead to the induction of flashbacks.

To continue the search for key neurotransmitter systems involved in dissociation in PTSD patients, we studied the effects of the benzodiazepine antagonist flumazenil in PTSD patients. This drug failed to precipitate flashbacks or panic attacks in PTSD patients (Randall et al. 1995). As with lactate, yohimbine, and m-CPP, flumazenil has been reported to produce panic attacks in patients with panic disorder (Woods et al. 1991). The absence of flumazenil-induced panic attacks and flashbacks in PTSD suggests that flumazenil is not associated with the overproduction of an endogenous benzodiazepine-inverse agonist, such as a diazepam-binding inhibitor, which might contribute to anxiety symptoms in other disorders (Costa and Guidotti 1987). Future studies will be needed to determine whether benzodiazepine-inverse agonists, such as FG 7142 or iomazenil, which precipitate anxiety in healthy subjects (Dorow et al. 1983; Randall et al. 1995) will produce flashbacks in PTSD patients.

Case reports suggest that alcohol and opiate withdrawal may increase PTSD symptoms, including flashbacks (Kosten and Krystal 1988; Salloway et al. 1990; J. P. Seibyl, personal communication, May 1994). Central noradrenergic systems are activated during alcohol and opiate withdrawal, suggesting a possible parallel between yohimbine- and withdrawal-induced flashbacks (Kosten and Krystal 1988).

Induction of Dissociative States in Healthy Individuals

Pathophysiological models that hypothesize a "final common pathway" for the neurobiology of dissociation presuppose that modulation of the activity of this pathway might produce dissociative states in healthy individuals. To date, three classes of drugs commonly produce dissociative-like states in healthy subjects: 1) antagonists of the NMDA subtype of glutamate receptor, 2) cannabinoids, and 3) serotonergic hallucinogens.

The non-competitive NMDA receptor antagonist anesthetics, phencyclidine and ketamine, produce a derealized and depersonalized state characterized by marked perceptual alterations and psychosis at subanesthetic doses (Domino et al. 1965; Javitt and Zukin 1991; Luby et al. 1959; Yamakura et al. 1993). The capacity of ketamine to produce dissociative-like states in healthy subjects has been rigorously evaluated in a series of studies (Krystal et al. 1994a, 1994b). In these studies, dissociative symptoms were rated using the Clinician-Administered Dissociative States Scale (CADSS; Bremner et al., in press). At low blood levels, ketamine produced a light-headed feeling. With higher blood levels of ketamine, subjects reported the slowing of time and alterations in the vividness, form, and context of sensory experiences. For example, subjects noted that objects appeared brighter or duller than expected, larger or smaller than usual, and distorted in shape or with altered proximity. Also, some subjects had difficulty hearing someone speaking close to them, although they reported that a radio playing quietly in the next room sounded unusually loud. Altered proprioceptive experiences were reported by subjects who felt that their limbs changed form or were floating in air.

Cognitive effects of ketamine also were prominent. Subjects reported constriction of their field of attention, resulting in the sensation of tunnel vision or the feeling that they were surrounded by fog. For example, subjects attending to a computer keyboard frequently lost track of events happening on the computer monitor. Ketamine also produced learning and memory impairments. Its effects increased proportionately to the dose administered and the duration of delay between stimulus presentation and testing. In addition, ketamine interfered with executive functions such as abstraction, assessed by proverb interpretation, and problem solving, evaluated by the Wisconsin Card Sorting Test (Heaton 1985). Although subjects felt that they had lost control of their thought processes, with effort they could focus on tasks.

Ketamine also produced emotional responses. At low doses, it had mild anxiolytic properties, whereas larger doses generally produced euphoria and anxiety. Anxiety stimulated by ketamine tended to follow perceptual alterations and thought disorganization and tended to be related to the subjects' degree of comfort with the drug-induced disturbances in thought and perception. Some subjects found the perceptual alterations produced by ketamine quite pleasurable, analogous to a ride in an amusement park, whereas others found the effects of ketamine frightening.

Ketamine-induced insight impairments and identity-related responses may have contributed to the elicitation of anxiety. Following drug infusion, some subjects lost the perspective that their mental status change was produced by ketamine, and they became concerned that they had contracted a mental illness. Transient identity alterations also were observed with ketamine. For example, a subject who received ketamine (0.26 mg/kg intravenous bolus followed by 0.65 mg/kg/hr) stated, "At first it seemed that I didn't exist, I couldn't process information; after a while, I was convinced that I was an organism, then I realized I was a human being, then after a longer while I remembered that I was a medical student." Ketamine did not lead to the emergence of multiple personalities, flashbacks, or vivid intrusive memories in research subjects. However, symptoms associated with psychosis, including delusions and thought disorder, were observed during ketamine infusion.

Two ongoing studies have attempted to pharmacologically alter ketamine-induced dissociative states by pretreating healthy subjects with lorazepam or haloperidol (Krystal et al. 1994a; (J. H. Krystal, L. P. Karper, D. C. D'Souza, et al., "Interactive effects of subanesthetic ketamine and lorazepam in humans," unpublished manuscript, 1997). Preliminary data from these studies suggested that lorazepam 2 mg administered orally 2 hours before ketamine administration tended to reduce altered environmental perceptions but had no effects on other dissociative symptoms or psychotic states produced by ketamine. Haloperidol failed to reduce dissociative symptoms, vigilance impairments, or amnestic effects produced by ketamine but reduced ketamine-induced distractibility, abstraction impairments, and bizarreness of thought processes. These data suggested that at the doses tested neither agent is a true ketamine antidote. They are also consistent with the literature suggesting that neuroleptics have limited efficacy in treating dissociative symptoms (Kluft 1987).

To date, there have not been formal evaluations of the effects of ketamine in PTSD patients or patients with other dissociative disorders. However, anecdotal data from Russian studies suggest that ketamine induces dissociative states and may promote guided recollection of traumatic material in Russian Afghanistan war veterans with PTSD (Krupitsky 1972, personal communication, January 1994).

Dissociative states also have been produced by psychoactive cannabinoids, such as tetrahydrocannabinol, the principal psychoactive component of marijuana and hashish. Cannabinoids bind to a specific G-protein-coupled receptor (Herkenham et al. 1990) through which they alter cellular functions, including blockade of N-type calcium channels, inhibition of cyclic adenosine monophosphate (cAMP) accumulation, and stimulation of arachidonic acid and intracellular calcium release (Felder et al. 1993). Some cannabinoid effects may be mediated by stimulation of glucocorticoid receptors (Eldridge and Landfield 1990) and blockade of NMDA receptors (Feigenbaum et al. 1989). At high doses, cannabinoid intoxication produces depersonalization, derealization, temporal disorientation, perceptual alterations, and insight impairments (Bromberg 1939; Dittrich et al. 1973; Melges et al. 1970). Depersonalization and temporal disorientation produced by marijuana smoking were associated with increased cortical regional cerebral blood flow assessed with the [133]xenon inhalation technique (Mathew et al. 1993). Cannabis has been reported to produce flashbacks that resemble cannabis intoxication in drug-free subjects (Hollister 1986). In one study (Stanton et al. 1976), 3% (1 of 31) of habitual marijuana users and 1% (3 of 348) of nonhabitual users reported flashbacks when drug-free, suggesting that flashbacks were not a frequent consequence of cannabis use. However, this study suggested that marijuana use also enhanced the likelihood of experiencing flashbacks following ingestion of the serotonergic hallucinogens.

Serotonergic hallucinogens, such as lysergic acid diethylamide (LSD), mescaline, and dimethyltryptamine (DMT), also produce dissociative symptoms. These agents stimulate serotonin-2 (5-HT$_2$) receptors (Rasmussen et al. 1986; Titeler et al. 1988). Serotonergic hallucinogens produce pronounced visual hallucinations, illusions, synesthesia, and expansive or portentous emotional responses (Freedman 1968; Strassman et al. 1994). Following ingestion of psychedelics, subjects report prominent feelings of derealization or depersonalization. Environmental stimuli may be experienced in a fragmented manner, body image distortion is common, and feelings of emotional detachment may arise (Freedman 1968; Klee 1963; Liebert et al. 1958; Rodin and Luby 1966; Savage 1955). Some clinicians also have reported that LSD may facilitate the recall of repressed memories (Freedman 1968), although this capacity has never been rigorously evaluated. Relative to the phencyclidine or ketamine experience, psychedelic hallucinogens tend to produce perceptual effects that predominate over dissociative effects and impairments in higher cognitive functions.

Flashbacks have been reported in healthy individuals following serotonergic hallucinogen use. Freedman (1968) and Horowitz (1969) suggested that LSD intoxication was traumatic for some users because it diminished control over awareness, resulting in intense emotional states experienced as beyond their control. In such cases, LSD flashbacks might have a traumatic etiology. However, some LSD-like experiences, such as synesthesia, may be reexperienced long after drug ingestion by individuals who find such experiences pleasant. These effects do not easily fit a trauma model, suggesting that sensitization, conditioning, or state-dependent learning also might apply (Freedman 1968, 1984; Horowitz 1969; McGee 1984). Subject expectancy also may play a role in druglike flashbacks. One study found that flashbacks may be produced in healthy subjects following placebo administration if subjects are coached to anticipate that a placebo will produce flashbacks (Heaton 1975). Heaton suggested that the expectancy of flashbacks led subjects to mislabel and selectively attend to aspects of normal experience that are consistent with a flashbacklike experience.

Lessons From Brain Stimulation Studies

Flashbacks are common to PTSD and conditions associated with local activation of cortical and limbic structures. Hughlings Jackson first described the complex polysensory reexperiencing of events that occurred in association with temporal lobe epilepsy as memory flashbacks (Taylor 1931). Patients with clinical and encephalographic evidence of temporal lobe epilepsy exhibited a range of dissociative symptoms, including depersonalization, derealization, auditory and visual hallucinations, and multiple personalities (Mesulam 1981b). Sacks (1985) also described a patient with seizure foci in her medial temporal structures that produced repetitive reexperiencing of Irish folk melodies. Anticonvulsant treatment eliminated the intrusive musical reexperiencing but also eliminated her ability to recall the melodies.

Penfield and Perot (1963) elicited dreamlike states, memories, and complex experiential phenomena through direct electrical stimulation of structures in the temporal lobe, temporoparietal association areas, hippocampus, and amygdala. Temporal lobe stimulation resulted in some individuals reexperiencing frightening events in a polysensory fashion, such as a possible thwarted kidnapping (see case 15 in Penfield and Perot 1963). However, neutral or pleasant experiences also were produced, such as hearing a choir sing "White Christmas" (see case 4 in Penfield and Perot 1963). The amygdala and hippocampus appear to be implicated in the experiential phenomena associated with temporal lobe activation. Gloor et al. (1982) found that experiential phenomena were associated with direct stimulation of the amygdala and the hippocampus. Moreover, memories, dreamlike states, or other complex experiential phenomena were produced only when temporal cortical stimulation was followed by afterdischarges in the amygdala or hippocampus. Results of this study were consistent with an earlier one that produced complex experiential phenomena through electrical stimulation of the hippocampus and amygdala (Halgren et al. 1978).

The brain stimulation studies suggest that the hippocampus and amygdala control the retrieval of memory in a highly specific manner, much as a program might control access to information stored on a computer. However, this interpretation appears overly simple. Complex experiential phenomena are usually associated with high-intensity stimuli or afterdischarges, suggesting that fairly large cortical areas must be activated (Halgren et al. 1978). Also, stimulation of the same location over several trials does not reliably reproduce experiential phenomena, whereas stimulation of disparate cortical regions may produce identical experiences (Halgren et al. 1978; Horowitz et al. 1968). In addition, surgical excision of an area that produces a memory when directly stimulated does not eliminate the memory (Baldwin 1960). A more circumspect interpretation of these data is that memory is stored within distributed networks and that the amygdala and hippocampus stimulations bias the retrieval of memories in a more general fashion, such as facilitating access to an associative network.

One of the striking similarities of flashback associated with PTSD and the brain stimulation studies are the inflexible nature of memory retrieval under these conditions. Dreams and memories often replay traumatic scenes in their entirety rather than being retrieved with the cognitive flexibility characteristic of declarative memory. The neurobiology underlying the loss of retrieval flexibility and efficiency associated with traumatic memory retrieval, limbic stimulation studies, and the developmental disorders is currently unclear. However, reduced mnemonic flexibility has been reported to characterize memory retrieval under conditions where the hippocampus is activated independently of the frontal cortex (Moscovitch 1992). Memory encoding by the hippocampus is modular, and organizing links between memories arise largely through cue association, as occurs during conditioning (Moscovitch 1992). Retrieval strategies involving the hippocampus are cue dependent and not strategic. In other words, the hippocampus cannot efficiently scan stored memories to retrieve a particular memory, even though it is involved in memory encoding. The organizing and strategizing component of memory retrieval appears to depend on the frontal cortex (Moscovitch 1989, 1992). Thus, flashbacks may share the qualities of memory retrieval exhibited by individuals during hippocampal stimulation because these conditions involve retrieval strategies that bypass the frontal component of memory retrieval despite relative preservation of the hippocampal component of memory retrieval.

Recollective processes that bypass frontal executive mechanisms controlling the strategic recollection of information also may share the quality of being reexperienced rather than recalled. Flashbacks produced by electrical stimulation in seizure patients (Penfield and Perot 1963) and those occurring in PTSD (Bremner et al. 1992; Southwick et al. 1991) were both described in this manner. Frontal cortical networks have been implicated in executive functions related to the control of memory retrieval (Baddeley 1986). Frontal lobe lesions, unlike hippocampal lesions, impair retrieval of autobiographical information (Baddeley and Wilson 1988). The frontal cortex also has been implicated in prioritizing responses, generating mental representations within working memory, self-monitoring, and editing of thought (Baddeley 1986; Goldman-Rakic 1987; Stuss 1992). The frontal cortex is nested within networks involving the amygdala, mediodorsal thalamic nucleus, hippocampus, and other regions that provide access to input regarding the nature and meaning of memories that are formed (Goldman-Rakic 1987). Sedative-hypnotic agents produce impairments on tests sensitive to frontal cortical impairment, as does ketamine (Krystal et al. 1994a; J. H. Krystal, L. P. Karper, D. C. D'Souza, et al., "Interactive Effects of Subanesthetic Ketamine and Lorazepam in Humans," unpublished manuscript, 1997).

Thalamic Networks and Dissociative States

Dissociative states occur normally in individuals without dissociative disorders when they are exposed to conditions of extremely low or high levels of sensory stimulation. Reductions in the intensity or variability of sensory stimulation, associated with hypnosis, sleep deprivation, and sensory deprivation, may produce altered states of consciousness with dissociative features (Bexton et al. 1954; Cappon and Banks 1960; Freud and Breuer 1892/1953; Lilly 1956; Krystal 1988). As an extreme illustration of this point, sensory polyneuropathies may cause marked depersonalization and derealization associated with feelings of being disembodied (Sacks 1985). Heightened sensory stimulation or arousal also may produce altered sensory processing. Significant levels of arousal and anxiety heighten the salience and vividness of environmental stimuli.

When individuals are under stress, attention is narrowed to the most salient aspects of the environment, consistent with the need to focus on the danger at hand. Thus, individuals fixate faster and longer on unusual or highly informative objects, such as weapons (Christianson 1992; Christianson and Loftus 1991), whereas less critical but important information about the context of the trauma may not receive much attention (Kramer et al. 1990). At extremely high levels of arousal, coherent integration of sensory information breaks down and dissociative symptoms emerge, even in individuals without dissociative disorders (Cappon and Banks 1961; Ludwig 1972; Krystal et al. 1988, 1991).

The thalamus plays a critical role in modulating responsivity to environmental stimuli associated with sleep and dreaming and may play a similar role in the genesis of dissociative states. As illustrated in Figure 11-1, the thalamus serves as a sensory gate or filter that directly and indirectly modulates the access of sensory information to the cortex, amygdala, and hippocampus (Amaral and Cowan 1980; McCormick 1992; Steriade and Llinás 1988; Turner and Herkenham 1991). During slow-wave sleep, for example, thalamic nuclei exhibit slow spindle oscillations that disrupt the transmission of sensory information to cortical and limbic structures (Steriade and Deschenes 1984). During wakefulness, thalamic neurons fire in a relay mode that facilitates transmission of sensory information to cortical regions. Rapid eye movement (REM) sleep, associated with dreaming, is characterized by phasic enhancement of the activity of glutamatergic thalamocortical cells (Steriade and McCarley 1990; Steriade et al. 1990). In this model, dreams and other sleep-related internally generated experiences may arise as thalamocortical or other direct cortical projections from the amygdala and hippocampus bypass the oscillatory thalamic processes that disrupt the flow of sensory information to the cortex (Llinás and Paré 1991; Swanson 1981). Thus, like dissociative states, sleep states may neurobiologically preserve associative and mnemonic functions while interrupting sensory processing. Sensory processing alterations associated with dissociative states could indicate the intrusion of sleep-related disturbances in sensory processing into the waking state. If so, then alterations in thalamic activity might link a spectrum of altered states of consciousness such as hypnosis, dreaming, and other conditions in which there is a combination of the features of sleep and waking states (Llinás and Paré 1991; Mahowald and Schenck 1991). Dissociative states also might be related to night terrors in which features of waking behavior intrude on sleep (Fisher et al. 1973; Kales et al. 1980; Oswald and Evans 1985). Evidence for a thalamic role in maintaining the boundary of sleeplike behavior and wakefulness is provided by patients with paramedian thalamic infarctions. These patients exhibit a profound sense of detachment, reduced responsivity to sensory stimuli, and sleeplike posturing throughout the circadian cycle without the electrophysiological correlates of non-REM sleep (Guilleminault et al. 1993). The hypothesis that the thalamus contributes to dissociation-like alterations in consciousness is further supported by thalamic activation during absence seizures (Prevett et al. 1995).

A role of the thalamus in dissociation also is suggested by its distinctive function in modulating the onset of night terrors. Posttraumatic nightmares occur within REM sleep and are not generally associated with motor behaviors, although they may repetitively review aspects of the trauma (Fisher et al. 1970, 1973; Greenberg et al. 1972). In contrast, posttraumatic night terrors bear a closer resemblance to flashbacks occurring in the waking state. Night terrors are associated with confusion upon awakening, reduced responsivity to environmental stimuli, displays of intense emotion, significant autonomic activation, increased sleep motility, complex motor activity, and somnambulism (Fisher et al. 1970, 1973; Hafez et al. 1987; Lavie and Hertz 1979; van der Kolk et al. 1984). Despite behavioral evidence that traumatic incidents are being reexperienced during night terrors, such as calls for help and appearing to act out physical struggles, individuals are generally amnestic for the content of their experiences. As with flashbacks and nightmares, night terrors may be precipitated in PTSD patients by reminders of the trauma or environmental stress (Fisher et al. 1970; Krystal 1968). Unlike nightmares, night terrors occur during deep sleep, particularly stage 4, and generally within the

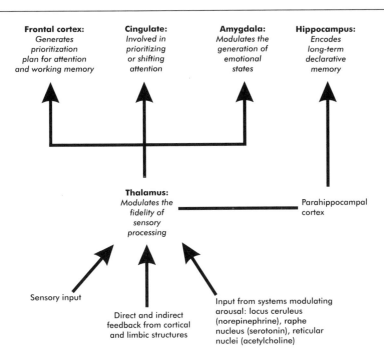

Figure 11–1. Position of the thalamus within networks that may be involved in the generation of dissociative states. Sensory information reaches the thalamus and is transmitted to limbic and cortical regions responsible for modulating thought, attention, learning and memory, and emotion. The thalamus receives input from limbic regions, such as the amygdala, and brain stem regions involved in stress-related arousal. It also receives direct and indirect feedback from cortical regions involved in prioritizing attention. When functioning in relay mode, the thalamus facilitates the accurate transmittal of sensory information. However, when slow oscillatory firing patterns predominate, the thalamus impedes the flow of sensory information to cortical and limbic regions associated with the predominate focus on internally generated thought processes and sensory experiences associated with dreaming, night terrors, and perhaps dissociation.

Krystal JH, Bennett A, Bremner JD, et al: "Toward a Cognitive Neuroscience of Dissociation and Altered Memory Functions in Post-Traumatic Stress Disorder," in *Neurobiological Consequences of Stress From Adaptation to Post-Traumatic Stress Disorder*. Edited by Friedman M, Charney DS, Deutch AY. New York, Raven, 1995. Reprinted with permission.

first hour after falling asleep (Fisher et al. 1973; Kales et al. 1980). Nightmares and night terrors may be further distinguished by the effects of paramedian thalamic lesions. These lesions eliminate the stages of sleep that contain night terrors but do not alter REM sleep and dreaming (Guilleminault et al. 1993).

Sensory distortions associated with stress may develop, in part, as a consequence of the thalamic role in modulating sensory processing. Thalamic nuclei appear to work both in series and in parallel with brain regions involved in traumatic stress response. One region that may be critical for fear learning and traumatic stress response is the central nucleus of the amygdala (Charney et al. 1993; M. Davis 1992; LeDoux 1987). Once activated by uncontrollable stressors, the central nucleus of the amygdala facilitates the thalamic relay of sensory information to cortical and limbic structures (Clugnet and LeDoux 1990; Steriade et al. 1990).

Central noradrenergic systems also are activated by significant uncontrollable stressors and have been linked to traumatic stress response (Krystal et al. 1989; Bremner et al. 1996a, 1996b). Stress-induced noradrenergic activation would be expected to facilitate thalamic transduction of sensory information by stimulating thalamic α_1-adrenergic receptors that increase thalamic activity associated with wakefulness and to inhibit slow thalamic oscillations (Buzsáki et al. 1990; McCormick and Wang 1991). Postsynaptic α_2 receptors promote thalamic slow oscillations. Thus yohimbine, an α_2 antagonist, could increase thalamic bursting by increasing norepinephrine release and blocking the stimulation slow oscillations produced by postsynaptic α_2 receptors (Buzsáki et al. 1990).

Serotonergic systems, linked to PTSD symptoms by the m-CPP study described previously (Southwick et al. 1993), also heighten sensory processing via the 5-HT_2 receptor (McCormick and Wang 1991). Both m-CPP and the serotonergic hallucinogens stimulate subtypes of this receptor (Sheldon and Aghajanian 1991). Perceptual alterations associated with extreme or uncontrollable stress suggest that massive activation of monoamine systems under these conditions may modulate thalamic function, resulting in interference rather than enhancement of the fidelity of sensory transmission.

Alterations in thalamic glutamatergic function also could contribute to sensory gating disturbances. Glutamate is the primary excitatory neurotransmitter within the thalamus (McCormick 1992) and the neurotransmitter involved with thalamic afferents from the amygdala, cerebral cortex, and hippocampus (Aggleton and Mishkin 1984; Aggleton et al. 1986; Giguere and Goldman-Rakic 1988; LeDoux and Farb 1991; McCormick 1992). Indirect cortical thalamic modulation also occurs via a circuit involving the striatum, globus pallidus, subthalamic nucleus, and thalamus (Carlsson and Carlsson 1990). Both NMDA and non-NMDA glutamate receptors are localized to the thalamus, where they have complementary functions (McCormick 1992). Previous reviews have suggested that alterations of the sensory filter function of the thalamus via blockade of NMDA receptors could contribute to the psychotomimetic effects of the NMDA antagonists (Carlsson and Carlsson 1990). These hypotheses may be consistent with electrophysiological evidence indicating that the thalamus may be particularly sensitive to the proconvulsant effects of subanesthetic doses of NMDA antagonists (Ferrer-Allado et al. 1973).

Given the prominent role of non-NMDA glutamate receptors in corticostriatothalamic circuitry, subanesthetic doses of selective NMDA antagonists might be predicted to produce distortions rather than complete blockade of thalamic sensory gating functions. This prediction is consistent with clinical observations suggesting that ketamine produces a state of detachment or withdrawal rather than sleep. Also, ketamine produces sensory distortions and illusions rather than blockade of sensory perceptions or pure hallucinatory experiences (Krystal et al. 1994b). The capacity of sensory deprivation to reduce rather than augment the behavioral effects of phencyclidine further suggests that NMDA antagonists alter rather than block sensory processing (B. D. Cohen et al. 1960). Future research is needed to clarify the extent of thalamic contributions to dissociative states.

The thalamus is a heterogeneous structure, and component thalamic nuclei have distinctive cortical afferents and efferents and different patterns of synaptic organization (M. L. Schwartz et al. 1991). For example, the reticular nuclei of the thalamus function in some ways as an extension of brain stem and mid-brain reticular activating systems (Steriade and Llinás 1988). However, other thalamic nuclei, such as the anteroventral and mediodorsal nuclei, appear to be involved in associative processes, such as learning (Gabriel et al. 1987, 1991; Orona and Gabriel 1983).

Sensory processing alterations and changes in attention may be linked in dissociative states. Clinically, the bridge between sensory gating and attention modulation is evident in the reduced responsivity to environmental stimuli exhibited by dissociated individuals and their reported focus on peripheral sensory stimuli or internal mental processes (Carlson and Putnam 1989). This connection also is suggested by the convergence of corticolimbic networks on the anterior cingulate gyrus, a brain region implicated in the capacity to shift and focus attention (Bench et al. 1993; Pardo et al. 1990). Anterior cingulate lesions may produce symptoms reminiscent of thalamic, limbic, and cortical lesions, including confusion, vivid daydreaming, apathy, impairments in sustained attention, and learning impairments (Laplane et al. 1981; Whitty and Lewin 1957). Direct projections to the anterior cingulate gyrus from midline and intralaminar thalamic nuclei suggest that the cingulate gyrus is responsive to shifts in thalamic sensory processing functions (Vogt et al. 1979). As suggested by the clinical case reports of patients with cingulate lesions, the cingulate gyrus also may be involved in the attribution of salience and the acquisition and retrieval of learned information (Gabriel et al. 1991; Gaffan et al. 1993). The contributions of the cingulate gyrus to sensory processing, emotional regulation, and learning are facilitated by its connectivity to other brain regions. For example, hippocampal and anteroventral thalamic inputs converge upon the anterior cingulate gyrus via the posterior cingulate gyrus (Gabriel and Sparenborg 1987; Gabriel et al. 1987). Similarly, the anterior cingulate gyrus is an important point of convergence for a network involving the amygdala, prefrontal cortex, and mediodorsal thalamic nucleus (Aggleton and Mishkin 1984; Gaffan and Murray 1990; Gaffan et al. 1993; Goldman-Rakic and Porrino 1985; Orona and Gabriel 1983).

Cortical Dysconnectivity and Dissociation

Geschwind (1980) wrote, "there is no evidence for the existence of any all-purpose computer in the brain." Consistent with this view, cortical functions are highly distributed across several cortical regions that require integration to generate coherent conscious experience. For example, frontoparietal interactions help to locate memories or mental representations in space, frontohippocampal interactions appear to contribute contextual information regarding these memories, and frontotemporal interactions contribute to working memory for shapes and features (A. Belger, G. McCarthy, J. Gore, "FMRI Studies of Working Memory Networks: Parietal and Temporal Lobe Studies," unpublished manuscript, 1996; Goldman-Rakic 1987). Also, the frontal cortex itself contains many functionally heterogeneous regions. Distinct frontal cortex loci mediate the generation of iconic or working memories for the location and features of environmental stimuli. Brain lesions of one region of the frontal cortex result in memory gaps for spatial features, whereas lesions of the other region produce an inability to recall faces (Goldman-Rakic 1987; Wilson et al. 1993). If corticocortical interactions were disturbed or disrupted, experiences and cognitive functions that depend on integrated cortical activity might be distorted. For example, if frontal cortical regions processing features of objects and their spatial attributes were interacting dysfunctionally, one might generate mental representations for stimuli in which features were not correctly matched to their spatial locations (i.e., objects could be experienced out of context or in bizarre or incoherent ways). Disturbances in function arising from abnormal integration of cortical function may be similar, by analogy, to conduction aphasias. In conduction aphasias, both comprehension and fluency are preserved, but speech is paraphasic because information cannot be effectively transmitted from association to motor cortices (Geschwind 1970).

Drugs that produce dissociative states disturb cortical integration at several levels. The key output neurons of the cortex are pyramidal neurons that use glutamate as their primary neurotransmitter. These neurons are regulated locally by modulatory

GABAergic neurons. Pyramidal neurons also receive distant input from subcortical monoaminergic, glutamatergic, and peptidergic systems and glutamatergic input from pyramidal neurons in other cortical areas (Goldman-Rakic 1987; Lewis et al. 1992). In the piriform cortex, serotonergic hallucinogens inhibit pyramidal neuronal activity by stimulating GABAergic interneurons via the 5-HT$_{2A/2B}$ receptors. However, these drugs also activate pyramidal neurons through stimulating 5-HT$_{2C}$ receptors (Sheldon and Aghajanian 1991).

Subanesthetic doses of ketamine distort the functional connectivity within the cortex by blocking the NMDA receptor-mediated component of glutamatergic corticocortical connectivity. One study, for example, suggested that blockade of NMDA receptors allowed sensory information to reach the cortex but interfered with the coherent transmission of this information from receptive areas to association cortices (Corssen and Domino 1966). Ketamine may produce these disturbances by altering the balance of glutamate receptor stimulation, decreasing the stimulation of NMDA receptors, and increasing non-NMDA glutamate receptor stimulation. Subanesthetic doses of ketamine preferentially reduce the activity of inhibitory cortical interneurons, disinhibiting cortical pyramidal neurons and increasing glutamate release (Dingledine et al. 1986; Moghaddam and Bolinao 1994). Enhancing GABA function reduces the dissociative effects of ketamine, consistent with the hypothesis that facilitating GABA function might reduce the consequences of decreased interneuronal activation. Blockade of non-NMDA glutamate receptors also might be predicted to reduce ketamine effects because glutamate released as a result of ketamine administration will bind to those glutamate receptor subclasses not blocked by ketamine (i.e., non-NMDA receptors). Barbiturates weakly but significantly block two non-NMDA glutamate-receptor subclasses, the amino-3-hydroxy-5-methylisoxazole-4-propionic acid (AMPA)/kainate receptors (Collins and Anson 1987; Morgan et al. 1991), and might be evaluated for their capacity to reduce ketamine effects.

Recent data also may implicate shifts in interhemispheric processing in hypnotic and dissociative experiences. In particular, recent studies report that hypnosis is associated with performance reductions on tests sensitive to impairments of the left frontal cortex (Gruzelier and Warren 1993). Hypnosis also may be associated with lateralized shifts in electroencephalogram frequency and evoked potential amplitudes (Spiegel 1991). The hypothesis that interhemispheric processing alterations contribute to dissociative states also is supported by a recent report of two cases in which alternate personalities were differentially elicited in patients with multiple personality disorder with temporal lobe epilepsy through administration of intracarotid amobarbital selectively to the two cortical hemispheres (Ahern et al. 1993).

Alteration in Glutamatergic Function: A Final Common Pathway for Dissociation?

Clinical studies related to the neurobiology of dissociative states are summarized in Table 11-1. Yohimbine and m-CPP produce dissociative states only in PTSD patients, who are prone to have these experiences. These drugs primarily produce dissociative states while stimulating anxiety or traumatic recollections. Thus, yohimbine and m-CPP may not directly induce dissociation but rather contribute to the modulation of networks, resulting in a dissociative state in vulnerable individuals. In the amygdala, hippocampus, thalamus, and cortex, noradrenergic and serotonergic systems serve to modulate the activity of glutamatergic neurons (Goldman-Rakic 1987; Lewis et al. 1992). Given the central role of glutamate in corticocortical, thalamocortical, amygdalocortical, and hippocampocortical connectivity, glutamatergic systems in the brain may be considered the framework on which higher cognitive functions rest. Thus, it may not be surprising that a drug, such as ketamine, that alters glutamatergic neurotransmission produces dissociative states in healthy individuals. The possibility that glutamate systems might be fundamentally involved in generating dissociative states is consistent with the observation that dissociative states produced by ketamine in healthy people arise as a direct consequence of drug administration and are not dependent on gener-

Table 11–1.   Summary of pharmacologically facilitated dissociative states

Substance	Healthy subjects	PTSD patients
Yohimbine	–	+
m-CPP	–	+
Lactate	–	+
Sedative-hypnotics	–	+[a]
Benzodiazepine antagonists	–	–
NMDA antagonists	+	+[b]
Cannabinoids	+	?
Serotonergic hallucinogens	+	?

Note.   PTSD = posttraumatic stress disorder; m-CPP = metachlorophenyl-piperazine; NMDA = N-methyl-D-aspartate; – = not associated with dissociative state; + = associated with dissociative state; ? = unclear association with dissociative state.
[a]Facilitation of dissociation during guided recollection.
[b]Not formally evaluated in patients with PTSD.

ating intense emotional responses or memories. The direct evocation of dissociative states by an NMDA antagonist raises the possibility that reductions in NMDA receptor function contribute to dissociative states in humans. If so, then pharmacological agents that enhance NMDA receptor function might have antidissociative properties (Jones et al. 1991; Nicholls 1993; Saletu et al. 1986; B. L. Schwartz et al. 1991).

Implications for the Treatment of Posttraumatic Stress Disorder

Dissociative phenomena, traumatic memories, and affective regulation are highly interrelated in PTSD patients Bremner et al. 1993). Traumatic memories and intense emotions may trigger dissociative phenomena in PTSD patients. Similarly, traumatic memories become more accessible when emotional or dissociative states resembling those at the time of traumatization are produced. Completing the triangle, traumatic memories and dissociative phenomena may precipitate strong emotional responses. Thus, reducing the incidence of flashbacks and the intrusiveness and distress related to traumatic memories must be understood in the context of treating each of the three interactive processes.

The first step in treating dissociative states in traumatized individuals is to alleviate the marked depersonalization, derealization, and extreme emotional arousal. Barbiturates and benzodiazepines may be useful for this purpose (Kluft 1987). The long-term benefits of acute anxiolysis are currently unclear. However, Kardiner (1941) emphasized the importance of the peritraumatic period in creating a long-lasting appraisal of traumatic events. Acute anxiolysis may be helpful in reducing negatively valenced cognitive distortions. Thus, in the context of supportive therapy, benzodiazepine treatment may facilitate the development of a more adaptive appraisal of the traumatic stress, perhaps by altering pairing of emotions and memories. Benzodiazepines also may prevent other stress-related alterations in memory function (see Bremner et al., Chapter 12, in this volume). Anxiolysis may reduce or prevent the development of dissociative states, facilitating reflective reevaluation of information related to the trauma.

Once hyperarousal is controlled, a second challenge faced by clinicians is to reduce amnesia for traumatic events. Almost every psychotherapeutic strategy for treating acute psychological trauma has as a goal the integration of the traumatic experience within the conscious life of patients (Freud and Breuer 1892/1953; Krystal 1988). This task is difficult if patients are amnestic for the trauma. Several guided recollection strategies have been employed to facilitate patients' access to traumatic memories, including relaxation training, free association, dream interpretation, hypnosis, and narcosynthesis (Bartemeier et al. 1946; Grinker and Spiegel 1943; Keane et al. 1989; Krystal 1988). Each of these processes takes advantage of an altered state of consciousness, associated with increased suggestibility, in which there is a reduction in functions usually associated with the frontal cortex, such as reflection, self-monitoring, and editing of thought (Stuss 1992).

A potential risk associated with conducting guided recollection while the patient is in a compromised state is that ideas introduced by the clinician may be more readily incorporated into the memo-

ries of the patient. For example, under hypnosis or during cannabis intoxication, a subject may not be able to monitor accurately
the source or validity of recalled memories (Laurence and Perry
1983; Pfefferbaum et al. 1977). Concerns about "false memories"
are particularly relevant to narcosynthesis or other techniques in
which the therapist recreates the roles of people within the patient's traumatic memory in order to facilitate memory retrieval
(Grinker and Spiegel 1943, 1945). Furthermore, the use of pharmacological agents, such as Amytal, in narcosynthesis may produce
amnesia for remembered information (Ghoneim et al. 1984). Because a patient may not fully recall information produced during
narcosynthesis at later times (Grinker 1944), narcosynthesis may
be best viewed as an information-gathering procedure.

Once an individual has access to memories of the trauma, what
can the patient and clinician do with them to reduce the incidence
of intrusive memories or flashbacks? Most patients are tormented
by the intrusion of traumatic memories, and for these individuals,
merely reviewing them an additional time is not necessarily therapeutic. Freud and Breuer (1892/1953) initially suggested two
strategies for reducing dissociative or conversion symptoms associated with hysteria: abreaction and the formation of new associations to the traumatic memories. By abreaction, Freud and Breuer
meant the discharge, during therapy, of stored feelings that could
not be adequately expressed at the time of the trauma. This hy-
draulic view of emotions largely has been abandoned (Krystal
1978). Alternatively, modern cognitive, behavioral, and insight-
oriented therapies focus on altering cognitive, affective, and
identity-related associations to the trauma (Foa et al. 1989; Keane
et al. 1989; Krystal 1988). Psychotherapy may help to reduce the intrusiveness and distress related to traumatic memories by altering
associations to the traumatic events, essentially changing the
meaning of the trauma to the individual.

Managing the recollection of traumatic memories, dissociative
states, and intense affects is a tremendous challenge to the clinician treating PTSD patients. Guided reexperiencing of the trauma
could evoke dissociative states that interfere with associative
learning and with generalizing therapeutic gains beyond the clini-

cal setting. Intense emotions evoked during such recollections could reinforce the association between traumatic memories and intolerable intense emotions, sensitizing patients to reminders, promoting a sense of helplessness or other negative appraisals of the trauma, and making patients more reluctant or unable to review traumatic material in subsequent therapy sessions (Pitman et al. 1991). Furthermore, by stimulating intense emotional responses and negative associations in some individuals, flooding may exacerbate depression or provoke impulsive behavior, including substance abuse (Pitman et al. 1991). These potential problems help to explain the need for extensive relaxation training prior to the initiation of guided reexposure therapies such as flooding (Keane et al. 1989). This step is probably a useful adjunct to all psychotherapies for PTSD patients (Hickling et al. 1986). Furthermore, one must carefully consider the level of arousal associated with guided recollection of traumatic memories and the patient's capacity to process the information. When in the course of a therapy session a patient provides clinical data consistent with the induction of dissociative states, further efforts to encourage him or her to process traumatic material seem unlikely to be fruitful.

The concern that interference with higher cognitive functions limits the clinical utility of altered states of consciousness applies equally to proposed pharmacological adjuvants to psychotherapy, such as the serotonergic hallucinogens (compare Freedman 1968) and NMDA antagonists (compare Krystal et al. 1994b). Particularly in patients with chronic PTSD who have been in treatment for many years, there seems to be little benefit in guiding them to reexperience the trauma at the expense of repeated dissociative episodes. Carefully conducted flooding therapy, preceded by relaxation training, may reduce intrusive symptoms of PTSD but has no beneficial impact on numbing or avoidance (Keane et al. 1989). Keane et al. (1989) highlight significant psychological and social deficits that impair treatment response in patients with chronic PTSD. Thus, treatments aimed at reevaluating traumatic memories may have an important but focused role in their therapy. In addition, research is needed to characterize optimal strategies for integrating pharmacotherapy approaches with these cognitive and behavioral psychotherapies.

If, analogous to relaxation training, pharmacological strategies were developed that preserved cognitive functions despite strong affects and traumatic memories, the formation of new associations to traumatic memories might proceed more effectively and rapidly. Benzodiazepines, reportedly useful in treating some PTSD symptoms in patients with dissociative disorders (Loewenstein et al. 1988), might help by reducing affective distress, although their amnestic properties might be counterproductive at high doses. Alternatively, one could evaluate pharmacological approaches to enhancing cognitive processing. Drugs that facilitate NMDA receptor function via enhancement of the glycine site, such as cycloserine or milacemide (Saletu et al. 1986; B. L. Schwartz et al. 1991), should be evaluated for antidissociative and other cognitive enhancing properties in PTSD patients.

Antidepressants are the best studied pharmacotherapy for PTSD, and research suggests that they provide a moderate degree of relief from flashbacks and intrusive memories. Case reports suggest that tricyclic antidepressants may reduce flashbacks, night terrors, and distress related to intrusive memories of the trauma (Burnstein 1983; Marshall 1975). Similar findings have been reported in open-label trials of monoamine oxidase inhibitors (Hogben and Cornfield 1981; Lerer et al. 1987) and serotonin reuptake blockers (Davidson et al. 1991; McDougle et al. 1991; Nagy et al. 1993). Placebo-controlled trials of tricyclic antidepressants and monoamine oxidase inhibitors have supported the findings from the open-label trials, although variability between studies and small effect sizes have limited the optimism regarding the efficacy of these agents (Davidson et al. 1990; Kosten et al. 1991; Lerer et al. 1987; Reist et al. 1989). The few studies that reported reexperiencing symptoms individually indicated that antidepressants were most effective in reducing the intrusion of traumatic memories and nightmares and less effective in reducing dissociative phenomena such as flashbacks and amnesia (Lerer et al. 1987; Nagy et al. 1993). Case reports also support the use of serotonin reuptake blockers for other dissociative disorders (Fichtner et al. 1992; Hollander et al. 1990), although fluoxetine has been reported to exacerbate dissociative symptoms in some patients (Black and Wojcieszek 1991). The disparity between dissociative and other intrusive symptoms may indicate that antidepressants reduce flashbacks as a secondary consequence of the other effects of these drugs. One mechanism possibly related to the efficacy of these agents is their capacity to prevent or reduce the consequences of noradrenergic hyperreactivity in PTSD patients (Krystal et al. 1989). This hypothesis is consistent with the capacity of fluoxetine treatment to block yohimbine-induced panic attacks in patients with panic disorder (Goddard et al. 1993). The limited efficacy of agents based on monoaminergic transmission suggests that a new direction is need in the development of pharmacotherapies for dissociative disorders. This new direction may be based in the pharmacology of excitatory amino acid neurotransmission implicated in the genesis of dissociative states.

Carbamazepine also has shown utility in reducing hyperarousal, sleep disturbance, and flashbacks in some PTSD patients (Lipper et al. 1986). Despite limited investigation, carbamazepine has received particular attention because of its capacity to suppress a form of neural sensitization, kindling, that may provide a cellular model for the sensitization to repeated stressors (Post and Weiss 1989). Further studies with anticonvulsant agents appear to be warranted.

Cognitive-enhancing pharmacotherapies, such as arginine vasopressin, have been suggested as treatments for memory deficits associated with PTSD (Pitman 1989). Cognitive-enhancing pharmacotherapeutic strategies might be beneficial in reducing encoding deficits associated with short-term memory impairment in PTSD patients. Drugs that might be evaluated for this purpose include ones that facilitate glutamate and acetylcholine function, such as the glycine partial agonist, cycloserine (Jones et al. 1991), and the cholinesterase inhibitor, tacrine (K. L. Davis et al. 1992). Vasopressin has been used to facilitate memory retrieval in patients with PTSD (Pitman et al. 1993), based on preclinical studies suggesting that vasopressin may enhance memory consolidation and retrieval in animals. However, the preclinical foundation of the vasopressin studies has been questioned because subsequent studies have suggested that the promnestic effects of exogenous administration of this hormone are attributable to its enhancement of arousal (Dawson et al. 1992).

Cognitive-enhancing agents do not appear to be the appropriate pharmacotherapeutic approach for reducing amnesia for the trauma. Posttraumatic amnesia appears to arise from the suppression of retrieval rather than from an ongoing memory encoding deficit. There is no evidence to suggest that tacrine or cycloserine reduces the integrity of memory repression. Agents that do appear to facilitate the recollection of traumatic memories, such as lactate, yohimbine, vasopressin, and m-CPP, reduce posttraumatic amnesia via facilitating state-dependent retrieval. However, the sedative-hypnotic agents are the most commonly employed agents for this purpose, combined with some form of guided recollection, such as the Amytal interview.

Conclusion

Dissociative states have received relatively little attention from neurobiologists. However, the initial pharmacological challenge studies suggest that many neurotransmitter systems play important modulatory roles in the pathological development of dissociative states, as in PTSD. Glutamate systems are critically involved in the cortical and limbic circuitry of sensory processing, attention regulation, and strategic memory retrieval. Recent studies, employing ketamine, suggest that deficits in NMDA receptor function may produce dissociation-like states in healthy individuals. Further characterization of the neurobiology of these functions may facilitate the development of antidissociative pharmacotherapies.

References

Aggleton JP, Mishkin M: Projection of the amygdala to the thalamus in the cynomologous monkey. J Comp Neurol 222:56–68, 1984

Aggleton JP, Desimone R, Mishkin M: The origin, course and termination of the hippocampothalamic projections in the macaque. J Comp Neurol 243:409–421, 1986

Ahern GL, Herring AM, Tackenberg J, et al: The association of multiple personality and temporolimbic epilepsy: intracarotid amobarbital test observations. Arch Neurol 50:1020–1025, 1993

Amaral DG, Cowan WM: Subcortical afferents to the hippocampal formation in the monkey. J Comp Neurology 189:573–591, 1980

American Psychiatric Association: Diagnostic and Statistical Manual of Mental Disorders, 3rd Edition, Revised. Washington, DC, American Psychiatric Association, 1987

Baddeley AD: Working Memory. New York, Oxford University, 1986

Baddeley AD, Wilson B: Frontal amnesia and the dysexecutive syndrome. Brain Cogn 7:212–230, 1988

Baldwin M: Electrical stimulation of the mesial temporal region, in Electrical Studies on the Unanesthetized Brain. Edited by Ramey ER, O'Doherty DS. New York, Hoeber, 1960, pp 159–176

Bartemeier LH, Kubie LS, Menninger KA, et al: Combat exhaustion. J Nerv Ment Dis 104:489–525, 1946

Bench CJ, Frith CD, Grasby PM, et al: Investigations of the functional anatomy of attention using the Stroop test. Neuropsychologia 31:907–922, 1993

Bexton WH, Heron W, Scott TH: Effects of decreased variation in the sensory environment. Canadian Journal of Psychology 8:70–76, 1954

Black DW, Wojcieszek J: Depersonalization syndrome induced by fluoxetine. Psychosomatics 32:468–469, 1991

Bremner JD, Southwick S, Brett E, et al: Dissociation and posttraumatic stress disorder in Vietnam combat veterans. Am J Psychiatry 149:328–332, 1992

Bremner JD, Steinberg M, Southwick SM, et al: Use of the Structured Clinical Interview for DSM-IV Dissociative Disorders for systematic assessment of dissociative symptoms in posttraumatic stress disorder. Am J Psychiatry 150:1011–1014, 1993

Bremner JD, Krystal JH, Southwick SM, et al: Noradrenergic mechanisms in stress and anxiety, I: preclinic studies. Synapse 23:28–38, 1996a

Bremner JD, Krystal JH, Southwick SM, et al: Noradrenergic mechanisms in stress and anxiety, I: clinical studies. Synapse 23:39–51, 1996b

Bremner JD, Mazure CM, Putnam FW, et al: Measurement of dissociative states with the Clinician-Administered Dissociative States Scale (CADSS). Journal of Traumatic Stress, in press

Bromberg W: Marihuana: a psychiatric study. JAMA 113:4–12, 1939

Burnstein AT: Treatment of flashbacks by imipramine. Am J Psychiatry 140:509–512, 1983

Buzsáki G, Kennedy B, Solt VB, et al: Noradrenergic control of thalamic oscillation: the role of α_2 receptors. Eur J Neurosci 3:222–229, 1990

Cappon D, Banks R: Studies in perceptual distortion. AMA Archives of Neurology and Psychiatry 10:99–104, 1960

Cappon D, Banks R: Orientational perception: a review and preliminary study of distortion in orientational perception. Arch Gen Psychiatry 5:380–392, 1961

Carlson EB, Putnam FW: Integrating research on dissociation and hypnotizability: are there two pathways to hypnotizability? Dissociation 2:32–38, 1989

Carlsson M, Carlsson A: Schizophrenia: a subcortical neurotransmitter imbalance syndrome? Schizophr Bull 16:425–432, 1990

Charney DS, Heninger GR, Breier A: Noradrenergic function in panic anxiety: effects of yohimbine in healthy subjects and patients with agoraphobia and panic disorder. Arch Gen Psychiatry 41:751–763, 1984

Charney DS, Woods SW, Goodman WK, et al: Serotonin function in anxiety, II: effects of the serotonin agonist m-CPP in panic disorder patients and healthy subjects. Psychopharmacology 92:14–24, 1987

Charney DS, Deutch AY, Krystal JH, et al: Psychobiologic mechanisms of posttraumatic stress disorder. Arch Gen Psychiatry 50:294–305, 1993

Christianson SÅ: Emotional stress and eyewitness testimony: a critical review. Psychol Bull 112:284–309, 1992

Christianson SÅ, Loftus EF: Remembering emotional events: the fate of detailed information. Cognition and Emotion 5: 81–108, 1991

Clugnet MC, LeDoux J: Synaptic plasticity in fear conditioning circuits: induction of LTP in the lateral nucleus of the amygdala by stimulation of medial geniculate body. J Neurosci 10:2818–2824, 1990

Cohen BD, Luby ED, Rosenbaum G, et al: Combined sernyl and sensory deprivation. Compr Psychiatry 1:345–348, 1960

Collins GGS, Anson J: Effects of barbiturates on responses evoked by excitatory amino acids in slices of rat olfactory cortex. Neuropharmacology 26:161–171, 1987

Corssen G, Domino EF: Dissociative anesthesia: further pharmacologic studies and first clinical experience with phencyclidine derivative CI-581. Anesth Analg 45:29–40, 1966

Costa E, Guidotti A: Neuropeptides as cotransmitters: modulatory effects at GABAergic synapses, in Psychopharmacology: The Third Generation of Progress. Edited by Meltzer HY. New York, Raven, 1987, pp 425–435

Davidson JRT, Kudler HS, Smith RD, et al: Treatment of post-traumatic stress disorder with amitriptyline and placebo. Arch Gen Psychiatry 47:259–266, 1990

Davidson JRT, Roth S, Newman E: Fluoxetine in post-traumatic stress disorder. J Trauma Stress 4:419–423, 1991

Dawson GR, Heyes CM, Iverson SD: Pharmacological mechanisms and animal models of cognition. Behavioral Pharmacology 3:285–297, 1992

Davis KL, Thal LJ, Gamzu ER, et al: A double-blind, placebo-controlled multicenter study of tacrine for Alzheimer's disease. N Engl J Med 327:1253–1259, 1992

Davis M: The role of the amygdala in fear-potentiated startle: implications for animal models of anxiety. Trends Pharmacol Sci 13:35–41, 1992

Dingledine R, Hynes MA, King GL: Involvement of N-methyl-D-aspartate receptors in epileptiform bursting in the rat hippocampal slice. J Physiol (Lond) 380:175–189, 1986

Dittrich A, Bättig K, von Zeppelin I: Effects of (-)Δ^9-transtetrahydrocannabinol (Δ^9-THC) on memory, attention and subjective state: a double blind study. Psychopharmacologia (Berl) 33:369–376, 1973

Domino EF, Chodoff P, Corssen G: Pharmacologic effects of CI-581, a new dissociative anesthetic, in man. Clin Pharmacol Ther 6:279–291, 1965

Dorow R, Horowski R, Paschelke G, et al: Severe anxiety induced by FG7142, a β-carboline ligand for the benzodiazepine receptor. Lancet 2:98–99, 1983

Eldridge JC, Landfield PW: Cannabinoid interactions with glucocorticoid receptors in rat hippocampus. Brain Res 534:135–141, 1990

Erickson MH: Hypnotic treatment techniques for the therapy of acute psychiatric disturbances in war. Am J Psychiatry 101:668–672, 1945

Feigenbaum JJ, Bergmann F, Richmond SA, et al: Nonpsychotropic cannabinoid acts as a functional N-methyl-D-aspartate receptor blocker. Proc Natl Acad Sci U S A 86:9584–9587, 1989

Felder CC, Briley EM, Axelrod J, et al: Anandamide, an endogenous cannabimimetic eicosanoid, binds to the cloned human cannabinoid receptor and stimulates receptor-mediated signal transduction. Proc Natl Acad Sci USA 90:7656–7660, 1993

Ferrer-Allado T, Brechner VL, Dymond A, et al: Ketamine-induced electroconvulsive phenomena in the human limbic and thalamic regions. Anesthesiology 38:333–344, 1973

Fichtner CG, Horevitz RP, Braun BG: Fluoxetine in depersonalization disorder. Am J Psychiatry 149:1750–1751, 1992

Fisher C, Byrne J, Edwards A, et al: A psychophysiological study of nightmares. J Am Psychoanal Assoc 18:747–782, 1970

Fisher C, Kahn E, Edwards A, et al: A psychophysiological study of nightmares and night-terrors, I: physiological aspects of the stage 4 night terror. J Nerv Ment Dis 157:75–98, 1973

Fitzgerald SG, Gonzalez E: Dissociative states induced by relaxation training in a PTSD combat veteran: failure to identify trigger mechanisms. J Trauma Stress 7:111–116, 1994

Foa EB, Steketee G, Olasov Rothbaum B: Behavioral/cognitive conceptualizations of post-traumatic stress disorder. Behavior Therapy 20:155–176, 1989

Freedman DX: On the use and abuse of LSD. Arch Gen Psychiatry 18:330-347, 1968

Freedman DX: LSD: the bridge from human to animal, in Hallucinogens: Neurochemical, Behavioral, and Clinical Perspectives. Edited by Jacobs BL. New York, Raven, 1984, pp 203–226

Freud S, Breuer J: On the psychical mechanism of hysterical phenomena (1892), in Sigmund Freud, M.D., LL.D.: Collected Papers, Vol 1. Edited by Jones E. London, Hogarth Press, 1953, pp 24–41

Gabriel M, Sparenborg S: Posterior cingulate cortical lesions eliminate learning-related unit activity in the anterior cingulate cortex. Brain Res 409:151–157, 1987

Gabriel M, Sparenborg SP, Stolar N: Hippocampal control of cingulate cortical and anterior thalamic information processing during learning in rabbits. Exp Brain Res 67:131–152, 1987

Gabriel M, Vogt BA, Kubota Y, et al: Training-stage related neuronal plasticity in limbic thalamus and cingulate cortex during learning: a possible key to mnemonic retrieval. Behav Brain Res 46:175–185, 1991

Gaffan D, Murray EA: Amygdalar interaction with the mediodorsal nucleus of the thalamus and the ventromedial prefrontal cortex in stimulus-reward associative learning in the monkey. J Neurosci 10:3479–3493, 1990

Gaffan D, Murray EA, Fabre-Thorpe M: Interaction of the amygdala with the frontal lobe in reward memory. Eur J Neurosci 5:968–975, 1993

Geiselman RE, Bjork RA, Fishman DL: Disrupted retrieval in directed forgetting: a link with posthypnotic amnesia. J Exp Psychol Gen 112:58–72, 1983

Geschwind N: The organization of language and the brain. Science 170: 940–944, 1970

Geschwind N: Neurological knowledge and complex behaviors. Cognitive Sciences 4:185–193, 1980

Ghoneim MM, Mewaldt SP: Benzodiazepines and human memory: a review. Anesthesiology 72:926–938, 1990

Ghoneim MM, Hinrichs JV, Mewaldt SP: Dose-response analysis of the behavioral effects of diazepam, I: learning and memory. Psychopharmacology 82:291–295, 1984

Giguere M, Goldman-Rakic PS: Mediodorsal nucleus: areal, laminar, and tangential distribution of afferents and efferents in the frontal lobe of rhesus monkeys. J Comp Neurol 277:195–213, 1988

Gloor P, Olivier A, Quesney LF, et al: The role of the limbic system in experiential phenomena of temporal lobe epilepsy. Ann Neurol 12: 129–144, 1982

Goddard A, Woods SW, Sholomskas DE, et al: Effects of the serotonin reuptake inhibitor fluvoxamine on yohimbine-induced anxiety in panic disorder. Psychiatry Res 48:119–133, 1993

Goldman-Rakic PS: Circuitry of primate prefrontal cortex and regulation of behavior by representational memory, in Handbook of Physiology, Section I: Higher Functions of the Brain. Edited by Plum F. New York, Oxford University Press, 1987, pp 373–417

Goldman-Rakic PS, Porrino LJ: The primate mediodorsal (MD) nucleus and its projections to the frontal lobe. J Comp Neurol 242:535–560, 1985

Greenberg R, Pearlman CA, Bampel D: War neuroses and the adaptive function of REM sleep. Br J Med Psychol 45:27–33, 1972

Grinker RR: Treatment of war neuroses. JAMA 126:142–145, 1944

Grinker RR, Spiegel JP: War Neuroses in North Africa. New York, Josiah Macy Jr Foundation, 1943

Grinker RR, Spiegel JP: War Neuroses. Philadelphia, Blakiston, 1945

Gruzelier J, Warren K: Neuropsychological evidence of reductions on left frontal tests with hypnosis. Psychol Med 23:93–101, 1993

Guilleminault C, Quera-Salva M-A, Goldberg MP: Pseudo-hypersomnia and pre-sleep behavior with bilateral paramedian thalamic lesions. Brain 116:1549–1563, 1993

Hafez A, Metz L, Lavie P: Long-term effects of extreme situational stress on sleep and dreaming. Am J Psychiatry 144:344–347, 1987

Halgren E, Walter RD, Cherlow DG, et al: Mental phenomena evoked by electrical stimulation of the human hippocampal formation and amygdala. Brain 101:83–117, 1978

Heaton RK: Subject expectancy and environmental factors as determinants of psychedelic flashback experiences. J Nerv Ment Dis 161:157–165, 1975

Heaton RK: Wisconsin Card Sorting Test. Odessa, TX, Psychological Assessment Resources, 1985

Herkenham M, Lynn AB, Little MD, et al: Cannabinoid receptor localization in brain. Proc Natl Acad Sci U S A 87:1932–1936, 1990

Hickling EJ, Sison GFP Jr, Vanderploeg RD: Treatment of posttraumatic stress disorder with relaxation and biofeedback training. Biofeedback Self Regul 11:125–134, 1986

Hogben GL, Cornfield RB: Treatment of war neurosis with phenelzine. Arch Gen Psychiatry 38:440–445, 1981

Hollander E, Liebowitz MR, Decaria C, et al: Treatment of depersonalization with serotonin uptake blockers. J Clin Psychopharmacol 10: 200–203, 1990

Hollister LE: Health aspects of cannabis. Pharmacol Rev 38:2–20, 1986

Horowitz MJ: Flashbacks: recurrent intrusive images after the use of LSD. Am J Psychiatry 126:565–569, 1969

Horowitz MJ, Adams JE, Rutkin BB: Visual imagery on brain stimulation. Arch Gen Psychiatry 19:469–486, 1968

Javitt DC, Zukin SR: Recent advances in the phencyclidine model of schizophrenia. Am J Psychiatry 148:1301–1308, 1991

Jones RW, Wesnes KA, Kirby J: Effects of NMDA modulation in scopolamine dementia. Ann N Y Acad Sci 640:241–244, 1991

Kales JD, Kales A, Soldatos CR, et al: Night terrors: clinical characteristics and personality patterns. Arch Gen Psychiatry 37:1413–1417, 1980

Kardiner A: Psychosomatic Monographs II-III: The Traumatic Neuroses of War. Washington, DC, National Research Council, 1941

Kardiner A, Spiegel H: War Stress and Neurotic Illness. New York, Hoeber, 1947

Keane TM, Fairbank JA, Caddell JM, et al: Implosive (flooding) therapy reduces symptoms of PTSD in Vietnam combat veterans. Behavior Therapy 20:245–260, 1989

Kirk T, Roache JD, Griffiths RR: Dose-response evaluation of the amnestic effects of triazolam and pentobarbital in normal subjects. J Clin Psychopharmacol 10:160–167, 1990

Klee GD: Lysergic acid diethylamide (LSD-25) and ego functions. Arch Gen Psychiatry 8:57–70, 1963

Kluft RF: An update on multiple personality disorder. Hospital and Community Psychiatry 38:363–373, 1987

Kopelman MD, Christensen H, Puffett A, et al: The great escape: a neuropsychological study of psychogenic amnesia. Neuropsychologia 32: 675–691, 1994

Kosten TR, Krystal JH: Biological mechanisms in post traumatic stress disorder: relevance for substance abuse. Recent Dev Alcohol 6: 49–68, 1988

Kosten TR, Frank JB, Dan E, et al: Pharmacotherapy for posttraumatic stress disorder using phenelzine or imipramine. J Nerv Ment Dis 179:366–370, 1991

Kramer TH, Buckhout R, Eugenio P: Weapon focus, arousal, and eyewitness memory: attention must be paid. Law and Human Behavior 14:167–184, 1990

Krupitsky EM: Ketamine psychedelic therapy (KPT) of alcoholism and neuroses. Multidisciplinary Association for Psychedelic Studies Newsletter 3:24–28, 1972

Krystal H: Massive Psychic Trauma. New York, International Universities Press, 1968

Krystal H: Trauma and affects. Psychoanal Stud Child 33:81–116, 1978

Krystal H: Integration and Self-Healing: Affect, Trauma, Alexithymia. Hillsdale, NJ, Analytic Press, 1988

Krystal JH, Woods SW, Hill CL, et al: Characteristics of self-defined panic attacks, in 1988 New Research Programs and Abstracts (NR 263). Washington, DC, American Psychiatric Association, 1988

Krystal JH, Kosten TR, Perry BD, et al: Neurobiological aspects of PTSD: review of clinical and preclinical studies. Behavior Therapy 20:177–198, 1989

Krystal JH, Woods SW, Hill CL, et al: Characteristics of panic attack subtypes: assessment of spontaneous panic, situational panic, sleep panic, and limited symptom attacks. Compr Psychiatry 32:474–478, 1991

Krystal JH, Karper LP, Bennett A, et al: Modulation of frontal cortical function by glutamate and dopamine antagonists in healthy subjects and schizophrenic patients: a neuropsychological perspective. Neuropsychopharmacology 10 (suppl 3):230S, 1994a

Krystal JH, Karper LP, Seibyl JP, et al: Subanesthetic effects of the NMDA antagonist, ketamine, in humans: psychotomimetic, perceptual, cognitive, and neuroendocrine effects. Arch Gen Psychiatry 51:199–214, 1994b

Krystal JH, Bennett A, Bremner JD, et al: Toward a cognitive neuroscience of dissociation and altered memory functions in post-traumatic stress disorder, in Neurobiological Consequences of Stress from Adaptation to Post-Traumatic Stress Disorder. Edited by Friedman M, Charney DS, Deutch AY. New York, Raven, 1995, pp 239–270

Laplane D, Degos JD, Baulac M, et al: Bilateral infarction of the anterior cingulate gyri and the fornices: report of a case. J Neurol Sci 51: 289–300, 1981

Laurence J-R, Perry C: Hypnotically created memory among highly hypnotizable subjects. Science 222:423–524, 1983

Lavie P, Hertz G: Increased sleep motility and respiration rates in combat neurotic patients. Biol Psychiatry 14:983–987, 1979

LeDoux JE: Emotion, in Handbook of Physiology: The Nervous System. Edited by Plum VF. Washington, DC, American Physiological Society, 1987, pp 419–459

LeDoux JE, Farb CR: Neurons of the acoustic thalamus that project to the amygdala contain glutamate. Neurosci Lett 134:145–149, 1991

Lerer B, Bleich A, Kotler M, et al: Post-traumatic stress disorder in Israeli combat veterans: effect of phenelzine treatment. Arch Gen Psychiatry 44:976–981, 1987

Lewis DA, Hayes TL, Lund JS, et al: Dopamine and the neural circuitry of primate prefrontal cortex: implications for schizophrenia research. Neuropsychopharmacology 6:127–134, 1992

Liebert RS, Werner H, Wapner S: Studies on the effects of lysergic acid diethylamide (LSD-25). AMA Archives of Neurology and Psychiatry 79:580–584, 1958

Lilly JC: Mental effects of reduction of ordinary levels of physical stimuli on intact healthy persons. Psychiatry Res 5:1–9, 1956

Lipper S, Davidson JRT, Grady TA, et al: Preliminary study of carbamazepine in post-traumatic stress disorder. Psychosomatics 27: 849–854, 1986

Llinás RR, Paré D: Of dreaming and wakefulness. Neuroscience 44: 521–535, 1991

Loewenstein RJ, Hornstein N, Farber B: Open trial of clonazepam in the treatment of post-traumatic stress symptoms in multiple personality disorder. Dissociation 1:3–12, 1988

Luby ED, Cohen BD, Rosenbaum G, et al: Study of a new schizophre-nomimetic drug—sernyl. AMA Archives of Neurology and Psychiatry 81:363–369, 1959

Ludwig AM: "Psychedelic" effects produced by sensory overload. Am J Psychiatry 128:1294–1297, 1972

Mahowald MW, Schenck CH: Status dissociatus: a perspective on states of being. Sleep 14:69–79, 1991

Marshall JR: The treatment of night terrors associated with the posttrau-matic syndrome. Am J Psychiatry 132:293–295, 1975

Mathew RJ, Wilson WH, Humphreys D, et al: Depersonalization after marijuana smoking. Biol Psychiatry 33:431–441, 1993

McCormick DA: Neurotransmitter actions in the thalamus and cerebral cortex and their role in the neuromodulation of thalamocortical activ-ity. Prog Neurobiol 39:337–388, 1992

McCormick DA, Wang Z: Serotonin and noradrenaline excite GABAergic neurons of the guinea pig and cat nucleus reticularis thalami. J Physiol (Lond) 442:235–255, 1991

McDougle CJ, Southwick SM, Charney DS, et al: An open trial of fluoxet-ine in the treatment of posttraumatic stress disorder. J Clin Psycho-pharmacol 11:325–327, 1991

McGee R: Flashbacks and memory phenomena: a comment on "flash-back phenomena-clinical and diagnostic dilemmas." J Nerv Ment Dis 172:273–278, 1984

Melges FT, Tinklenberg JR, Hollister LE, et al: Temporal disintegration and depersonalization during marihuana intoxication. Arch Gen Psy-chiatry 23:204–210, 1970

Mesulam MM: Dissociative states with abnormal temporal lobe EEG: multiple personality and the illusion of possession. Arch Neurol 38: 176–181, 1981b

Moghaddam B, Bolinao ML: Stimulatory effects of sub-anesthetic doses of ketamine, a psychotogenic NMDA receptor antagonist, on the out-flow of dopamine and glutamate in the prefrontal cortex. Society for Neuroscience Abstracts 20:(#524.12), 1994

Morgan WW, Bermudez J, Chang X: The relative potency of pentobarbi-tal in suppressing the kainic acid or the N-methyl-D-aspartic acid-induced enhancement of cGMP in cerebellar cells. Eur J Pharmacol 204:335–338, 1991

Moscovitch M: Confabulation and the frontal systems: strategic versus associative retrieval in neuropsychological theories of memory, in Varieties of Memory and Consciousness: Essays in Honour of Endel Tulving. Edited by Roediger HL III, Craik FIM. Hillsdale, NJ, Lawrence Erlbaum, 1989, pp 133–160

Moscovitch M: Memory and working-with-memory: a component process model based on modules and central system. Journal of Cognitive Neurosciences 4:257–267, 1992

Nagy LM, Morgan CA III, Southwick SM, et al: Open prospective trial of fluoxetine for posttraumatic stress disorder. J Clin Psychopharmacol 13:107–113, 1993

Nicholls DG: The glutamatergic nerve terminal. Eur J Biochem 212:613–631, 1993

Olsen RW: GABA-benzodiazepine-barbiturate receptor interactions. J Neurochem 37:1–13, 1981

Orona E, Gabriel M: Multiple-unit activity of the prefrontal cortex and mediodorsal thalamic nucleus during acquisition of discriminative avoidance behavior in rabbits. Brain Res 263:295–312, 1983

Oswald I, Evans J: On serious violence during sleep-walking. Br J Psychiatry 147:688–691, 1985

Paller KA: Recall and stem-completion priming have different electrophysiological correlates and are modified differentially by directed forgetting. J Exp Psychol Learn Mem Cogn 16:1021–1032, 1990

Pardo JV, Pardo PJ, Janer KW, et al: The anterior cingulate cortex mediates processing selection in the Stroop attentional conflict paradigm. Proc Natl Acad Sci U S A 87:256–259, 1990

Penfield W, Perot P: The brain's record of auditory and visual experience: a final summary and discussion. Brain 86:595–696, 1963

Pfefferbaum A, Darley CF, Tinklenberg JR, et al: Marijuana and memory intrusions. J Nerv Ment Dis 165:381–386, 1977

Pitman RK: Posttraumatic stress disorder, conditioning and network theory. Psychiatric Annals 18:182–189, 1988

Pitman RK, Altman B, Greenwald E, et al: Psychiatric complications during flooding therapy for posttraumatic stress disorder. J Clin Psychiatry 52:17–20, 1991

Pitman RK, Orr SP, Lasko NB: Effects of intranasal vasopressin and oxytocin on physiologic responding during personal combat imagery in Vietnam veterans with posttraumatic stress disorder. Psychiatry Res 48:107–117, 1993

Pitts FN, McClure JN: Lactate metabolism in anxiety neurosis. N Engl J Med 277:1329–1336, 1967

Post RM, Weiss SRB: Sensitization, kindling, and anticonvulsants in mania. J Clin Psychiatry 59 (suppl):23–30, 1989

Prevett MC, Duncan JS, Jones T, et al: Demonstration of thalamic activation during typical absence seizures using $H_2^{15}O$ and PET. Neurology 45:1396–1402, 1995

Rainey JM Jr, Aleem A, Ortiz A, et al: A laboratory procedure for the induction of flashbacks. Am J Psychiatry 144:1317–1319, 1987

Randall PK, Bremner JD, Krystal JH, et al: Effects of the benzodiazepine antagonist, flumazenil, in PTSD. Biol Psychiatry 38:319–324, 1995

Rasmussen K, Glennon RA, Aghajanian GK: Phenethylamine hallucinogens in the locus coeruleus: potency of action correlates with rank order of 5-HT_2 binding affinity. Eur J Pharmacol 32:79–82, 1986

Reist C, Kauffmann CD, Haier RJ, et al: A controlled trial of desipramine in 18 men with posttraumatic stress disorder. Am J Psychiatry 146:513–516, 1989

Rodin E, Luby E: Effects of LSD-25 on the EEG and photic evoked responses. Arch Gen Psychiatry 14:435–441, 1966

Rosen H., Meyers HJ: Abreaction in the military setting. AMA Archives of Neurology and Psychiatry 57:161–172, 1947

Sacks O: The Man Who Mistook His Wife for a Hat. New York, Summitt Books, 1985

Saletu B, Grünberger J, Linzmayer L: Acute and subacute CNS effects of milacemide in elderly people: double-blind placebo-controlled quantitative EEG and psychometric investigations. Archives of Gerontology and Geriatrics 5:165–181, 1986

Salloway S, Southwick S, Sadowsky M: Opiate withdrawal presenting as posttraumatic stress disorder: a case of malingering following the L'Ambiance Plaza Building disaster. Hospital and Community Psychiatry 41:666–667, 1990

Sargent W, Slater E: Acute war neuroses. Lancet 2:1–2, 1940

Savage C: Variations in ego feeling induced by D-lysergic acid diethylamide (LSD-25). Psychoanal Rev 42:1–16, 1955

Schwartz BL, Hashtroudi S, Herting RL, et al: Glycine prodrug facilitates memory retrieval in humans. Neurology 41:1341–1343, 1991

Schwartz ML, Dekker JJ, Goldman-Rakic PS: Dual mode of corticothalamic synaptic termination in the mediodorsal nucleus of the rhesus monkey. J Comp Neurol 309:289–304, 1991

Sheldon PW, Aghajanian GK: Excitatory responses to serotonin (5-HT) in neurons of the rat piriform cortex: evidence for mediation by 5-HT$_{1C}$ receptors in pyramidal cells and 5-HT$_2$ receptors in interneurons. Synapse 9:208–218, 1991

Southwick SM, Krystal JH, Morgan A, et al: Yohimbine and m-chlorophenylpiperazine in PTSD, in 1991 New Research Programs and Abstracts (NR 348). Washington, DC, American Psychiatric Association, 1991

Southwick SM, Krystal JH, Morgan CA, et al: Abnormal noradrenergic function in post-traumatic stress disorder. Arch Gen Psychiatry 50: 266–274, 1993

Spiegel D: Neurophysiological correlates of hypnosis and dissociation. J Neuropsychiatry Clin Neurosci 3:440–445, 1991

Stanton MD, Mintz J, Franklin RM: Drug flashbacks, II: some additional findings. International Journal of Addictions 11:53–69, 1976

Starke K, Borowski E, Endo T: Preferential blockade of presynaptic α-adrenoceptors by yohimbine. Eur J Pharmacol 34:385–388, 1975

Steriade M, Deschenes M: The thalamus as a neuronal oscillator. Brain Res Brain Res Rev 8:1–63, 1984

Steriade M, Llinás RR: The functional states of the thalamus and the associated neuronal interplay. Physiol Rev 68:649–741, 1988

Steriade M, McCarley RW: Brainstem Control of Wakefulness and Sleep. New York, Plenum, 1990

Steriade M, Datta S, Paré D, et al: Neuronal activities in brain-stem cholinergic nuclei related to tonic activation in thalamocortical systems. J Neurosci 19:2541–2559, 1990

Strassman RJ, Qualls CR, Uhlenhuth EH, et al: Dose-response study of N,N-dimethyltryptamine in humans, II: subjective effects and preliminary results of a new rating scale. Arch Gen Psychiatry 51:98–108, 1994

Stuss DT: Biological and psychological development of executive function. Brain Cogn 20:8–23, 1992

Swanson LW: A direct projection from Ammon's horn to prefrontal cortex in the rat. Brain Res 217:150–154, 1981

Taylor J (ed): Selected Writings of John Hughlings Jackson on Epilepsy and Epileptiform Convulsions. London, Hodder and Stroughton, 1931

Titeler M, Lyon RA, Glennon RA: Radioligand binding evidence implicates the brain 5-HT$_2$ receptor as a site of action for LSD and phenylisopropylamine hallucinogens. Psychopharmacology 94:213–216, 1988

Turner BH, Herkenham M: Thalamoamygdaloid projections in the rat: a test of the amygdala's role in sensory processing. J Comp Neurol 313:295–325, 1991

van der Kolk B, Blitz R, Burr W, et al: Nightmares and trauma: a comparison of nightmares after combat with lifelong nightmares in veterans. Am J Psychiatry 141:187–190, 1984

Vogt BA, Rosene DL, Pandya DN: Thalamic and cortical afferents differentiate anterior from posterior cingulate cortex in the monkey. Science 204:205–207, 1979

Whitty CWM, Lewin W: Vivid day-dreaming: an unusual form of confusion following anterior cingulectomy. Brain 80:72–76, 1957

Wilson FAW, Scalaidhe SPO, Goldman-Rakic PS: Dissociation of object and spatial processing domains in primate prefrontal cortex. Science 260:1955–1958, 1993

Woods SW, Charney DS, Silver JM, et al: Benzodiazepine receptor responsivity in panic disorder, II: behavioral, biochemical, and cardiovascular responses to the benzodiazepine receptor antagonist flumazenil. Psychiatry Res 36:115–127, 1991

Yamakura T, Mori H, Masaki H, et al: Different sensitivities of NMDA receptor channel subtypes to non-competitive antagonists. Neuroreport 4:687–690, 1993

Chapter 12

Trauma, Memory, and Dissociation: An Integrative Formulation

J. Douglas Bremner, M.D., Eric Vermetten, M.D.,
Steven M. Southwick, M.D., John H. Krystal, M.D., and
Dennis S. Charney, M.D.

S everal theoretical papers published in 1989 introduced a new phase in trauma research. Nemiah (1989), Putnam (1989), and van der Kolk and van der Hart (1989) (see also Nemiah, Chapter 1; Putnam and Carlson, Chapter 2; van der Hart et al., Chapter 9, in this volume) published reviews that highlighted the contribution Pierre Janet (1889, 1920) has made to the field of psychological trauma. Janet gave the first description of symptoms associated with extreme stress, including both what is known today as symptoms of posttraumatic stress disorder (PTSD) and symptoms of dissociation. He also pointed out that individuals who dissociated in response to a single trauma were at increased risk to dissociate with subsequent stressors. Whether this subsequent dissociation is due to a constitutional predisposition to dissociate or whether psychological trauma has an effect on the individual that results in long-term susceptibility to dissociation is an open question. Janet himself felt that there was in fact a contribution of both factors. The renewed focus on the theoretical contributions of Janet stimulated empirical research in this area, which is represented by the chapters in this volume.

Recently, alterations in memory (which are an important component of dissociation) have been the subject of considerable interest. In addition to the obvious role that alterations in memory play in amnesia, they also are involved in other dissociative symptoms. For example, amnestic episodes often involve symptoms of derealization and depersonalization, and traumatic memories are typically recalled in a state of derealization or depersonalization. Identity alterations can involve gaps in memory and are intimately related to alterations in autobiographical memory, which recently have received appropriately increased attention in the field of traumatic stress (see van der Hart et al., Chapter 9, in this volume). It is clear that understanding the relationship between stress-induced alterations in memory and dissociation will contribute to our understanding of the effects of traumatic stress on the individual. In this chapter, we review the relationship between dissociation and alterations in memory in traumatized individuals, using both theoretical and biological frameworks (Bremner et al. 1993c, 1995a; Charney et al. 1993) in an attempt to develop a more comprehensive understanding of the effects of stress on the individual.

Is There Specificity for the Dissociative Disorders, Posttraumatic Stress Disorder, and Other Trauma-Spectrum Psychiatric Disorders?

Some authors have questioned whether there is specificity to diagnoses such as PTSD. Implicit in this criticism is the idea that if PTSD cannot be shown to have specificity in relation to other disorders, such as depression, that are commonly held to have validity as constructs, then this indicates that PTSD does not have validity as a diagnosis. Taking the other side of this argument, clinicians who commonly treat patients with PTSD have concluded, based on their clinical experience, that PTSD does indeed have validity as a diagnosis. They therefore attempt to argue for the specificity of the disorder, which they feel is needed to support their viewpoint that PTSD has validity as a diagnosis. Both lines of reasoning, of course, are based on the assumption that PTSD should have specificity in relation to other diagnoses to be valid as a diagnosis.

   The current diagnostic nomenclature has contributed to this issue of specificity, in addition to in many ways inhibiting a broader understanding of the relationship between traumatic stress and psychiatric symptomatology. The editions of the *Diagnostic and*

Statistical Manual of Mental Disorders written since the original recognition of PTSD as a diagnostic entity in 1980 have separated PTSD from dissociative disorders and other disorders that are believed to be related to traumatic stress, such as depression or borderline personality disorder. Most people focus on a particular disorder, such as PTSD or the dissociative disorders, to the exclusion of the rest. Clinicians tend to ask about the symptoms with which they are most familiar. If patients have a wide range of trauma-related symptoms in a PTSD-dissociative-anxiety spectrum, they will therefore be diagnosed as having PTSD by a PTSD-focused clinician, a dissociative disorder by a dissociation-focused clinician, and so on. What is missing is an appreciation for the central role that traumatic stress plays in these psychiatric disorders.

PTSD is the only disorder that has the requirement for diagnosis of exposure to a traumatic stressor. Clinicians and investigators therefore were focused from the outset on the primacy of the traumatic experience in the symptoms of patients with PTSD. Investigators working in other trauma-related disorders, such as the dissociative disorders, discovered that psychological trauma also was an important part of the presenting symptoms of their patients (Putnam et al. 1986; Spiegel and Cardena 1991). As clinicians and researchers began communicating with each other more, and as studies were conducted addressing these issues of traumatic exposure, they realized that there was considerable overlap between their patient populations. Converging evidence now suggests that traumatic exposure results in a range of symptom outcomes that go beyond DSM-IV (American Psychiatric Association 1994) criteria for PTSD. For instance, there are a number of studies that have examined the relationship between the onset of depression and exposure to stressful life events (Mazure 1994). More than 80% of patients with the diagnosis of borderline personality disorder have been found to have a history of exposure to extreme childhood abuse (Herman et al. 1989); 90% of patients with the diagnosis of multiple personality disorder (what is termed today by DSM-IV as dissociative identity disorder) have been found to have a history of exposure to extreme childhood abuse (Putnam et al.

1986). Childhood abuse also has been associated with alcoholism, substance abuse, panic disorder, and eating disorders (Finkelhor 1986).

There is considerable overlap between the symptoms listed in the diagnostic criteria for psychiatric disorders associated with traumatic stress. For instance, many symptoms of depression are equivalent to symptoms of PTSD. Psychomotor agitation can be rephrased as hyperarousal, and hopelessness as a sense of fore-shortened future. Other symptoms that are identical in the criteria for depression and PTSD include decreased sleep, decreased concentration, and feeling cut off from others. In fact, the only symptom of depression that is not included in the criteria for PTSD is depressed mood, and most clinicians who work with PTSD patients feel that these patients are frequently anhedonic. The only symptoms of PTSD that are not a part of depression are increased startle, feeling on guard, flashbacks, and amnesia.

These symptoms also overlap with other psychiatric disorders. For instance, flashbacks and amnesia are part of PTSD but essentially represent dissociative phenomena (Spiegel 1984). Flashbacks in PTSD patients would potentially qualify diagnostically for panic attacks in 100% of cases (Mellman and Davis 1985), and dissociative symptoms such as derealization and depersonalization form part of the spectrum of symptoms that occur during panic attacks in patients with panic disorder. Disturbances of identity are captured by the borderline personality disorder symptom of feeling empty inside, are part of dissociative identity disorder, and are also commonly seen in PTSD patients (although not part of the diagnostic criteria for PTSD). Patients with borderline personality disorder are also commonly observed to have dissociative symptoms during self-mutilation or express the desire to use self-mutilation to break out of states of depersonalization or derealization. Figure 12–1 shows the range of overlap of symptomatology existing among psychiatric disorders that have been linked with trauma, including PTSD, depression, dissociative disorders, borderline personality disorder, alcoholism, substance abuse, and anxiety disorders. This overlap suggests that PTSD and dissociation are part of a continuum of trauma-spectrum psychiatric disor-

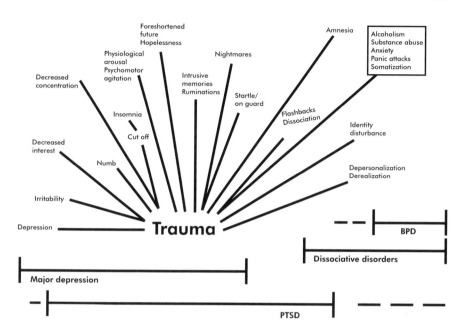

Figure 12–1. Range of symptomatology among psychiatric disorders linked with trauma. *Note.* BPD = borderline personality disorder. PTSD = posttraumatic stress disorder.

ders. According to this model, clinicians should not be focusing on whether PTSD has specificity as a diagnosis but should be thinking about the range of psychiatric symptoms that can be part of the outcome of exposure to traumatic stress.

Dissociative Responses to Trauma

Empirical findings are consistent with an overlap between PTSD and the dissociative disorder. In 1992, we studied Vietnam combat veterans with and without PTSD by using the Dissociative Experiences Scale (DES) of Bernstein and Putnam (1986). Vietnam combat veterans with the diagnosis of PTSD ($N = 53$) were compared with Vietnam combat veterans without PTSD ($N = 32$) who were recruited from a Veterans Administration outpatient medical clinic. PTSD patients in that study had a significantly higher score on the

DES (27.0 [18.0 SD]) than Vietnam veterans without PTSD (13.7 [SD = 16.0]). This difference persisted after statistically controlling for differences in level of traumatic exposure in the form of combat stress for combat veterans with and without PTSD. Dissociative symptoms as measured with the DES were correlated with PTSD symptoms measured with the Mississippi Scale for Combat-Related Posttraumatic Stress Disorder (Keane et al. 1988) ($r = 0.34$, $P < .05$). PTSD patients reported higher levels of dissociation at the time of combat-related traumatic events than did non-PTSD subjects. The magnitude of difference was substantial, suggesting an all-or-none type of phenomenon. On a 13-point scale for the measurement of dissociative states (a modification of the PDEQ by Marmar et al. [see Chapter 8 of this volume]) mean score for the PTSD patients was 11.5 (1.6 SD) compared with 1.8 (2.1 SD) for the non-PTSD subjects. In addition, dissociation at the time of combat trauma was strongly related to current PTSD symptomatology (as measured with the Mississippi Scale), after adjusting for level of combat exposure, participation in atrocities, and number of months in Vietnam, with multiple linear regressions (Bremner et al. 1992). We also have found an increase in baseline dissociative states as measured with the Clinician-Administered Dissociative States Scale (CADSS) in PTSD patients in comparison with patients with other psychiatric disorders and control subjects (Bremner et al., in press). The CADSS was found to have good interrater reliability, test-retest reliability, and convergent validity with the DES and SCID-D. [1]

In addition, consistent with Janet's formulation that dissociation due to extreme trauma increased the risk for dissociative responses to subsequent traumas, as well as for long-term psychopathology (Janet 1889, 1920), Vietnam combat veterans with PTSD who dissociated at the time of trauma had an increase in dissociative responses to subsequent postmilitary stressful events. We also found that PTSD patients had an increase in dissociative states

---

[1] The CADSS is available on the Internet at the following address: http://info.med.yale.edu/psych/org/ypi/trauma/cadss.txt

during traumatic recall (reading scripts of their traumatic events) as measured with the CADSS (Bremner et al., in press).

Other studies have reported an association between trauma and dissociative symptomatology. These studies have found an increase in hypnotizability (Spiegel et al. 1988) and dissociative symptomatology (Bremner et al. 1992, 1993e; Carlson and Rosser-Hogan 1991; Loewenstein and Putnam 1988; Marmar et al. 1994) in patients with PTSD. In addition, individuals exposed to childhood abuse (Chu and Dill 1990; Putnam et al. 1986) and the acute stressors of natural disasters (Cardena and Spiegel 1989; Koopman et al. 1994) have been observed to have an increase in dissociative symptomatology. Other studies have found a relationship between dissociation at the time of trauma and long-term psychopathology (Koopman et al. 1994; Marmar et al. 1994).

Patients with trauma-related dissociation experience a wide range of dissociative symptomatology. We examined dissociative symptoms with the Structured Clinical Interview for DSM-IV Dissociative Disorders (SCID-D; Steinberg 1993) in patients with Vietnam combat-related PTSD ($N = 40$) in comparison with Vietnam veterans without PTSD ($N = 15$). Vietnam veterans with PTSD had markedly increased levels of dissociative symptomatology in comparison with non-PTSD subjects. For instance, mean score on the amnesia subscale of the SCID-D, which measures gaps in memory that are not due to ordinary forgetting, in PTSD patients was 3.7 (0.8 SD) on a scale of 1–4, compared with 1.1 (0.3 SD) in the non-PTSD patients. Other symptoms also were increased in PTSD patients compared with non-PTSD subjects as measured on the subscales of the SCID-D (Bremner et al. 1993d), including derealization (3.2 [1.2 SD] versus 1.1 [0.3 SD]), a measure of changes in the perception of one's environment; depersonalization (3.4 [1.1 SD] versus 1.1 [0.4 SD]), a measure of distortions in one's perception of one's body; and identity confusion and identity alteration. In summary, these studies are consistent with a high degree of overlap between PTSD and the dissociative disorders and suggest that dissociative responses to trauma are often seen in patients who later develop psychopathology related to traumatic stress.

We have raised a number of questions about the current diagnostic separation of PTSD from other psychiatric disorders, including dissociative disorders, depression, and anxiety disorders. One therefore might ask, Should the diagnostic schema be changed and PTSD included as one of the dissociative disorders, or should all of these disorders be collapsed into a single "disorder of stress"? The answer is that currently there are not sufficient data to justify any particular reformulation of the psychiatric consequences of traumatic stress.

Is Dissociation a Sign of Pathology or Part of a Normal Continuum?

If PTSD and dissociative disorders are part of a spectrum of disorders related to psychological trauma, dissociation should be a pathological outcome of trauma. There is currently debate, however, about whether dissociation is part of a normal spectrum of personality traits or a marker of psychopathology. Dissociation could be an adaptive response to trauma, and increases in dissociation in traumatized populations could be a by-product of the defenses of those individuals. A second possibility is that individuals who are born with a capacity for dissociation are more likely to develop psychiatric disorders. In this situation, dissociation would represent a risk factor for the development of psychiatric disorders in response to traumatic stress. A third possibility is that dissociation during trauma and dissociative responses to subsequent stressors are markers of psychopathology related to traumatic stress. A fourth possibility is that dissociation is a normal personality trait that varies in the general population, is nonspecifically associated with psychiatric disorders, but is not related to the development of psychopathology.

One strategy in approaching these four possibilities is to examine the relationship between dissociation and constructs that are a part of normal personality. Constructs that appear to be phenomenologically similar to dissociation include hypnotizability, absorption, fantasy proneness, and openness to experience (Kihlstrom 1992; Kihlstrom et al. 1994). Because these constructs occur normally in the general population, a relationship between them and dissociation would suggest that dissociation may be a healthy personality trait rather than a marker of psychopathology. Absorption occurs in healthy individuals and involves the ability to become completely involved in something to the point where everything else is excluded. The Tellegen Absorption Scale (TAS; Tellegen and Atkinson 1974), which is used to measure absorption, includes items such as "sometimes when I am reading poetry I feel a chill of excitement" and "I enjoy concentrating on a fantasy or daydream and exploring all its possibilities, letting it grow and develop." Absorption, as measured by the TAS, is strongly related to other constructs that are healthy personality traits, such as openness to experience ($r = .62-.85$ [Glisky et al. 1991; Radtke and Stam 1991]) and daydreaming ($r = .57$ [Hoyt et al. 1989]). Absorption has been shown to be modestly correlated with hypnotizability (Tellegen and Atkinson 1974), which is normally distributed in the population ($r = .3$ [Frischholz et al. 1987]; $r = .15$ [Glisky and Kihlstrom 1993]; $r = .22$ [Glisky et al. 1991; Radtke and Stam 1991]; $r = .24$ [Hoyt et al. 1989]). Absorption also has been shown to be modestly correlated with dissociation as measured by the DES (Nadon et al. 1991). However, the relationship between the TAS and the DES weakens significantly when absorption-like items are removed from the DES (Kihlstrom et al. 1994). This finding raises the question of whether absorption is really related to the "core" symptoms of dissociation. Dissociation and hypnotizability, as reviewed by Putnam and Carlson (Chapter 2, in this volume), are only weakly correlated ($r = .1-.2$) in healthy populations, although Spiegel et al. (1988) have found increases in hypnotizability in traumatized psychiatric populations, who also have been found to have increases in dissociative symptomatology. Hypnotizability also has been shown to be weakly correlated with openness to experience and fantasy proneness (daydreaming) ($r = .1-.2$ [Glisky and Kihlstrom 1993]). In summary, these findings do not provide convincing evidence that dissociation is related to nonpathological personality traits, although they do not necessarily provide evidence for the opposite view that dissociation is a construct of pathology.

The determination of pathology is based on the presence of symptoms that result in disability and distress. To judge whether dissociative symptoms are disabling, it is important to have an appreciation for how the symptoms manifest themselves in patients. In the following discussion, we describe some clinical cases of Vietnam veterans with PTSD and high levels of dissociative symptomatology.

Clinical Presentations of Dissociation in Patients With Posttraumatic Stress Disorder

Case Example 1

D is a 44-year-old white male who came from a working-class neighborhood in Connecticut. His childhood was without incident, and he described himself as an "average American kid." He was drafted out of high school and served in the army in Vietnam from 1967 to 1968.

D drove a "track," a mobile artillery unit that fired rounds at the enemy, during his frequent combat missions into enemy territory. He became good friends during his tour with a man named Bobby, and they would help each other out during times of need. One day D's unit was on a patrol, and Bobby was driving his track just in front of D, when the unit was suddenly ambushed by the Vietcong. An artillery round hit Bobby's track, and Bobby started screaming for help. D jumped out of his track and ran to help Bobby. As D pulled him out of the track, Bobby emitted a chilling moan, and he realized that the lower part of Bobby's body was missing. Suddenly, it seemed to D as if everything around him was slowing down. Sounds were disappearing, even though the battle continued, and D's perception of the world around him changed. Everything seemed foggy, as if it were far away, and it seemed as if he were looking through a tunnel, with the periphery of his vision gone. The world seemed strange or foreign, and D could not recognize his friends or his surroundings (symptoms of derealization). He felt like he had no idea who he was (depersonalization). After the battle, D sat immobile and was unresponsive to others. Some of his friends protected him by hiding him in a Vietnamese hooch (straw house) for 2 days. He sat on the floor, not knowing who he was or being able to recognize his surroundings, only looking at the glint coming off a knife that he held in his lap.

After his discharge from the army, D returned to his hometown where he married, started working at the local factory, and later had a son. D continued to have discrete episodes, usually during times of stress, of suddenly being unable to recognize familiar surroundings or people close to him, such as his wife and son. D said that during these episodes, he would look at his wife and be able to recognize her facial features but be completely without the sensation of familiarity. During one episode, D was on a family vacation in Florida, and he, his wife, and son were walking through crowded Disney World. He suddenly had the sensation that all of the people around him were strange or foreign. Looking at his family, he felt as if he did not know who they were. Colors in the environment seemed blurred, and his surroundings seemed foreign or strange. He said that his wife had to lead him by the hand out of Disney World, and they could not spend any more time there during their vacation.

Case Example 2

B is a 44-year-old white male who served in the army from 1963 to 1966. He was a jokester who was everybody's friend in high school. After graduation from high school, a group of his friends went down to the army recruiter to get information about enlisting, and so he went along. He enlisted to have the opportunity of being with his friends.

Soon after his enlistment, the United States became involved in the Vietnam War. B was sent over as a combat infantryman. One time, B was killing wounded enemies with a bayonet instead of a gun to prevent the gunfire from revealing their position to enemy reinforcements. B described the experience in this way:

> As I was bayoneting the wounded, I had the sensation of separating from myself and looking down from a distance at the "killer" who was bayoneting the enemy soldiers. I first had this feeling when I noticed some pleasure within myself at killing the enemy, which filled me with horror and disgust and which seemed unconnected with my conception of myself and of what I felt I was capable of doing. From that time

on, in combat situations I would separate from myself and watch while the killer would carry out combat missions. The killer was better able to do the job, as he was without concern for others or fear, unlike myself.

After his discharge from the army in 1966, B reported continued episodes of separating from his body in times of stress, usually when he became angry or felt physically threatened. These episodes occurred during situations such as barroom brawls, which recreated the experience of being in combat. B came for treatment with the chief complaint of "blackouts," which were increasing in frequency and which he felt he had no control over (amnesia). A seizure disorder had been ruled out with electroencephalogram and computed tomography of the head. After a careful history, it was discovered that these blackouts were actually episodes in which he would separate from his body and watch while the killer would do something harmful or destructive that would get him into trouble. During the most recent episode, B had become angry at someone during the course of an argument and ran home to get a knife. While running back to the site of the dispute, B separated from his body (depersonalization) and watched with consternation the activity of the killer (identity alteration). B ran up to the other person and put the knife to his throat, while B tried to urge the killer not to do anything that would get him into trouble. B eventually was able to get control of himself (or the other side of himself) and the other person was not hurt.

Case Example 3

P was born and raised in a small town in Connecticut. At the age of 18, he joined the Marines and was sent to Vietnam for active combat duty. He was a member of the 101st cavalry, General Custer's division.

In 1969, while on patrol in Vietnam, P's unit was ambushed and his best friends, Johny, Willy, and Mack, were killed. Willy walked into a claymore mine and it blew his legs off and blew his body into P, knocking him down. Then the Vietcong opened fire. They shot Mack in the face. P saw it happen as if in slow motion (derealization). He saw his arm moving and the glitter of his watch. Then he saw Johny with a bullet in his head. He had a strange look, with his eye blown out of the socket. P related the event in the following way:

Johny was screaming. I held him in my arms, rocking him. He told me to tell his mother he was sorry and that it hurt real bad. Then he told me to shoot him, and I did.

I felt like the experience was drawn out over a long period of time. I had moments of losing track of what was happening, and things happened during the event that I later couldn't account for. At first, things became extremely bright, like under the floodlights at night in a baseball field, and then suddenly, colors became very dull as if I were looking at the world through a fog. It seemed like I was looking at things through a tunnel or as if there were a pair of binoculars turned backwards. I could hear the moaning of my dying friends, but it sounded long and drawn out. Things seemed unreal, as if I were in a dream or as if I were watching the situation as a spectator. I felt disconnected from my own body, like I could look back at myself and see my own reaction. My own body felt much larger than normal, like a giant, and I thought that I would get hit by a bullet. I felt like I was "in shock."

P started having episodes where he saw his dead buddies soon after returning from the war. The first time he saw them it was dusk, and he was sitting on his porch. There was a field behind the house. They were out there, on patrol, walking in full combat gear. He started calling them. His sister said, "Who are you calling?" He said, "Call, you can get them back." He remembered her calling for them there on the porch, even though she could not see them.

P would sit at the bar in his basement and drink with his dead buddies. He walked into the house one day, and they were sitting there at the bar. They drank beer together. They told him to go back to Vietnam with them and that they would be together again. They would fight together again, but this time they would win the war. They had the smell of the Mekong delta, a damp smell.

P was at his sister's house walking through a field in the backyard. It looked like a landing zone. He had the sensation of walking through a bubble. He heard a fleet of helicopters. His daughter came and hugged him and asked what was wrong—did he hear helicopters? He said, "Yeah, can't you hear them?" She said, "Let them land; don't go with them." He went out and got in his car. Then he saw his dead buddies. Johny was sitting next to him. He was young and had freckles, he was only 18. He started driving.

Willy and Mack were in the back seat. They did not say anything; they were like zombies. They were wearing combat fatigues, and their faces were real white. You could see their freckles like they were glowing. P said to himself, "It's not real, it's in my mind." They were not talking, but he felt he could read their minds. He felt scared. They had been with him a long time, and he was getting scared of them. Then Johny grabbed the wheel and yanked it. The car drove off the road onto someone's lawn. He felt light-headed and was having a hard time breathing. He drove home, parked the car, and ran up to see his girlfriend. He said, "Get them out of my car." She went down and looked and said that there was no one there.

These case examples illustrate the wide range of dissociative symptoms that can be associated with exposure to psychological trauma. They also show how dissociative symptoms occur at the time of the original trauma and then recur, often in a similar form, during exposure to subsequent stressors. These stressors, as seen in the case examples, often involve something as trivial as a trip to Disney World and have an important impact on patient functioning. Dissociation is a part of the daily lives of these patients, which makes it difficult for them to interact socially with family and friends and to cope with challenges in their environment.

There are important interrelationships between individual symptoms of dissociation. For example, amnesia can be associated with depersonalization or identity alteration, and depersonalization and derealization can occur simultaneously. Consistent with these interrelationships, we have found a high degree of correlation between individual symptoms of dissociation as measured with the CADSS (Bremner et al., in press). These data suggest that the individual symptoms of dissociation do not have validity as separate constructs. As shown in the previous case examples, patients typically experience dissociative symptoms in combination with one another.

Dissociation and Memory

Dissociation can be conceptualized as being related to alterations in memory function. Psychogenic amnesia is characterized by gaps in memory lasting from minutes to days. Pathological recall of traumatic memories typically occurs in a dissociated state, with symptoms of derealization and depersonalization. Dissociative identity disorder essentially involves the transition between different collections of autobiographical memories that have coherence as separate entities. Patients with disorders such as PTSD have a variety of other manifestations of alterations in memory, including deficits in explicit and implicit memory function. In addition, hypnosis, which is phenomenologically similar to dissociation, involves many features that resemble alterations in memory function. Individuals undergoing hypnosis are subject to posthypnotic amnesia, in which the hypnotist can suggest to them that they will have no memory for what occurred while they were under hypnosis. Hypnosis has been described, in fact, as "an interaction in which one person experiences subjectively compelling responses to suggestions offered by another person, the hypnotist, of imaginative alterations in *perception and memory*" (Kihlstrom 1992, p. 307, italics added).

Mechanisms of Normal Memory Function

To fully understand how stress-related alteration in memory function relates to dissociation and PTSD, it is useful to review mechanisms of healthy memory function. Memory formation involves encoding, storage (or consolidation), and retrieval. Encoding is the initial laying down of the memory trace. Storage involves the keeping of the memory trace over time. A related concept is consolidation, which refers to the process, occurring over several weeks or more, of establishing the permanence of a memory trace, during which time the memory trace is theoretically susceptible to modification. Retrieval is the process of bringing out a memory from storage into consciousness.

Memory function can be divided into explicit (declarative) and implicit (nondeclarative or "procedural") (Squire and Zola-Morgan 1991). Explicit memory includes free recall of facts and lists, as well as working memory, which is the ability to store information in a visual or verbal buffer while performing a particular operation using that information. In contrast, implicit memory is demonstrated only through tasks or skills in which the knowledge is embedded. Forms of implicit memory include priming, conditioning, and tasks or skills. Priming involves providing the first few letters of a word and asking the subject to say the first word that comes to mind. Conditioning refers to the development of consistent physiological and emotional responses to a previously neutral stimulus. The most common animal model of conditioning (reviewed in the following discussion) involves pairing a tone or a light (the conditioned stimulus) with an electric shock (the unconditioned stimulus). With repeated trials, the conditioned stimulus alone will be evoke responses, such as an increase in startle amplitude, that were previously only elicited by the unconditioned stimulus. This paradigm implies that a form of learning has occurred that is embedded in the conditioned response and is not available for conscious recall.

Neuroanatomical Basis of Memory

Several brain structures are involved in a mutually interrelated network in the mediation of memory function. The hippocampus and adjacent cortex (entorhinal, perirhinal, parahippocampal cortex) and dorsomedial nucleus of the thalamus mediate explicit memory function (Mishkin 1978; Murray and Mishkin 1986; Squire and Zola-Morgan 1991; Zola-Morgan et al. 1989). The dorsolateral prefrontal cortex (also known as the principle sulcus or middle frontal gyrus) is involved in explicit recall as measured by working memory tasks (Goldman 1971; Goldman-Rakic 1988). Parietal cortex plays an important role in spatial memory and attention (Posner et al. 1988; Save et al. 1992). Memories are stored in the primary neocortical sensory and motor areas and later evoked in those same cortical areas (Damasio 1990; Zola-Morgan and Squire 1990). Visual information is stored in the occipital cortex, tactile information in the sensory cortex, auditory information in the middle temporal gyrus, and olfactory information in the orbitofrontal cortex. It has been hypothesized (Zola-Morgan and Squire 1990) that the role of the hippocampus is to bring together memory elements from diverse neocortical areas at the time of retrieval of explicit memory.

Implicit memory function is mediated by the amygdala, neocortex, and hippocampus. Conditioned fear responses are a type of implicit memory mediated by the amygdala, and these responses are measured with the acoustic startle response. The acoustic startle response is a primitive reflex that is part of an animal's response to threat. The startle response can be potentiated by the addition of something aversive, such as electric shock. The neuroanatomy and neurophysiology of emotional memory (measured by the conditioned fear response in animals) have been well characterized (Davis 1992). Lesions of the central nucleus of the amygdala have been shown to completely block fear-potentiated startle (Hitchcock and Davis 1986; Hitchcock et al. 1989), whereas electrical stimulation of the central nucleus increases acoustic startle (Rosen and Davis 1988). The amygdala integrates information that is necessary for the proper execution of the stress response, including (internal) emotion and information from the external environment (Turner and Herkenham 1991; Turner et al. 1980). The central nucleus of the amygdala projects to a variety of brain structures that are involved in effecting the stress response (Rosen et al. 1991). The hippocampus is involved in emotional memory for the context of a fear-inducing situation. Reintroduction to the context of the shock or the environment where the shock took place (i.e., the testing box), even in the absence of the shock, will result in conditioned fear responses. Lesions of the hippocampus interfere with acquisition of conditioned emotional responses to the environment where the shock was received (reviewed in Bremner et al. 1995a).

Effects of Stress on Memory Function

Evidence from a variety of studies shows a relationship between exposure to traumatic stress and deficits in explicit memory function. Concentration camp survivors from World War II have been found to have high rates of impairment in explicit memory function (Helweg-Larsen et al. 1952; Thygesen et al. 1970). Korean prisoners of war have been found to have an impairment on explicit

memory tasks of free verbal recall measured with the Logical component of the Wechsler Memory Scale—Revised (WMS-R; Russell
1975) in comparison with Korean veterans without a history of containment (Sutker et al. 1990, 1991). We have measured explicit
memory function with the WMS-R Logical (verbal memory) and
Figural (visual memory) components in Vietnam combat veterans
with PTSD ($N = 26$) and control subjects matched for factors that
could affect memory function ($N = 15$). PTSD patients had a significant decrease in free verbal recall (explicit memory) (Bremner et
al. 1993b) as measured by the WMS-R Logical component, without
deficits in IQ as measured by the Wechsler Adult Intelligence
Scale—Revised (WAIS-R; Wechsler 1981). PTSD patients also had
deficits in explicit recall as measured with the Selective Reminding
Test (SRT; Hannay and Levin 1985for both verbal and visual components. We have subsequently found deficits in explicit memory
tasks of free verbal recall measured by the WMS-R Logical component in adult survivors of childhood abuse seeking treatment for
psychiatric disorders (Bremner et al 1995b). Studies have found
deficits in explicit short-term memory as assessed with other measures in Vietnam combat veterans with PTSD in comparison with
National Guard veterans without PTSD (Uddo et al. 1993) and in
Vietnam combat veterans with PTSD in comparison with control
subjects (Yehuda et al. 1995). Studies are currently in progress in female Vietnam combat nurses with PTSD (J. Wolfe, personal communication, October 1994). Deficits in academic performance also
have been shown in Beirut adolescents with PTSD in comparison
with Beirut adolescents without PTSD (P. Saigh, personal communication, August 1994). These studies suggest deficits in encoding
on explicit memory tasks. Other studies in patients with PTSD have
shown enhanced recall on explicit memory tasks for trauma-related
words relative to neutral words in comparison with control subjects (Zeitlin and McNally 1991). In summary, the findings are consistent with deficits in encoding on explicit memory tasks and
deficits in retrieval, as well as enhanced encoding or retrieval for
specific trauma-related material.

Studies are needed to examine the effects of unconscious cognitive material (Kihlstrom 1987), also referred to as implicit memory

function (Kihlstrom 1987; Schacter 1995), on mental life in patients with PTSD. Alterations in implicit memory in PTSD patients include conditioned fear responding and alterations in priming effects in comparison with control subjects. PTSD patients have been shown in preliminary studies to have an enhancement of implicit recall (i.e., recall following priming) for trauma-related words relative to neutral words in comparison with control subjects (Zeitlin and McNally 1991). The Stroop Test (cited in Foa et al. 1991) is a measure of nonexplicit (i.e., not available for conscious recall) cognitive processes that has been used in the study of PTSD. This test involves presenting words in different colors and asking subjects to name the color. Delays in color naming can be interpreted as a measure of interference from unconscious cognitive processes. Vietnam combat veterans with PTSD have been found to take longer to color-name "PTSD" words, such as "body bag," than obsessive words, positive words, and neutral words (McNally et al. 1990, 1993), and this delay was correlated with severity of PTSD symptomatology as measured by the Mississippi Scale for Combat-Related Posttraumatic Stress Disorder (Keane et al. 1988). Stroop interference also has been shown in patients with PTSD related to the trauma of rape (Cassiday et al. 1992; Foa et al. 1991). The cognitive processes that are part of the performance of the Stroop Test are associated with activation of the cingulate cortex. These studies therefore make Stroop interference one of the more replicated findings in PTSD.

Patients with PTSD commonly report an increase in startle responsiveness (used in the measurement of conditioned fear responding). Increased startle magnitude has been found in Vietnam combat veterans with PTSD in comparison with control subjects for 90–100 dB noise (Butler et al. 1990; see also Paige et al. 1990). Other studies have shown no difference in trials to habituation of startle response (Ross et al. 1989). An increase in heart rate and skin conductance during the startle paradigm has been reported in patients with civilian PTSD in comparison with control subjects (Shalev et al. 1992). Conditioned fear responding also is measured clinically in PTSD patients with the psychophysiology paradigm. As reviewed in Prins et al. (1995), PTSD patients have shown an increase in heart rate and blood pressure responsiveness to traumatic cues in the form of both trauma-related slides and scripts. Clinically, PTSD patients commonly become physiologically aroused when they encounter trauma-related cues in their environment, such as hearing a car backfire or smelling cut grass. These findings are consistent with increased conditioned responding in patients with PTSD.

Effects of Stress on Brain Regions
Involved in Memory

Stress has long-term effects on brain regions involved in memory. Stress-induced alterations in these brain regions may underlie many symptoms of PTSD, such as pathological recall of traumatic memories and deficits in free recall (Bremner et al. 1995a). In addition, brain regions involved in memory include many regions described as part of the "limbic brain," which includes the hypothalamus, thalamus, hippocampus, amygdala, orbitofrontal cortex, and cingulate. Limbic brain regions have long been believed to be involved in emotionality, fear responses, and effecting the stress response. These brain regions are in turn affected by exposure to traumatic stress.

Studies of monkeys who died spontaneously following exposure to severe stress because of improper caging and overcrowding were found on autopsy to have damage to the CA2 and CA3 subfields of the hippocampus (Uno et al. 1989). Follow-up studies showed that hippocampal damage was associated with direct exposure of glucocorticoids to the hippocampus (Sapolsky et al. 1990). Studies in a variety of animal species have shown that direct glucocorticoid exposure results in a loss of pyramidal neurons and dendritic branching (McEwen et al. 1992; Packan and Sapolsky 1990; Sapolsky et al. 1985; Uno et al. 1989; Watanabe et al. 1992; Wooley et al. 1990) that is associated with deficits in memory (Luine et al. 1994).

We compared hippocampal volume measured with magnetic resonance imaging (MRI) in Vietnam combat veterans with PTSD

($N = 26$) and healthy subjects ($N = 22$) matched for factors that could affect hippocampal volume, including age, sex, race, years of education, height, weight, handedness, and years of alcohol abuse. Patients with combat-related PTSD had an 8% decrease in right hippocampal volume in comparison with control subjects ($P < .05$) but no significant decrease in volume of comparison structures, including temporal lobe and caudate. Deficits in free verbal recall (explicit memory) as measured by the WMS-R (Wechsler 1987) Logical component, percent retention, were associated with decreased right hippocampal volume in the PTSD patients ($r = 0.64$; $P < .05$) but not in the control subjects. There was not a significant difference between PTSD patients and control subjects in left hippocampal volume or in volume of the comparison regions measured in this study, the left or right caudate and temporal lobe volume (minus hippocampus) (Bremner et al. 1995b). Recently, we found a statistically significant 12% reduction in left hippocampal volume in 17 adult survivors of childhood physical and sexual abuse in comparison with 17 control subjects who were matched on a case-by-case basis for age, sex, race, handedness, years of education and years of alcohol abuse (Bremner et al. 1997b).

The amygdala plays an important role in conditioned fear responses and exaggerated startle, which are prominent features of the clinical presentation of PTSD. We present here previously unpublished data from measurements of the amygdala in patients with combat-related PTSD ($N = 19$) and matched control subjects ($N = 15$). PTSD patients were Vietnam combat veterans in inpatient and outpatient treatment programs for PTSD. Healthy control subjects were free of psychiatric or medical disorders and were selected to be similar to the patients in several demographic factors. All of the subjects were part of a previously reported study of hippocampal volume in combat-related PTSD patients and control subjects (Bremner et al. 1995b). There was no difference between patients and control subjects for age (47.8 [3.6 SD] versus 46.3 [8.5 SD]), sex (all male), race (95% white and 5% black versus 80% white, 13% black, 7% Hispanic), years of education (12.9 [1.9 SD] versus 13.9 [3.2 SD]), handedness (79% right-handed versus 87% right-handed), years of alcohol abuse (9.9 [8.5 SD] versus 6.9 [10.3

SD]), height, and weight. Coronal MRI scans were obtained on a 1.5 Tesla scanner with TR = 25, TE = 5, and slice thickness 3 mm. Volume of the amygdala was determined by measuring the cross-sectional area of the amygdala in all coronal slices, including and anterior to the bifurcation of the basilar artery; summing the cross-sectional areas; and multiplying by the slice thickness. Inter-rater reliability for the amygdala was determined using the intra-class correlation coefficient with one-way analysis of variance (ANOVA) (with values of the coefficient approaching one, repre-senting a high level of agreement between two raters) for volumet-ric assessments of amygdala with two raters (JDB and EV). Intraclass correlation coefficients (ICC) for interrater reliability (R) were as follows: left amygdala ICC = 0.56 (F = 3.56; df = 33,34; P < .01) and right amygdala ICC = 0.56 (F = 3.55; df = 33,34; P< .01). These results demonstrate excellent interrater reliability for the amygdala. We did not find a difference between patients and con-trol subjects for the left amygdala (2,047 [470 SD] versus 2,018 [332 SD] mm^3) or right amygdala volume (1,992 [392 SD] versus 1,950 [425 SD] mm^3). Our findings are not consistent with a difference in amygdala volume in PTSD patients compared with control sub-jects. Of course, alterations in amygdala function in PTSD will not necessarily be reflected in a change in volume of the amygdala.

We also have used positron-emission tomography (PET) and [^{18}F]2-fluoro-2-deoxyglucose (FDG) in the measurement of cere-bral glucose metabolic rate following administration of yohimbine and placebo in Vietnam combat veterans with PTSD (N = 10) and healthy control subjects (N = 10). We previously have found evi-dence for alterations in noradrenergic function—as demonstrated with increased PTSD symptoms, intrusive memories, flashbacks, and anxiety—following administration of the α_2 antagonist, yo-himbine, which stimulates brain norepinephrine release, in PTSD patients in comparison with control subjects (Southwick et al. 1993). Animal studies have shown a decrease in metabolism in cerebral cortex following high levels of norepinephrine release. We found that administration of yohimbine resulted in a differen-tial effect on brain metabolism in PTSD patients in comparison with control subjects in orbitofrontal, temporal, parietal, and prefrontal cortex, with PTSD patients showing a tendency to decrease brain metabolism, whereas control subjects showed a tendency to increase brain metabolism with yohimbine in comparison with placebo. PTSD patients also had a decrease in hippocampal metabolism, which was not seen in the control subjects (Bremner et al. 1997c). These findings are consistent with an increased release of norepinephrine in the brain following yohimbine in PTSD. Considering the role of norepinephrine in the hippocampus as a neuromodulator that affects memory encoding and retrieval, enhanced norepinephrine release in the hippocampus with stressors may be associated with the pathological recall that is typical of traumatic memories in patients with PTSD.

The studies previously summarized are consistent with alterations in brain regions involved in memory with associated deficits in memory function. It is also important to consider the effects on memory function of neurotransmitters and neuropeptides released during stress.

Modulation of Memory by Neurotransmitters and Neuropeptides Released During Stress

Brain chemicals released during stress, which are highly concentrated in brain regions involved in memory such as the hippocampus, amygdala, and prefrontal cortex, play a role in the modulation of memory function. These chemicals include norepinephrine, epinephrine, adrenocorticotropic hormone (ACTH), glucocorticoids, dopamine, acetylcholine, endogenous opiates, vasopressin, oxytocin, and gamma-aminobutyric acid (GABA) (for a review, see De Wied and Croiset 1991; McGaugh 1989, 1990). For instance, removal of the adrenal medulla, site of most of the body's epinephrine, results in an impairment in new learning, which is restored by administration of adequate amounts of epinephrine (Borrell et al. 1983). Posttraining administration of epinephrine after a learning task influences retention with an inverted U-shaped curve: retention is enhanced at moderate doses and impaired at high doses (Gold and van Buskirk 1975; Liang et al. 1986; McGaugh 1990). In one recent study (Cahill et al. 1994), the α-adrenergic antagonist, propranolol, or placebo was administered to healthy human subjects 1 hour before a neutral or an emotionally arousing (stress-related) story. Propranolol, but not placebo, interfered with recall of the emotionally arousing story but not the neutral story, suggesting that activation of α-adrenergic receptors in the brain enhances the encoding of emotionally arousing memories (Cahill et al. 1994). We have found an increase in corticotropin-releasing factor (CRF), a neuropeptide that modulates memory function and plays an important role in the stress response in patients with PTSD (Bremner et al. 1997a). Vasopressin has been shown to facilitate traumatic recall in patients with PTSD (Pitman et al. 1993). It is hoped that extending preclinical findings about the effects of stress-related neuromodulators on memory function to clinical populations will enhance our understanding of memory alterations in PTSD.

Neural Mechanisms Mediating the Effects of Stress on Memory

The neural mechanisms of stress sensitization, fear conditioning, and extinction are useful in understanding the effects of stress on brain systems involved in memory. Stress sensitization refers to the phenomenon wherein repeated exposure to a stressor results in an amplification of responsiveness to subsequent stressors. For example, acute stress results in an increased release of norepinephrine in the hippocampus as well as other brain regions. In comparison with animals that have no history of exposure to stress, animals with a history of exposure to prior stressors become sensitized to exposure to subsequent stressors so that there is an accentuation of norepinephrine release in the hippocampus with a subsequent stressor. Norepinephrine (in addition to other neurotransmitters and neuropeptides) modulates memory formation and retrieval. This fact raises the possibility that stress sensitization, acting through neuromodulators, such as norepinephrine, may be associated with alterations in memory encoding and retrieval, which may have implications for understanding the mechanisms of traumatic recall in PTSD. Stress sensitization is clinically applicable to PTSD. Patients with PTSD have a difficult time with ordinary stressful events that healthy persons can tolerate without too much trouble. For instance, the stress of having a fender bender or having an argument with one's spouse can lead to a total decompensation in these patients. We have found that exposure to the stressor of childhood physical abuse increases the risk for the development of combat-related PTSD. Bremner et al. (1993a) suggest that sensitization resulting from early childhood stress may increase the vulnerability for the development of psychopathology in response to a subsequent stressor (i.e., combat stress in Vietnam).

We have reviewed the mechanism of fear conditioning, in which a pairing of a normally neutral stimulus with an aversive stimulus, such as electric shock, eventually results in fear responding to the light alone. Conditioned responding to cues in the environment that are reminiscent of the original trauma is a major source of disability for PTSD patients. Patients with PTSD have a heightened physiological responsiveness (increased heart rate and blood pressure) to reminders of the original trauma (e.g., combat films and sounds, scripts of traumatic events) relative to control subjects as measured with the psychophysiology paradigm. This increase in responsiveness resembles conditioned fear responding in animals.

Extinction refers to an inhibition of conditioned responses to cues associated with a fearful stimulus that takes place gradually over time following the removal of the original fearful stimulus. Extinction involves neocortical (Jarrell et al. 1987; LeDoux 1993) and orbitofrontal (Morgan and LeDoux 1994) inhibition of amygdala function. A failure of extinction is a prominent aspect of PTSD, which may explain why these patients continue to have conditioned responses to trauma-related cues for many years after exposure to the original trauma.

We have reviewed healthy memory function and how stress affects brain regions involved in memory and healthy memory function. In the following discussion, we review possible brain mechanisms for dissociation from the standpoint of the neurobiology of memory.

Brain Mechanisms in Dissociation

The neural basis for dissociative states may be found in the neurobiology of memory. The intimate relationship between dissociation and alterations in memory logically suggests that the biological basis for dissociative states may be found in brain structures that mediate memory function. Consistent with this idea, electrical stimulation of the hippocampus and adjacent cortex results in symptoms that are similar to dissociation (Halgren et al. 1978). As reviewed by Krystal et al. (Chapter 11, in this volume), administration of ketamine hydrochloride, a noncompetitive antagonist of the N-methyl-D-aspartate (NMDA) receptor, results in an increase in dissociative symptomatology, as measured with the CADSS (Bremner et al., in press), and in a disruption of delayed word recall in healthy subjects. The NMDA receptor, which is highly concentrated in the hippocampus, is involved in memory function at the molecular level through long-term potentiation (LTP). Subjects who took ketamine in the Krystal et al. (1994) study had a wide range of dissociative symptoms, including out-of-body experiences, feeling as if their arms were toothpicks, having gaps in time, feeling that time stood still, disturbances in the sense of self-identity, and derealization. Considering the role that the hippocampus plays in memory, dysfunction of the hippocampus may result in a breakdown of healthy integration of memory and consciousness. This breakdown may entail abnormalities of memory encoding, consolidation, or storage or some combination of the three. Dissociative states at the time of psychological trauma may represent a marker of pathological processes affecting brain structures involved in memory, such as the hippocampus. Traumatic events that are encoded when an individual is in a deficient state would be expected to be retrieved when the individual is in a similar deficient state. This theory may explain the phenomenon of how traumatic recall often occurs when the individual is in a dissociative state that is similar to the dissociative state that was experienced at the time of the original trauma.

Validity of Childhood Memories of Abuse: Relevance of Stress-Induced Changes in Brain Regions Involved in Memory

Recently, there has been considerable controversy concerning the validity of memories related to childhood abuse. The controversy is in part related to the vast increase in reported incidents of childhood abuse. Some authors have claimed that psychotherapists are suggesting to their patients abuse incidents that never occurred, using the term *false memory syndrome* to describe the alleged development of memories for abuse in suggestible individuals (Loftus et al. 1994a). As many as 38% of individuals who had been abused to an extent severe enough to require a visit to the emergency room (with full documentation that the abuse had indeed taken place) have been found to have no recall of the abuse up to 20 years later (Loftus et al. 1994b; Williams 1994a). A central issue in this debate is whether the lack of recall is because of "normal forgetting" (Loftus et al. 1994b) or memory-related mechanisms specific to psychological trauma, such as "repression" or, its synonymous appellation, dissociative amnesia (Williams 1994b). A mechanism such as amnesia could explain why individuals have a delayed recall of abuse for up to 20 years after the event.

Some authors have pointed to studies from cognitive psychology to support the claim that memory is subject to distortions over time and that this mechanism is operative in individuals who claim delayed recall of abuse. For example, in one of these studies, subjects viewed a series of slides that included a slide with a stop sign. After the slide presentation, the subjects received misleading verbal information that included reference to a yield sign. When given a test of recall of material from the slides, which involved a forced choice between a stop sign and a yield sign, subjects who received misleading verbal information performed more poorly than subjects who did not receive misleading information. The authors concluded from these results that misleading information can result in a modification, or "rewriting," of the original memory trace (Loftus and Loftus 1980). Other studies, however, have provided evidence that is not consistent with the idea that misleading information can result in a modification of the original memory trace. In one study, slides that included a hammer were followed by misleading verbal information that made reference to a wrench. Subjects were then tested for recall of the slide material, but the forced choice test involved a hammer and a screwdriver (i.e., not the item from the misleading verbal information, which was a wrench). Subjects in this experiment who received misleading verbal information performed equally to subjects who did not receive misleading verbal information. The authors concluded that there is not convincing evidence for the idea that misleading information can result in a modification of the original memory trace (McCloskey and Zaragoza (1985a). McCloskey and Zaragoza (1985a, 1985b) suggested that other factors, such as forgetting the source of the original information, may be involved in the findings of E. F. Loftus and G. R. Loftus (1980).

These studies also involved memories of typical events and did not address whether memories of events such as abuse are subject to distortion. One then might wonder, Are memories for stress-related events similar to those experienced by victims of childhood abuse equally vulnerable? A study addressing this question focused on 5- and 7-year-old children's recall of the details of a doctor's examination. Half of the children received anal and genital examinations as part of a routine checkup, whereas the other half received a scoliosis examination (nongenital examination). There were no cases of free recall of genital touching in children who received the nongenital examination; with direct questioning, only one child incorrectly reported being genitally touched. Accuracy of recall was better for the genital examination than for the nongenital exam. Children were highly resistant to misleading questions regarding details of the examination (Saywitz et al. 1991). This study suggests that the types of events forming the basis of childhood abuse may not be as subject to distortions, insertions, and deletions as may be more "mundane" memories.

Alterations in neural mechanisms in memory with stress exposure may result in a difference in memory function in abused patients. Some authors have criticized the statement that memories of abuse could be unavailable to consciousness for many years, only to return to active consciousness years after the fact. It should be considered that alterations in brain regions involved in memory could result in unusual manifestations of memory function, such as long-term amnesia. Certain emotional or physiological states, which are triggered in psychotherapy, also could lead to state-dependent recall, in effect cueing recall of abuse events for which there had been long-term amnesia. Future studies on the effects of stress on the neurobiology of memory should provide useful additional information to help clarify this issue.

Principles of Treatment for Alterations in Memory and Symptoms of Dissociation Related to Psychological Trauma

Understanding trauma, memory, and dissociation has the potential to be useful in the treatment of traumatized patients. Many authors have advocated a reintegration of splintered aspects of memory and experience in the treatment of traumatized patients (Kluft 1993). This type of therapy is often long term because many traumatized individuals have a weakening of the identity and personality structure, making it difficult for them to tolerate the intense affect that comes with the reintegration of traumatic memories (Fine 1991). Patients often have an increase in recall of traumatic events as they proceed through therapy. This recall of events may be upsetting, and sometimes, patients will become symptomatically worse. Clinical judgment is required to determine if the patients have a strong enough personality structure to tolerate the added anxiety associated with discussing traumatic memories. Sometimes, developing a long-term relationship with the therapist before discussing traumatic events in detail can be beneficial in these situations.

Considering the current controversy regarding issues such as false memory syndrome, how should the therapist treat patients who are experiencing a delayed recall of traumatic events? We have reviewed questions regarding the effects of misleading and suggestive information on memory recall. It is clear that a therapist should not push patients to remember abuse events that the therapist feels may exist. On the other hand, studies in children have clearly shown that if one does not ask specific questions, chances are the patients will not volunteer information about abuse events, probably because of shame. Therefore, the psychiatric interview and history, with specific inquiries about abuse experiences, should not be abandoned. On the other hand, the therapist should exercise great caution not to suggest to patients events that may not have happened.

Conclusion

Traumatic stress results in a variety of symptom outcomes, as well as long-term effects on brain systems involved in memory. In this chapter, we have argued for a comprehensive approach to the effects of stress on the individual, emphasizing the fact that psychological trauma is associated with increased symptoms of PTSD, as well as dissociation, depression, and other outcomes such as alcohol and substance abuse. The variety of possible outcomes of psychological trauma may explain why there is considerable overlap in the symptomatology of these different disorders. Alterations in brain regions involved in memory may provide a link between dissociation and other symptoms related to traumatic stress. Stress results in long-term changes in these brain regions, and there is evidence that dysfunction of these brain regions may mediate symptoms of dissociation as well as symptoms of PTSD. A biological approach to stress and memory can provide some useful insights into the current controversy surrounding false memory syndrome. Understanding the effects of stress on memory, and the relationship between alterations in memory and dissociation, is also useful in planning treatment approaches for traumatized patients.

References

American Psychiatric Association: Diagnostic and Statistical Manual of Mental Disorders, 4th Edition. Washington, DC, American Psychiatric Association, 1994

Bernstein E, Putnam T: Development, reliability, and validity of a dissociation scale. J Nerv Ment Dis 174:727–735, 1986

Borrell J, De Kloet ER, Versteeg DHG, et al: Inhibitory avoidance deficit
following short-term adrenalectomy in the rat: the role of adrenal
catecholamines. Behav Neural Biol 39:241, 1983

Bremner JD, Southwick SM, Brett E, et al: Dissociation and posttraumatic
stress disorder in Vietnam combat veterans. Am J Psychiatry 149:
328–333, 1992

Bremner JD, Southwick SM, Johnson DR, et al: Childhood physical abuse
in combat-related posttraumatic stress disorder. Am J Psychiatry 150:
235–239, 1993a

Bremner JD, Scott TM, Delaney RC, et al: Deficits in short-term memory
in post-traumatic stress disorder. Am J Psychiatry 150:1015–1019,
1993b

Bremner JD, Davis M, Southwick SM, et al: The neurobiology of posttraumatic stress disorder, in American Psychiatric Press Review of Psychiatry, Vol 12. Edited by Oldham JM, Riba MG, Tasman A.
Washington, DC, American Psychiatric Press, 1993c, pp 182–204

Bremner JD, Steinberg M, Southwick SM, et al: Use of the Structured
Clinical Interview for DSM-IV Dissociative Disorders for systematic
assessment of dissociative symptoms in posttraumatic stress disorder.
Am J Psychiatry 150:1011–1014, 1993d

Bremner JD, Vermetten E, Krystal JH, et al: Functional neuroanatomical
correlates of the effects of stress on memory. J Trauma Stress 8:
527–554, 1995a

Bremner JD, Randall P, Scott TM, et al: MRI-based measurement of hippocampal volume in combat-related posttraumatic stress disorder.
Am J Psychiatry 152:973–981, 1995b

Bremner JD, Lichio J, Darnell A, et al: Elevated DSF corticotropic releas-
ing factor concentrations in posttraumatic stress disorder. Am J Psychiatry 154:624–629, 1997a

Bremner JD, Randall P, Vermetten E, et al: MRI based measurement of
hippocampal volume in posttraumatic stress disorder related to childhood physical and sexual abuse: a preliminary report. Biol Psychiatry
41:23–32, 1997b

Bremner JD, Innis RB, Ng CK, et al: PET measurement of central metabolic correlates of yohimbine administration in posttraumatic stress
disorder (abstract). Arch Gen Psychiatry 54:246–256, 1997c

Butler RW, Braff DL, Rausch JL, et al: Physiological evidence of exagger-
    ated startle response in a subgroup of Vietnam veterans with
    combat-related PTSD. Am J Psychiatry 147:1308–1312, 1990
Cahill L, Prins B, Weber M, et al: β-adrenergic activation and memory for
    emotional events. Nature 371:702–703, 1994
Cardena E, Spiegel D: Dissociative reactions to the San Francisco Bay
    area earthquake of 1989. Am J Psychiatry 150:474–478, 1989
Carlson EB, Rosser-Hogan R: Trauma experiences, posttraumatic stress,
    dissociation, and depression in Cambodian refugees. Am J Psychiatry
    148:1548–1552, 1991
Cassiday KL, McNally RJ, Zeitlin SB: Cognitive processing of trauma cues
    in rape victims with posttraumatic stress disorder. Cognitive Therapy
    and Research 16:283–295, 1992
Charney DS, Deutch AY, Krystal JH, et al: Psychobiologic mechanisms of
    posttraumatic stress disorder. Arch Gen Psychiatry 50:294–299, 1993
Chu JA, Dill DL: Dissociative symptoms in relation to childhood physical
    and sexual abuse. Am J Psychiatry 147:887–892, 1990
Damasio AR: Category-related recognition defects as a clue to the neural
    substrates of knowledge. Trends Neurosci 13:95–98, 1990
Davis M: The role of the amygdala in fear and anxiety. Annu Rev Neuro-
    sci 15:353–375, 1992
De Wied D, Croiset G: Stress modulation of learning and memory pro-
    cesses. Methods and Achievements in Experimental Pathology 15:
    167–199, 1991
Fine CG: Treatment stabilization and crisis prevention: pacing the ther-
    apy of the multiple personality disorder patient. Psychiatr Clin North
    Am 14:661–675, 1991
Finkelhor D: A Sourcebook on Child Sexual Abuse. Newbury Park, CA,
    Sage, 1986
Foa EB, Feske U, Murdock TB, et al: Processing of threat related informa-
    tion in rape victims. J Abnorm Psychol 100:156–162, 1991
Frischholz EJ, Spiegel D, Trentalange MJ, et al: The Hypnotic Induction
    Profile and absorption. Am J Clin Hypn 30:87–93, 1987
Glisky ML, Kihlstrom JF: Hypnotizability and facets of openness. Int J
    Clin Exp Hypn 41:112–123, 1993
Glisky ML, Tataryn DJ, Tobias BA, et al: Absorption, openness to experi-
    ence, and hypnotizability. J Pers Soc Psychol 60:263–272, 1991
Gold PE, van Buskirk R: Facilitation of time-dependent memory pro-
    cesses with posttrial epinephrine injections. Behavior and Biology
    13:145–153, 1975

Goldman PS: Functional development of the prefrontal cortex in early life and the problem of neuronal plasticity. Exp Neurol 32:366–387, 1971

Goldman-Rakic PS: Topography of cognition: parallel distributed networks in primate association cortex. Annu Rev Neurosci 11:137–156, 1988

Halgren E, Walter RD, Cherlow DG, et al: Mental phenomena evoked by electrical stimulation of the human hippocampal formation and amygdala. Brain 101:83–117, 1978

Hannay HJ, Levin HS: Selective Reminding Test: an examination of the equivalence of four forms. J Clini Exp Neuropsychol 7:251–263, 1985

Helweg-Larsen P, Hoffmeyer H, Kieler J, et al: Famine disease in German concentration camps: complications and sequels. Acta Medica Scandinavica 274:235–460, 1952

Herman JL, Perry JC, van der Kolk BA: Childhood trauma in borderline personality disorder. Am J Psychiatry 146:490–495, 1989

Hitchcock JM, Davis M: Lesions of the amygdala, but not of the cerebellum or red nucleus, block conditioned fear as measured with the potentiated startle paradigm. Behav Neurosci 100:11–22, 1986

Hitchcock JM, Sananes CB, Davis M: Sensitization of the startle reflex by footshock: blockade by lesions of the central nucleus of the amygdala or its efferent pathway to the brainstem. Behav Neurosci 103:509–518, 1989

Holen A: The North Sea oil rig disaster, in International Handbook of Traumatic Stress Syndromes. Edited by Wilson JP, Raphael B. New York, Plenum, 1993

Janet P: l'Automatisme Psychologique. Paris, Balliere, 1889

Janet P: The Major Symptoms of Hysteria. New York, Macmillan, 1920

Jarrell TW, Gentile CG, Romanski LM, et al: Involvement of cortical and thalamic auditory regions in retention of differential bradycardiac conditioning to acoustic conditioned stimuli in rabbits. Brain Res 412:285–294, 1987

Keane T, Caddell JM, Taylor KL: The Mississippi Scale for Combat-Related Posttraumatic Stress Disorder: three studies in reliability and validity. J Consult Clin Psychol 56:85–90, 1988

Kihlstrom JF: The cognitive unconscious. Science 237:1445–1451, 1987

Kihlstrom JF: Hypnosis: a sesquicentennial essay. Int J Clin Exp Hypn 11:301–314, 1992

Kihlstrom JF, Glisky ML, Angiulo MJ: Dissociative tendencies and dissociative disorders. J Abnorm Psychol 103:117–124, 1994

Kluft RP: Basic principles in conducting the treatment of multiple personality disorder, in Clinical Perspectives on Multiple Personality Disorder. Edited by Kluft RP, Fine CG. Washington, DC, American Psychiatric Press, 1993, pp 53–73

Koopman C, Classen C, Spiegel D: Predictors of posttraumatic stress symptoms among survivors of the Oakland/Berkeley, California, firestorm. Am J Psychiatry 151:888–894, 1994

Krystal JH, Dkarper LP, Seibyl JP, et al: Subanesthetic effects of the noncompetitive NMDA antagonist, ketamine, in humans. Arch Gen Psychiatry 51:199–214, 1994

LeDoux JL: Emotional memory: in search of systems and synapses. Ann N Y Acad Sci 702:149–157, 1993

Liang KC, Juler RG, McGaugh JL: Modulating effects of posttraining epinephrine on memory: involvement of the amygdala noradrenergic system. Brain Res 368:125–133, 1986

Loewenstein R, Putnam F: A comparison study of dissociative symptoms in patients with complex partial seizures, MPD, and PTSD. Dissociation 1:17–23, 1988

Loftus EF, Loftus GR: On the permanence of stored information in the human brain. Am Psychol 35:409–420, 1980

Loftus EF, Garry M, Feldman J: Forgetting sexual trauma: what does it mean when 38% forget? J Consult Clin Psychol 62:1177–1181, 1994a

Loftus EF, Polonsky S, Fullilove MT: Memories of childhood sexual abuse: remembering and repressing. Psychology of Women Quarterly 18:67–84, 1994b

Luine V, Villages M, Martinex C, et al: Repeated stress causes reversible impairments of spatial memory performance. Brain Res 639:167–170, 1994

Marmar CR, Weiss DS, Schlenger DS, et al: Peritraumatic dissociation and posttraumatic stress in male Vietnam theater veterans. Am J Psychiatry 151:902–907, 1994

Mazure CM (ed): Stress and Psychiatric Disorders. Washington, DC, American Psychiatric Press, 1994

McCloskey M, Zaragoza M: Misleading postevent information and memory for events: arguments and evidence against memory impairment hypotheses. J Exp Psychol Gen 114:1–16, 1985a

McCloskey M, Zaragoza M: Postevent information and memory: reply to Loftus, Schooler and Wagenaar. J Exp Psychol Gen 114:381–387, 1985b

McEwen BS, Gould EA, Sakai RR: The vulnerability of the hippocampus to protective and destructiveeffects of glucocorticoids in relation to stress. Br J Psychiatry 160:18–24, 1992

McGaugh JL: Involvement of hormonal and neuromodulatory systems in the regulation of memory storage: endogenous modulation of memory storage. Annu Rev Neurosci 12:255–287, 1989

McGaugh JL: Significance and remembrance: the role of neuromodulatory systems. Psychological Sciences 1:15–25, 1990

McNally RJ, Kaspi SP, Riemann BC, et al: Selective processing of threat cues in posttraumatic stress disorder. J Abnorm Psychol 99:398–402, 1990

McNally RJ, English GE, Lipke HJ: Assessment of intrusive cognition in PTSD: use of the modified Stroop paradigm. J Trauma Stress 6:33–41, 1993

Mellman TA, Davis GC: Combat-related flashbacks in posttraumatic stress disorder: phenomenology and similarity to panic attacks. J Clin Psychiatry 46:379–382, 1985

Mishkin M: Memory in monkeys severely impaired by combined but not separate removal of amygdala and hippocampus. Nature 173: 297–298, 1978

Morgan MA, LeDoux JE: Medial orbital lesions increase resistance to extinction but do not affect acquisition of fear conditioning (abstract). Proceedings of the Society for Neuroscience 2:1006, 1994

Murray EA, Mishkin M: Visual recognition in monkeys following rhinal cortical ablations combined with either amygdalectomy or hippocampectomy. J Neurosci 6:1991–2003, 1986

Nadon R, Hoyt IP, Register PA, et al: Absorption and hypnotizability: context effects re-examined. J Pers Soc Psychol 60:144–153, 1991

Nemiah JC: Janet redivivus: the centenary of l'Automatisme Psychologique. Am J Psychiatry 146:1527–1530, 1989

Packan DR, Sapolsky RM: Glucocorticoid endangerment of the hippocampus: tissue, steroid and receptor specificity. Neuroendocrinology 51:613–618, 1990

Paige SR, Reid GM, Allen MG, et al: Psychophysiological correlates of posttraumatic stress disorder in Vietnam veterans. Biol Psychiatry 27:419–425, 1990

Pitman RK, Orr SP, Lasko NB: Effects of intranasal vasopressin and oxytocin on physiologic responding during personal combat imagery in Vietnam veterans with posttraumatic stress disorder. Psychiatry Res 48:107–117, 1993

Posner MI, Petersen SE, Fox PT, et al: Localization of cognitive operations in the human brain. Science 240:1627–1631, 1988

Prins A, Kaloupek DG, Keane TM: Psychophysiological evidence for autonomic arousal and startle in traumatized adult populations, in Neurobiological and Clinical Consequences of Stress: From Normal Adaptation to Posttraumatic Stress Disorder. Edited by Friedman MJ, Charney DS, Deutch AY. New York, Raven, 1995, pp 291–314

Putnam FW: Pierre Janet and modern views of dissociation. J Trauma Stress 2:413–429, 1989

Putnam FW, Guroff JJ, Silberman EK, et al: The clinical phenomenology of multiple personality disorder: a review of 100 recent cases. J Clin Psychiatry 47:285–293, 1986

Radtke HL, Stam HJ: The relationship between absorption, openness to experience, anhedonia, and susceptibility. Int J Clin Exp Hypn 39:39–56, 1991

Randall PK, Bremner JD, Krystal JH, et al: Effects of the benzodiazepine antagonist, flumazenil, in PTSD. Biol Psychiatry 38:319–324, 1995

Rosen JB, Davis M: Enhancement of acoustic startle by electrical stimulation of the amygdala. Behav Neurosci 102:195–202, 1988

Rosen JB, Hitchcock JM, Sananes CB, et al: A direct projection from the central nucleus of the amygdala to the acoustic startle pathway: anterograde and retrograde tracing studies. Behav Neurosci 105: 817–825, 1991

Ross RJ, Ball WA, Cohen ME, et al: Habituation of the startle reflex in posttraumatic stress disorder. J Neuropsychiatry Clin Neurosci 1: 305–307, 1989

Russell E: A multiple scoring method for the assessment of complex memory functions. J Consult Clin Psychol 43:800–809, 1975

Sapolsky R, Krey L, McEwen B: Prolonged glucocorticoid exposure reduces hippocampal neuron number: implications for aging. J Neurosci 5:1221–1226, 1985

Sapolsky RM, Uno H, Rebert CS, et al: Hippocampal damage associated with prolonged glucocorticoid exposure in primates. J Neurosci 10:2897–2902, 1990

Save E, Poucet B, Foreman N, et al: Object exploration and reactions to spatial and nonspatial changes in hooded rats following damage to parietal cortex or hippocampal formation. Behav Neurosci 106: 447–456, 1992

Saywitz KJ, Goodman GS, Nicholas E, et al: Children's memories of a physical examination involving genital touch: implications for reports of child sexual abuse. J Consult Clin Psychol 59:682–691, 1991

Schacter DL: Implicit memory: a new frontier for cognitive neuroscience, in The Cognitive Neurosciences. Edited by Gazzaniga MS. Cambridge, MA, MIT Press, 1995

Shalev AY, Orr SP, Peri T, et al: Physiologic responses to loud tones in Israeli patients with posttraumatic stress disorder. Arch Gen Psychiatry 49:870–874, 1992

Southwick SM, Krystal JH, Morgan CA, et al: Abnormal noradrenergic function in posttraumatic stress disorder. Arch Gen Psychiatry 50:266–274, 1993

Spiegel D: Multiple personality as a posttraumatic stress disorder. Psychiatr Clin North Am 7:101–110, 1984

Spiegel D, Cardena E: Disintegrated experience: the dissociative disorders revisited. J Abnorm Psychol 100:366–378, 1991

Spiegel D, Hunt T, Dondershine HE: Dissociation and hypnotizability in posttraumatic stress disorder. Am J Psychiatry 145:301–305, 1988

Squire LR, Zola-Morgan S: The medial temporal lobe memory system. Science 253:1380–1386, 1991

Steinberg M: Structured Clinical Interview for DSM-IV Dissociative Disorders (SCID-D). Washington, DC, American Psychiatric Press, 1993

Sutker PB, Galina H, West JA, et al: Trauma-induced weight loss and cognitive deficits among former prisoners of war. Am J Psychiatry 147: 323–328, 1990

Sutker PB, Winstead DK, Galina ZH, et al: Cognitive deficits and psychopathology among former prisoners of war and combat veterans of the Korean conflict. Am J Psychiatry 148:67–72, 1991

Tellegen A, Atkinson G: Openness to absorbing and self-altering experiences (" absorption"), a trait related to hypnotic susceptibility. J Abnorm Psychol 83:268–277, 1974

Thygesen P, Hermann K, Willanger R: Concentration camp survivors in Denmark: persecution, disease, disability, compensation. Dan Med Bull 17:65–108, 1970

Turner BH, Herkenham M: Thalamoamygdaloid projections in the rat: a test of the amygdala's role in sensory processing. J Comp Neurol 313:295–325, 1991

Turner BH, Mishkin M, Knapp M: Organization of amygdaloid projections from modality-specific association areas in the monkey. J Comp Neurol 191:515–543, 1980

Uddo M, Vasterling JT, Brailey K, et al: Memory and attention in post-traumatic stress disorder. Journal of Psychopathology and Behavioral Assessment 15:43–52, 1993

Uno H, Tarara R, Else JG, et al: Hippocampal damage associated with prolonged and fatal stress in primates. J Neurosci 9:1705–1711, 1989

van der Kolk BA, van der Hart O: Pierre Janet and the breakdown of adaptation in psychological trauma. Am J Psychiatry 146:1530–1540, 1989

Watanabe Y, Gould E, McEwen BS: Stress induces atrophy of apical dendrites of hippocampal CA3 pyramidal neurons. Brain Res 588:341–345, 1992

Wechsler D: Wechsler Adult Intelligence Scale—Revised. San Antonio, TX, Psychological Corporation, 1981

Wechsler D: Wechsler Memory Scale—Revised. San Antonio, TX, Psychological Corporation, 1987

Williams LM: Recall of childhood trauma: a prospective study of women's memories of child sexual abuse. J Consult Clin Psychol 62:1167–1176, 1994a

Williams LM: What does it mean to forget child sexual abuse? a reply to Loftus, Garry, and Feldman (1994). J Consult Clin Psychol 62:1182–1186, 1994b

Wooley CS, Gould E, McEwen BS: Exposure to excess glucocorticoids alters dendritic morphology of adult hippocampal pyramidal neurons. Brain Res 531:225–231, 1990

Yehuda R, Keefer RSE, Harvey PD, et al: Learning and memory in combat veterans with posttraumatic stress disorder. Am J Psychiatry 152:137–139, 1995

Zeitlin SB, McNally RJ: Implicit and explicit memory bias for threat in posttraumatic stress disorder. Behav Res Ther 29:451–457, 1991

Zola-Morgan SM, Squire LR: The primate hippocampal formation: evidence for a time-limited role in memory storage. Science 250:288–290, 1990

Zola-Morgan S, Squire LR, Amaral DG, et al: Lesions of perirhinal and parahippocampal cortex that spare the amygdala and hippocampal formation produce severe memory impairment. J Neurosci 9:4355–4370, 1989

Index

*Page numbers printed in **boldface** type refer to tables or figures.*

panic attacks induced by
pharmacological challenge
studies, 324–327
Anxiolytics, 272, 321, 323, 345
Arachidonic acid, 330
Arginine vasopressin, 349–350,
387, 388
"Artificial hysteria," 109
ASD. *See* Acute stress disorder
Association for the Advancement
of Behavior Therapy (AABT),
309
Attention, 340
Attorneys, 92
Auditory hallucinations, 30, 196
Autobiographical memory,
117–118, 366, 379
Autohypnotic model, 29–32, 46
hypnosis as metaphor for,
47–48
tests of
correlation between
measures of
hypnotizability and
dissociation, 35–36,
37–38, 131–133, **134**
postulated increase in
hypnotizability after
traumatic experiences,
40–41, **42**
Automatic writing, 30, 110
Automaticity, dissociation
compared with, 117–118
Autonomic arousal, 206, 219–221
Avoidance, 205, 207, 221, 266, 299
Awareness, continuum of, 136

Barber Suggestibility Scale (BSS),
124

Barbiturates, 322–323
BAT. *See* Behavioral Avoidance
Test
BCA case, 8
Beck Depression Inventory (BDI),
293, 299–302, 314
Behavioral avoidance, 205, 207,
221
Behavioral Avoidance Test (BAT),
293, 294, 297, 301, 314
Benzodiazepine antagonists, 327,
344
Benzodiazepines, 322–323, 345,
348
Bingeing and purging behavior,
71, 164. *See also* Bulimia
nervosa; Eating disorders
Blindness, 4–6, 9
Body dysmorphic disorder, 163
Body image distortion, 231,
331
Borderline personality disorder
(BPD), 68–71, 254, 367
childhood abuse and, 208, 230,
367
dissociative symptoms in,
368
eating disorders and, 166
factitious disorders and, 167
Boundary transgressions, 267
Bowers, Kenneth, 35
BPD. *See* Borderline personality
disorder
Brain regions involved in
memory, 380–381
neuroimaging studies of effects
of stress on, 384–387
Brain stimulation studies,
331–334